D0843222

Foundations

of

Modern Auditory Theory

VOLUME I

Foundations

of

Modern Auditory Theory

Edited by

Jerry V. Tobias

Federal Aviation Administration
Oklahoma City, Oklahoma

VOLUME I

1970

ACADEMIC PRESS   New York San Francisco London

A Subsidiary of Harcourt Brace Jovanovich, Publishers

ACADEMIC PRESS, INC.
111 Fifth Avenue, New York, New York 10003

United Kingdom Edition published by
ACADEMIC PRESS, INC. (LONDON) LTD.
24/28 Oval Road, London NW1

LIBRARY OF CONGRESS CATALOG CARD NUMBER: 78-91432

PRINTED IN THE UNITED STATES OF AMERICA

For

P. E. and W. K. R., among others

v

Table of Contents

Chapter Eight   **ENLARGED MECHANICAL MODEL OF THE COCHLEA
                 WITH NERVE SUPPLY**

   Georg von Békésy

Chapter Nine   **MONAURAL PROCESSING**

   F. Blair Simmons

Chapter Ten   **FUNCTIONAL MANIFESTATIONS OF LESIONS OF THE
                SENSORINEURAL STRUCTURES**

   Harold F. Schuknecht

Chapter Eleven **MUSICAL PERCEPTION**

W. Dixon Ward

List of Contributors

Numbers in parentheses indicate the pages on which authors' contributions begin.

Georg von Békésy, *Laboratory of Sensory Sciences, University of Hawaii, Honolulu, Hawaii* (305)

Donald N. Elliott, *Department of Psychology, Wayne State University, Detroit, Michigan* (115)

Winifred (Riach) Fraser, *Department of Psychology, Wayne State University, Detroit, Michigan* (115)

Lloyd A. Jeffress, *Applied Research Laboratories and Department of Psychology, University of Texas, Austin, Texas* (85)

Jan O. Nordmark, *Mathema AB, Stockholm, Sweden* (55)

Bertram Scharf, *Department of Psychology, Northeastern University, Boston, Massachusetts* (157)

Harold F. Schuknecht, *Harvard Medical School and Massachusetts Eye and Ear Infirmary, Boston, Massachusetts* (381)

F. Blair Simmons, *Division of Otolaryngology, Stanford University, Stanford, California* (343)

Arnold M. Small, *Psychology and Speech Pathology and Audiology Departments, University of Iowa, Iowa City, Iowa* (1)

Donald C. Teas, *Departments of Speech, Psychology, Physiology, and Electrical Engineering, University of Florida, Gainesville, Florida* (255)

Juergen Tonndorf, *Otolaryngology Department, College of Physicians and Surgeons, Columbia University, New York* (203)

W. Dixon Ward, *Department of Otolaryngology, University of Minnesota, Minneapolis, Minnesota* (405)

Preface

Once upon a time, a long time ago, there was a little girl who wanted to learn about rabbits. She was a bright little girl so she went to the library, where the librarian spent an hour searching out the very best rabbit book available for a child of that age. It was well illustrated, was written in clear, understandable terms, was filled with examples of rabbit-life and rabbit wisdom, and was, all in all, a perfect choice for the child.

A week passed and the little girl came back, carrying the book carefully to the woman who had given so much of her knowledge, her time, and her energy to selecting the perfect book. When she had reshelved it, the librarian asked, "How did you like it?" The little girl looked very serious for a minute, and finally found just the right phrase. She said, "It told me more about rabbits than I wanted to know."

For a long time now, I've been looking for a book that would tell me more about ears than I wanted to know. It doesn't exist. This book isn't it either, although it was devised for the purpose of filling more gaps than any of the others do. It is for the same sort of reader whom the long-lived standard references still attract.

When I first learned that there was nothing on my shelf to direct me, with a minimum of pain, toward the answers to the commonest questions about auditory function, structure, and response, I began a campaign to get one or more of my colleagues to do a book. Everyone refused. One experienced editor suggested that the easiest way would be to write the thing myself, but since I didn't know much then about being an editor, I didn't believe him. Now I can add my advice to his: anyone who attempts to compile a treatise of the magnitude of this one has to be an eccentric – if not when he starts, then certainly by the time he's done.

Still, I learned that anyone with a strong, selfish, good reason for continuing can do the editorial job. I had such a reason. This book was written for my personal instruction and convenience. It puts at my fingertips most of the kinds of information that I need when I'm working on a paper for a journal; it helps guide me through articles that are only peripherally within my area of expertise; and it often is adequate to warn me that my latest new insight is not really so new or so clever. Not till now has it been possible to consult with so many truly wise colleagues and to find such useful authoritative opinion on the vagaries of critical bands or of periodicity pitch, or on any of innumerable other topics, without spending too much time on attenuated literature searches or too much equipment money on long-distance phone calls.

The greatest discovery of all was that nearly everyone in the field had the same selfish interest that I did—they all wanted some handy sourcebook for their desks, and since the only way to get one was to compile one, I decided to edit, and the contributors decided to contribute.

This is Volume I of the two-volume result. In it, most of the kinds of information necessary to understand basic auditory processes is brought together. The exposition is intended to be clear, but the style is certainly not that of a primer. Readers ought to know enough about hearing (though not necessarily about all of the subspecialties) to feel competent to contribute a chapter themselves some day. The authors wrote their chapters for each other, so any reader is, in some sense, in the same category as a writer.

Some of the contents of this volume are a bit different from what one might find in a book designed only as a text: several writers have strong points of view and occasionally those biases are not popular. But, as with many theoretically founded prejudices, startling and useful conclusions sometimes result.

I have to offer one important apology to some readers. Several of the classical areas in the field of audition have been left out. The choice was mine and I accept the consequence. But such things as loudness perception, to pick one example, are well treated in the texts that, although 15 or 20 or 30 years old, are still available and are still important. This book is not designed to fill gaps that don't exist. As a result, it cannot successfully stand as the *only* sourcebook on your desk, but I hope it can come close.

In acknowledging the people who did most to make this book happen, I have to start with the most important ones, the contributors—von Békésy, Elliott, Fraser, Jeffress, Nordmark, Scharf, Schuknecht, Simmons, Small, Teas, Tonndorf, and Ward. Then there's Earl Schubert, who got me started in trying to figure out how auditory systems do all the things that they do. Lloyd Jeffress deserves special mention, too, for the continuing reminders he's given me and so many others that good research can be a joy both to see and to do.

Among my own people, a few deserve special mention for having turned a bibliographical holocaust into an orderly and correct referencing system. They checked every citation, proofread every reference, checked each article and book mentioned in any chapter against the original source material, arranged everything according to the British Museum's standard (the most universally acceptable for so wide a range of scientific writing), and finally rechecked it all after the type was set. They are Beth Burrus, Vic Jackson, Phyllis Ketchum, Pat Layard, Linda Osterhaus, Douglas Polk, and Jan Vorse.

Foundations

of

Modern Auditory Theory

VOLUME I

Chapter One

Periodicity Pitch

FOREWORD

Not long ago, auditory theory was only pitch theory. The critical questions being asked about the auditory system pertained to such things as whether the all-or-none principle of neural conduction meant that there could be no "telephone" transmission, whether the existence of diplacusis could be reconciled with the volley theory, or whether evidence of phase perception was too much for the place theory to account for. Some of these kinds of questions still arise, but the theories to which the issues are now taken are compound, eclectic statements that allow parts of the auditory process to be handled by a place mechanism in the end organ, part by a volleying neural network, part by mechanical and electrical inhibitory processes, and so on. Among the areas that still seem mysterious is periodicity pitch. The basic problem arises from data that show listeners are able to perceive modulation frequencies when energy at those frequencies is carefully kept out of the stimulus. The resolution of the periodicity pitch question leads necessarily to a resolution of the classic theoretical problems of audition. Is the phenomenon one based on demodulation by the ear? If so, then the analysis of an envelope frequency is identical to the analysis of any other similar frequency. If not, then what *is* the mechanism by which "nonexistent" tones are heard? Arnold Small has addressed himself to such questions for most of his research career.

Periodicity Pitch

Arnold M. Small*

I. HISTORICAL ANTECEDENTS

Many of the phenomena reviewed in this chapter are not new. Their basis—indeed, in some cases, their existence—has been debated and has stimulated research for well over 200 years. Often, there is a tendency to discount older research simply because of its age. For example, older work in hearing is discounted for its imprecision of stimulus specification. However, in the area of pitch perception, the limitations of older equipment may not be serious and become less so when only relative pitch or changes in pitch are considered. In this light, it is instructive to review some older data and their interpretation.

Although periodicity pitch has gone by many names throughout the years, it may be defined by a particular stimulus configuration coupled with a specific listener response. Thus, periodicity pitch, operationally, is the pitch assigned to a complex stimulus and corresponding approximately to the rate of signal envelope variation. Under these circumstances, there is ordinarily little or no energy at the frequency that corresponds to the perceived pitch. One might well ask what class of signals fits this description.

In older research, several methods have been used to introduce periodic variations into waveform envelopes. One is by interruptions of a steady signal. König (1876), Dennert (1887), and Schaefer and

*Psychology and Speech Pathology and Audiology Departments, University of Iowa, Iowa City, Iowa.

Abraham (1901a, 1901b, 1902) were among the first to study stimuli of this type. They all found a pitch that was equal to the rate of interruption. For example, Schaefer and Abraham used a siren with four holes followed by four blank spaces in a repetitive fashion around its disc. They found two pitches: one was the same as would have been produced if there had been all holes and no blanks, and the other corresponded to the rate at which the groups of four open holes appeared — three octaves lower.

A second way to generate envelope periodicities is by adding together two sinusoids whose frequencies are similar. The envelope of such a combination undergoes amplitude changes at a rate equal to the frequency difference between the sinusoids. With small frequency separations, loudness changes, or beats, occur at the same rate as the envelope amplitude changes. For larger separations and under proper intensity conditions, a *pitch* is perceived — also corresponding to the rate of envelope change. Such a pitch is called a beat note or difference tone and, according to Jones (1935), was first reported by Sorge, Romineu, and Tartini in 1744, 1751, and 1754, respectively. Young (1800) and König (1876), expanding a suggestion originally made by Smith (1749), proposed that the same envelope changes that, when sufficiently slow, are heard as beats will, when sufficiently rapid, be perceived as difference tones. This hypothesis represents an early attempt to relate pitch perception to the waveform of the stimulus. These authors regarded any periodic change in the stimulus as a basis for the perception of a tone. However, the precise nature and the location of the central mechanism responsible for the interpretation of waveform periodicity were never specified.

Helmholtz and his followers vigorously opposed this periodicity point of view. Rather than accept the notion that the auditory system may perceive pitch on the basis of waveform periodicity, they defended a resonance theory wherein the ear performs a frequency analysis. In his theory, Helmholtz (1863) provided an explicit physiological basis for Ohm's (1843) acoustic law. Ohm's law, in essence, states that the ear performs a Fourier analysis upon the stimulus; that is, the sinusoidal components of a complex sound are individually perceived. Curiously enough, Ohm formulated his statement largely on the basis of some experiments by Seebeck (1841), and Seebeck, as will be seen, disagreed vigorously with Ohm's law.

Helmholtz postulated a series of individual resonators consisting of stretched transverse fibers on the basilar membrane. Each resonator along the membrane was tuned to a different frequency by virtue of its differential tension, length, and mass. Upon stimulation of the ear by a pure tone, a single stretched fiber would be set into vibration, which in turn would activate the neuron associated with it. Neurons associated with different resonant fibers then would be recognized at some higher neural center as representing specific pitches. (The neural aspects of this theory draw heavily upon Müller's 1826 doctrine of specific nerve energies.) Inasmuch as the active fibers were presumed to have an orderly spatial arrangement, this theory is a type of place theory.

There were immediate objections to Helmholtz's theory. Many revolved around the stated specificity of action. It was conceded, even by Helmholtz, that damping in the cochlea must be considerable, and for that reason, as Wien (1905), among others, pointed out, no resonator can be completely unresponsive to any input frequency. Why is it then, it was asked, that if more than one resonator is active, only one pitch is perceived?

It was in response to this criticism that Gray (1900) advanced his principle of maximum stimulation. He contended that, by virtue of some unspecified mechanism, the action of the basilar membrane gives rise to a specific pitch corresponding to the point at which stimulation is largest. An objection to this principle was that the burden of analysis is thrown upon the higher neural centers. Consequently a chief distinction between a place theory and other theories (that explicitly depend upon higher centers) seemed to have disappeared.

As a matter of fact, both before and after Gray's enunciation, the place theory had some of its greatest difficulty in explaining the pitch of complex stimuli. In general, according to Ohm's law, one would expect the components of a complex signal to be perceived separately – each with an appropriate and distinctive pitch. Further, the loudness of such components should be closely related to their relative intensity. To the extent that these statements are not substantiated one might question the underlying assumption, i.e., Ohm's law. And indeed, there are circumstances, many reported years ago, in which these statements seem not to hold.

For example, Seebeck (1841) used a siren for several experiments in which the loudness of the various components assumed values that were not in keeping with their actual physical magnitude. In one experiment a row of holes in a siren disc were arranged to give impulses as shown in Fig. 1a. A second row of holes, concentric to the first row provided impulses at twice the rate of the first and, of course, yielded a pitch one octave higher (Fig. 1*b*). A third row had holes that were not

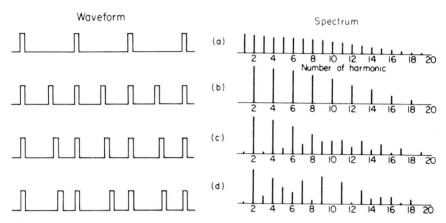

Figure 1   Seebeck's experiment. Waveform *b* has a repetition rate twice as great as waveform *a*, and its pitch is an octave higher. Waveform *c* has alternate pulses displaced slightly from the middle position, and waveform *d* has similar displacement of greater magnitude. In *c* and *d*, two pitches are heard—one corresponds to that heard with *a*, and the other to that heard with *b*, in spite of the fact that very little energy exists at the fundamental frequency as shown in the spectrum at the right. (Schouten, 1940a. By permission from *Proceedings Koninklijke Nederlandse Akademie van Wetenschappen.*)

spaced at equal intervals, but at the separations shown in Fig. 1*c*. In this case, two pitches were prominent—one the same as *b*, and the other, an octave lower, the same as *a*. Yet the actual magnitude of the component at this lower frequency was extremely small. The fourth condition, shown in Fig. 1*d*, was similar to the third except that the alternate pulses were displaced to even a greater degree. In this last case, the lower octave, corresponding to that heard in Fig. 1*a*, was far more prominent in spite of the very small amplitude of the spectral component.

  Stumpf (1926) also observed similar phenomena in his studies of synthetic vowels. When various harmonics of a given frequency were sounded simultaneously, he found the pitch of the complex to be equal to that of the fundamental — even when the fundamental was not physically present. Actually, many natural vowel sounds possess little energy at the fundamental frequency, yet the fundamental pitch is the predominant one.

II. PSYCHOACOUSTIC DATA

A. Periodicity Pitch—An Artifact?

Since the time of Helmholtz, the hypothesis most commonly advanced to account for the perception of a pitch corresponding to the envelope periodicity has been that a difference tone is generated.

Recall that in the case of a two-sinusoid complex, envelope modulation occurs at a rate equal to the frequency difference, or in the case of a complex of harmonics without a fundamental, it occurs at the common difference frequency. Consequently, if in fact a difference tone is generated by the ear, it must correspond in frequency to the rate of envelope modulation and thus to the pitch usually assigned to these stimuli. The generation of a difference tone has been linked to the nonlinearity of the auditory system. Writers have variously suggested that the locus of nonlinearity is the tympanic membrane (Helmholtz, 1863), the ossicular chain (Békésy, 1934), the hydromechanical action of the basilar membrane (Tonndorf, 1958), or the nervous system (Licklider, 1959).

That a difference tone may be generated under certain circumstances is scarcely open to doubt. But whether a difference tone accounts for the perception of periodicity pitch may be seriously questioned.

Low-level Stimulation. A number of investigators have addressed themselves to the problem of determining under what conditions evidence of nonlinearity may be detected. It is generally conceded that in the case of two or more input signals both harmonics and sum and difference frequencies may be generated. Consequently, existence of any of these frequencies in the auditory system can be interpreted as evidence of nonlinearity.

Many systems have a region of input values for which their amplitude response is linear. Usually, when the input is sufficiently large, however, system amplitude response becomes nonlinear. Thus, one of the most important conditions leading to a manifestation of nonlinearity is the magnitude of the input signal. Unfortunately, there are limited data on the relations between the *detection* of difference tones or the relative *amplitude* of the difference tones, and the magnitude of the input signals. Békésy (1934) observed that the amplitude of the first-order difference tone (as determined by the method of best beats) is 40 dB below that of the primaries when the primaries are between 800 and 4000 Hz and the difference tones are between 200 and 800 Hz.

For a difference tone as low as 100 Hz, the relative level is greater —
28 dB below the primaries. Moe (1942), using the same method, found
that with primaries of 950 and 690 Hz, the first-order difference tone
is about 20 dB below the level of the primaries.

Neither Békésy nor Moe nor Plomp (1965) could detect the presence
of a difference tone when the primaries were less than about 60 dB
re 0.0002 microbar. Plomp (1965) addressed himself directly to the
question of the minimum sound level at which the fundamental appears perceptually in a signal that, though devoid of fundamental,
gives rise to periodicity pitch. His subjects listened alternately to the
complex signal and to either one of two sinusoids — one equal to the
fundamental frequency, and the second, ten percent higher. The sound
level was then increased until they reported the presence of a tone of
the same pitch as the sinusoid that was equated to the fundamental.
Plomp reported that a level of about 65 dB SPL is required before a
difference tone equal to the common difference frequency between
components is detected. It is not clear to me how Plomp's subjects
were able to differentiate between the periodicity pitch and the
difference tone, both of which, in this case, would be equal to the
pitch of the fundamental frequency. In any event, Plomp concluded
that the perception of a difference tone is not the basis for the perception of periodicity pitch.

If periodicity pitch is nothing more than a difference tone resulting
from common spacing between components and generated by the
amplitude nonlinearity of the auditory system, then periodicity pitch
should cease to exist at low sound levels. In fact, it does not.

A number of studies have been conducted using low sound levels.
Thurlow and Small (1955) for example, used amplitude modulated
signals at 20 dB SL with the energy confined to frequencies above
1000 Hz. At this level, the sound pressure of any component is considerably less than 20 dB re 0.0002 microbar; yet periodicity pitch is
clearly audible under the conditions of their study. Small and Campbell (1961b) determined which frequencies mask the periodicity pitch
associated with an amplitude-modulated signal. Their lowest-level
signal — 20 dB SL — is well below the ear's region of nonlinearity and
their highest-level signal — 70 dB SL — has a distinct possibility of
being in a region of nonlinearity. Their results indicate that subjects
have little difficulty in perceiving periodicity pitch at low signal
levels. Further, there is no difference in the shape of the masking
function at low versus high signal levels. This latter finding may be
interpreted as indicating that the same mechanism is operating in the

perception of periodicity pitch at low and at high levels. Since, on
the basis of many studies (for example, Békésy, 1934; Moe, 1942; and
Plomp, 1965), a manifestation of difference tones is most unlikely at
this low level, periodicity pitch must not be based on a difference tone
even at relatively high levels.

Cancellation. Schouten (1938, 1940a) provided a series of studies
that demonstrate the independence of periodicity pitch (or *residue,*
as he has called it) from nonlinearity as manifested in the form of a
difference tone. In general, if a sinusoidal signal is present, this signal
may be completely cancelled by adding a second sinusoid having
precisely the same amplitude and a phase difference of 180 degrees.
Schouten reasoned that cancellation should work whether the first
sinusoid were generated externally by an oscillator or within the ear
as a difference tone.

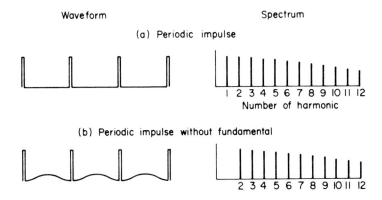

Figure 2 Cancellation of the fundamental frequency of a complex signal. Figure *a*
shows a periodic impulse or dc pulse train and its spectrum. By appropriate adjustment
of phase and amplitude, the fundamental may be cancelled as shown in Figure *b*. In
both cases, however, the pitch of the signal corresponds to the fundamental. (Schouten,
1938. By permission from *Proceedings Koninklijke Nederlandse Akademie van Wetenschappen.*)

Thus, if a difference tone is generated by a complex stimulus, it
should be possible to cancel it by means of an externally supplied
sinusoid. If the pitch of the complex is due to the presence of the
difference tone, then upon its cancellation, the pitch should change.
Schouten used this technique with a complex signal consisting of a
200-Hz fundamental and its harmonics (Fig. 2). In this situation, the
component at the fundamental frequency possesses an amplitude and

phase that are the resultant of the original component at that frequency and the "subjectively" generated difference tone. He found that "if we now cancel the fundamental tone we find that a sharp note of pitch 200 remains unchanged present in the perceived sound." Schouten concluded therefore that the pitch of a series of harmonic components is not determined by the presence of a fundamental frequency provided by the generation of a difference tone.

Beats. Fletcher (1934) in his "case of the missing fundamental" found that the fundamental frequency of a complex signal can be removed without altering the pitch of the complex. This effect is a manifestation of periodicity pitch since the envelope periodicity of the waveform is unchanged by the removal of the lower components (see Fig. 22). If this phenomenon is due to the regeneration of the fundamental in the form of a difference tone, then it should be possible to detect the presence of the difference tone by means of beats. For example, if the fundamental frequency is 200 Hz, the presence of a sinusoidal component of frequency 200 within the ear can be determined by introducing a probe tone whose frequency is slightly mistuned from 200 Hz. If beats are heard, then energy is presumed to be present at the fundamental frequency and thus the perceived pitch is accounted for. However, no beats are perceived in this situation. It is important to note that the signal level must be kept reasonably low, since there is ample evidence of nonlinear distortion at moderate and high stimulus levels.

Schouten (1938), you remember, took a somewhat different approach: he used a complex signal complete with fundamental, then cancelled the fundamental by a subjective manipulation of the phase and amplitude of an externally generated sinusoid. In order to ascertain whether in fact the fundamental had been successfully eliminated, he introduced a sinusoid to beat with the fundamental. No beats were perceived, so he concluded that there was no energy at the frequency to which the pitch of the complex stimulus was assigned.

Selective Masking. Selective masking is one of the most powerful arguments in ruling out the importance of low-frequency energy in determining periodicity pitch. If a difference tone is responsible for periodicity pitch, then a masking stimulus whose energy is centered in the spectral region of the difference tone should effectively mask the difference tone. As a result, the periodicity pitch should disappear; that is, the pitch of the stimulus should change. Conversely, a masking stimulus that contains only high-frequency energy should have very little influence on the audibility of a low-frequency difference tone; consequently, with a masker of this type, no change in periodicity pitch might be expected.

Working independently, Licklider (1954) and Thurlow and Small (1955) found that a low-frequency masker that saturates the low-frequency channels of the ear has essentially no effect upon the low periodicity pitch. They concluded therefore that periodicity pitch is being carried by the "wrong" neurons — the ones that respond to high frequencies and ordinarily give rise to a sensation of a high pitch. Davis *et al.* (1951) drew a similar conclusion from electrophysiological evidence.

Small and Campbell (1961b) repeated and extended these earlier studies on the effects of masking on periodicity pitch. They used two

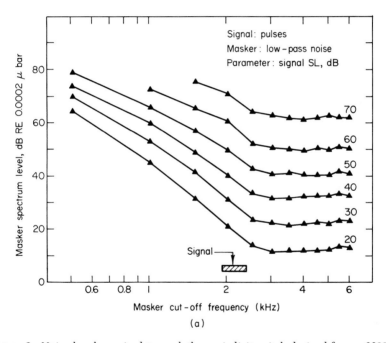

(a)

Figure 3 Noise level required to mask the periodicity pitch derived from a 2200 Hz tone pulsed 150 times per sec as a function of the cutoff frequency of the noise band. Signal energy is located near 2200 Hz, but the pitch of the signal corresponds to 150 Hz. In *a* low-pass noise is used as the masker; in *b* high-pass noise is present. Circled data points are those at which some subjects were unable to mask the signal with the highest noise levels available. Each data point is based upon six judgments by each of ten subjects. Noise located only in the region of 150 Hz had little effect on periodicity pitch. (Small and Campbell, 1961b. By permission from *Journal of the Acoustical Society of America.*)

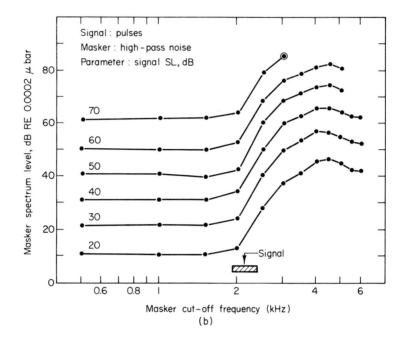

Signal : pulses
Masker : high-pass noise
Parameter : signal SL, dB

(b)

Masker cut-off frequency (kHz)

Masker spectrum level, dB RE 0.0002 μ bar

types of noise—high- and low-pass—as maskers. And they used two types of signals: (*a*) bursts of a 2200-Hz sinusoid repeated about 150 times per sec, and for comparison, (*b*) steady pure tones of 2200 and 150 Hz. The subject's task was to adjust the level of the masker until the periodicity pitch associated with the complex stimulus just disappeared. The authors hypothesized that if the periodicity pitch associated with the pulsed signal were the result of energy at the repetition rate (fundamental frequency), then the pattern of masking associated with the pulsed signal should be similar to that of a pure tone whose frequency equals the repetition rate. Conversely, if periodicity pitch were related to or were being carried by the high-frequency components of the signal, then the masking pattern for periodicity pitch should be similar to that arising from a steady pure tone whose frequency approximates that of the sinusoid being pulsed. Figure 3 shows their results for the pulsed signal that provided the periodicity pitch. Figure 3*a* which depicts the masking pattern provided by a low-pass noise masker, indicates that the masker level required to mask periodicity pitch decreases as the energy in the noise band is extended upward in frequency. This decrease occurs inde-

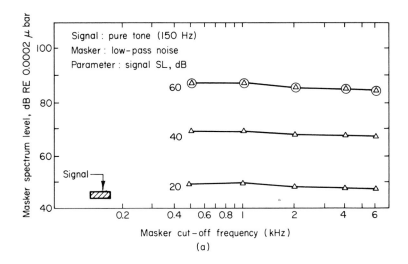

(a)

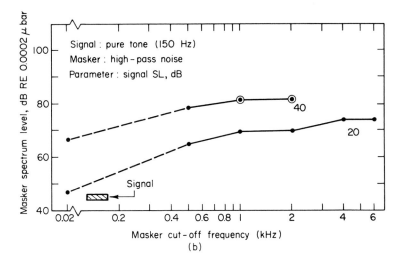

(b)

Figure 4 Noise level required to mask the pitch of a 150-Hz tone as a function of the cutoff frequency of the noise band. Signal energy is located in the crosshatched region of the spectrum. Circled data points have the same meaning as in Fig. 3. Low-pass noise was used for *a* and high-pass noise for *b*. Masking changes very little with cutoff frequency as long as the region of signal energy is contained within passband of the noise. (Small and Campbell, 1961b. By permission from *Journal of the Acoustical Society of America*.)

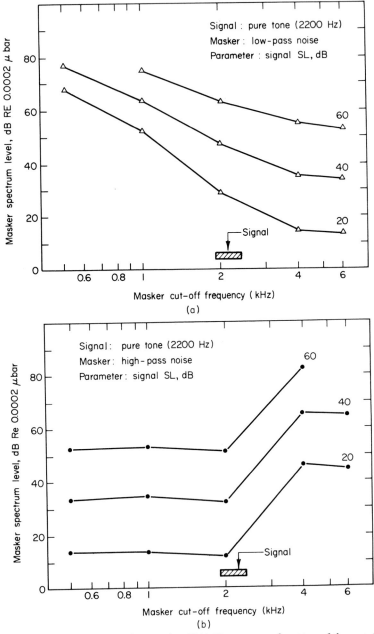

Figure 5 Noise level required to mask a 2200 Hz tone as a function of the cutoff frequency of the noise band. The figure format is identical to Figs. 3 and 4. (Small and Campbell, 1961b. By permission from *Journal of the Acoustical Society of America.*)

pendently of signal level and continues until the masker bandwidth is large enough to include the region of the spectrum that contains the nominal signal energy. For a high-pass noise masker (Fig. 3b), as the bandwidth is narrowed by raising the low-frequency cutoff, no change is seen in the masked threshold until the masker energy is above and nonoverlapping with the signal energy. Figures 4 and 5 show comparable results for 150- and 2200-Hz pure tones. Quite clearly, the pulse stimuli yield a masking pattern very similar to that of the 2200-Hz pure tone and quite unlike that of the 150-Hz pure tone. Yet the pitch of the pulse stimuli corresponds to that of 150 Hz. These data then support the hypothesis that periodicity pitch is mediated by high- rather than low-frequency components of the signal.

Selective Fatigue. Selective fatigue has been used in the same manner as masking to evaluate the contributions of various spectral regions to the perception of periodicity pitch. That is, if certain "channels" or neurons are rendered nonfunctional, then auditory thresholds in frequency regions specific to those channels or neurons will be degraded. Thus, if perception of periodicity pitch is the result of energy at the pulse repetition rate, a change in sensitivity in this frequency region should cause the energy at the repetition rate to become inaudible — with a consequent change in pitch. In the case of masking, the threshold depression is introduced by a simultaneously presented interfering stimulus; for fatigue, the threshold shift and the presumed nonfunctionality of certain auditory neurons is introduced by a stimulus that is terminated before the threshold of the test stimulus is assessed. (The degree to which fatigue spreads to frequencies other than that of the fatiguer is well documented by Munson and Gardner, 1950, and by Harris and Rawnsley, 1953.)

Small and Yelen (1962) made use of selective fatigue in investigating the periodicity pitch associated with a signal consisting of bursts of a 2200-Hz sinusoid repeated 150 times per sec. Their fatigue paradigm consisted of a fatiguer lasting 0.4 sec, a recovery interval of 0.02 sec, and a test stimulus of 0.05 sec. All three signals — ac pulses, and sinusoids of 150 and 2200 Hz — were used as fatiguer and as test stimulus in combination with themselves and with each other. Figure 6a illustrates, for a 55-dB SPL fatiguer, the amount that the post-fatigue test stimulus has to be increased relative to a prefatigue test stimulus for it to again become audible. Pulses produce fatigue for pulses and for the 2200-Hz tone, but not for the 150-Hz tone. These results are identical to those obtained when the 2200-Hz tone is the fatiguer. The 150-Hz pure tone does not affect the pitch threshold for either the pulses or the high tone, but does shift the threshold for

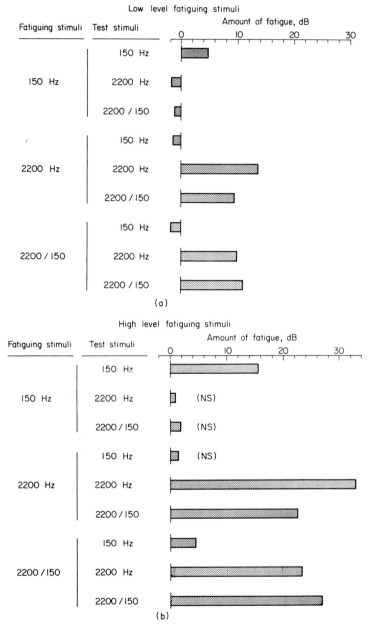

Figure 6 Increase in signal level required to hear pitch following exposure to a fatiguing stimulus of (a) 55 dB and (b) 100 dB re 0.0002 microbar. (Small and Yelen, 1962. By permission from *Journal of the Acoustical Society of America.*)

150 Hz. These results are in agreement with the masking studies: depression of the auditory system's sensitivity in the frequency region corresponding to the periodicity pitch has no effect upon the perception of this pitch. In fact, the data imply that the pitch information is carried by the part of the auditory system that is responsive to high frequencies. In Fig. 6b, the level of the fatiguing stimulus was deliberately increased to a level (100 dB SPL) that would give rise to nonlinear distortion with consequent envelope detection and the appearance of energy at the frequency corresponding to the repetition rate. Under these conditions, when fatigue is produced by sinusoids, the results are similar to those obtained with the low-level fatiguer. However, when the *pulses* are presented at high levels, there is indeed a threshold shift produced at the repetition frequency, indicating that although nonlinear distortion may be demonstrated, the presence of energy at the repetition rate is not influential in determining the pitch of the signal.

B. Parameters Influencing the Perception of Periodicity Pitch

The foregoing discussion has been negative; data have been reviewed that show that the presence of energy at the fundamental frequency is not a requisite condition for the perception of periodicity. Consequently it is of interest to consider those dimensions of the signal that *are* important.

Waveform Envelope. Most data suggest that the pitch of a complex tone corresponds to the fundamental frequency regardless of whether that frequency is physically present in the signal. In Schouten's (1938) early work this complex tone took the form of periodic dc pulses. Such a pulse train may be viewed as a series of harmonically related components. It might be reasoned that the same results would obtain if the complex tone were synthesized — built up of harmonically related components derived from discrete, independent sources. Indeed, if the important aspect of signals yielding periodicity pitch is their spectrum then such a prediction would necessarily follow. Hoogland (1953) tested this notion with a composite sound produced by five independent oscillators set to high-frequency harmonics (e.g., 3.0, 3.1, 3.2, 3.3, and 3.4 k Hz) of a low-frequency — and missing — fundamental. Only at high sound levels is a pitch corresponding to the fundamental perceived. When the level is reduced below that at which nonlinear distortion is expected, no low pitch is audible. Hoogland interpreted his results as a substantiation of the difference tone hypothesis and therefore as support for a place theory of pitch perception.

Mathes and Miller (1947) worked with somewhat similar stimulus conditions. Their principal concern was with phase effects in monaural perception, so they developed complex signals by modulation techniques that permitted phase control over the various spectral components. With sinusoidally amplitude modulated signals whose spectrum consists of three components, a low pitch corresponding to envelope periodicity is perceived. If, with this same signal, the central component or carrier is shifted 90°, the result approximates a frequency-modulated signal. Under this condition the envelope is smoother, but because there are only three components, periodic envelope maxima still occur; however, they are at a higher frequency than for the simple amplitude-modulated signal. With this FM signal, the "basic pitch", as Mathes and Miller called it, increased with the increase in envelope maxima. Further, they got similar results by tuning three oscillators for equal frequency spacing, e.g., 950, 1000, and 1050 Hz. In such situations, because of the instability of oscillators, the phase of the central component shifts with respect to the average of the other two. As it does, the envelope at times shows marked envelope periodicities and at other times presents a rather constant envelope amplitude. Periodicity pitch is not audible under the second condition, but is under the first, even when listening is carried out at levels that Mathes and Miller felt would give rise to little or no nonlinear distortion. These results do not support Hoogland's conclusion; they suggest that factors in addition to power spectrum per se are important in determining periodicity pitch.

Licklider (1955) questioned whether Hoogland's "negative" results might not be a function of the random phase relation of the signal components. Consequently he used a signal consisting of eight harmonically related components whose phase could be controlled. He found that the audibility of the periodicity pitch is directly related to the abruptness of periodic changes in the signal envelope. This abruptness is dependent upon phase relations among the components. When the phases are adjusted for maximum impulsiveness, periodicity pitch is clearly audible; the converse is true when the phases are adjusted for minimum impulsiveness. These results, together with those of Mathes and Miller, demonstrate that periodicity pitch is not determined simply by the presence of harmonically related components (or even equally spaced components), but by characteristics of the waveform envelope.

Small (1955) approached this problem of the temporal aspect of the signal directly. His stimuli, either sinusoids or noise, were gated on and off periodically at a rate of 100 interruptions per sec. Certain temporal aspects of the envelope were varied: the duty cycle (the ratio of the burst duration to the repetition period) and the rise-fall time of the burst. Since, as temporal aspects of a gated sinusoid are manipulated, changes are introduced into the signal spectrum, it is impossible to know whether perceptual changes are a result of temporal or of spectral effects. Wide-band noise undergoes no spectral change within the audible frequency range, when similarly gated and manipulated, so it was used in a control condition. For example, if rise-time altered the perceptibility of periodicity pitch for interrupted sinusoids, but not for interrupted noise, the implication would be that the change in perception occurred because of spectral rather than temporal effects. A portion of Small's results is summarized in Fig. 7 and is plotted as the percentage of pitch matches that fall within ten percent of the pulse repetition rate of the signal. Figure 7a indicates that, as duty cycle and rise-fall time are increased, the audibility of periodicity pitch decreases. On the other hand, with noise (Fig. 7b), although increasing duty cycle apparently lowers the perceptibility of periodicity pitch, rise-fall time has little effect.

Small's results support the idea that abruptness of envelope change is a characteristic that leads to a prominence of periodicity pitch, but this prominence, in his case at least, seems to be related to the increased number of audible spectral components. However, since duty cycle affects interrupted noise and sinusoids in the same manner, its influence must be largely temporal.

Often, but not always, investigators interested in periodicity pitch have used signals in which the repetition or modulation rate is inextricably bound to the fundamental period of the waveform. In such experiments, obviously, one cannot determine the relative contributions of the fundamental and the modulation. Schouten (1938), however, made an attempt to separate these effects, and Flanagan and Guttman (1960a) extended his work (Fig. 8 shows the signals they used — patterns 1 and 2 were also used by Schouten). The amplitude and phase spectra for each signal (Fig. 8 b and c) show that the use of variable-polarity pulses allows the independent manipulation of pulse repetition rate and fundamental period. The task of the five subjects was to match the pitch of each stimulus pattern by appropriate adjustments of the fundamental period of each of the other patterns. The results of these matches are shown in Fig. 9. For a long

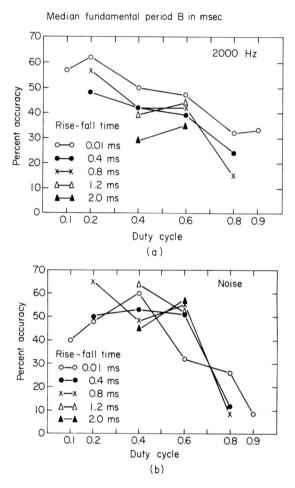

Figure 7 Percentage of pitch matches falling between 90 and 110 Hz as a function of stimulus duty cycle. The stimulus was a signal interrupted 100 times per sec. In *a*, the signal is a 2000 Hz tone; in *b*, it is wide-band thermal noise. The parameter is the rise-fall time of individual bursts. Each data point is based on six judgments from each of eleven subjects. (Small, 1955. By permission from *Journal of the Acoustical Society of America*.)

fundamental period, *T*, the curves vary systematically; indeed matches appear to be made on the basis of pulse repetition rate. For example, if pattern 1 is being matched to pattern 6, the fundamental period of pattern 6 must be six times as long as that of pattern 1 (in order for there to be an equal number of pulses per unit time). In

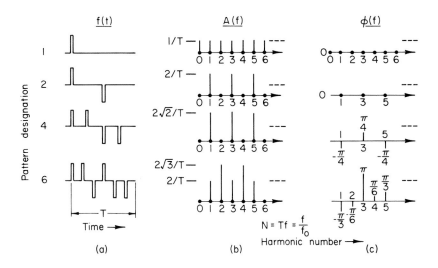

Figure 8 Signals in which pulse repetition rate and fundamental period are independent. Time waveforms are shown in *a* and amplitude and phase spectra in *b* and *c*, respectively. The fundamental period is *T* and the harmonic number *N*. (Flanagan and Guttman, 1960a. By permission from *Journal of the Acoustical Society of America*.)

contrast, at higher fundamental frequencies all the matching functions are identical – that is, the pitch match is apparently made on the basis of fundamental frequency and is independent of pulse repetition rate. It is of interest to note that Schouten (1940a) found the pitch of pattern 1 to be an octave lower than that of pattern 2, for pulse rates of 400 Hz, a result in agreement with these more recent findings.

Flanagan and Guttman (1960b) and Guttman and Flanagan (1964) also investigated the perception of the same signals under conditions of high-pass filtering – that is with no fundamental frequency. The signals and procedures used and the results obtained were similar to those of their first study except that (*a*) not all subjects made consistent fundamental frequency pitch matches on all patterns under those conditions that yielded such matches in their first study, and (*b*) at very high fundamental frequencies (greater than 1000 Hz), matches tended to be made to the lowest harmonic present in the signal spectrum. These authors attempted to explain their results in terms of temporal and spatial events on the basilar membrane. Flanagan (1960, 1962) then devised a descriptive mathematical model and its electrical analog, both of which are discussed in Section IV, C.

Fine Structure. Previous to 1956, most data indicated that period-

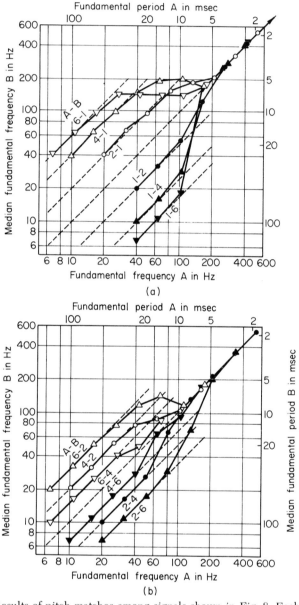

Figure 9 Results of pitch matches among signals shown in Fig. 8. Each function in *a* and *b* relates the fundamental frequency of the *B* signal necessary for a pitch match to the *A* signal presented at a particular fundamental frequency. Every data point represents the median of ten judgments obtained from five subjects. For low fundamental frequencies, pitches are matched to equate pulse rate. At fundamental frequencies above 200 Hz, pitches are matched to equate fundamentals. (Flanagan and Guttman, 1960a. By permission from *Journal of the Acoustical Society of America.*)

icity pitch corresponds to the frequency of envelope modulation. De Boer (1956) showed that this correspondence is true only approximately. In an amplitude-modulation situation he maintained a constant modulating frequency while varying the carrier frequency. Since envelope periodicity is determined by the modulating signal, if periodicity pitch were dependent simply upon the rate of envelope modulation, it would remain unchanged as carrier frequency was varied. Figure 10 shows the actual case. As carrier frequency increases, the pitch at first increases, then abruptly jumps to a lower value, rises again, and repeats the process. In general, this changing pitch value varies about the pitch corresponding to the modulating frequency.

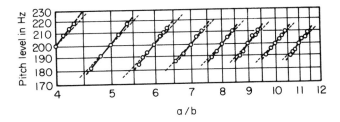

Figure 10 Pitch of sinusoidally amplitude-modulated signal as a function of carrier frequency *a*. Modulating frequency *b* was 200 Hz. The pitch match was effected by varying the modulating frequency of a complex in which the ratio of carrier to modulating frequency was an integer. Pitch does not remain constant even though the modulating frequency is unchanged. Each data point is the mean of five judgments from a single subject. (de Boer, 1956.)

If the carrier frequency remains constant, but the modulating frequency is increased, the general trend of periodicity pitch is upward as shown in Fig. 11. Periodicity pitch does not follow the modulating frequency exactly however. Rather, the pitch actually decreases, then jumps abruptly to a higher pitch from which it again decreases, with this sequence being repeated as the modulating frequency increases. De Boer pointed out that these results are consistent with the hypothesis that the pitch of the residue (periodicity pitch) corresponds only to those frequencies that are integral submultiples of the carrier frequency. It is as if, when the modulating frequency is close to one of these submultiples, periodicity pitch "locks in" on it. For example, when a carrier of 2000 Hz is used, integral submultiples exist at 1000 Hz (2), 667 Hz (3), 500 Hz (4), 400 Hz (5), 333 Hz (6), 286 Hz (7), 250 Hz (8), and so on. If the carrier frequency is now raised and the modulating frequency kept constant—perhaps at 250 Hz—the sub-

multiples move upward and the presumed consequence is that periodicity pitch does likewise. Then when the next lower submultiple —
(9) — is closer to the modulating frequency than is submultiple (8), the
pitch falls to the value corresponding to the frequency of that submultiple. The same reasoning holds for the results shown in Fig. 9 if
the downward tilt of the lines is ignored.

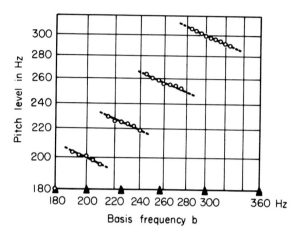

Figure 11 Pitch of a sinusoidally amplitude-modulated signal as a function of modulating or "basis" frequency *b*. Carrier frequency *a* was 1800 Hz. Pitch does not vary
continuously with modulating frequency; rather, it varies in a step-like fashion. Each
data point is based on five judgments by a single subject. (de Boer, 1956.)

Schouten *et al.* (1962) replicated and extended de Boer's work.
Figure 12 indicates a portion of their results and corresponds to de
Boer's data shown in Fig. 10. The results are similar except that, in
contrast to de Boer's findings, (*a*) pitch may be carried rather far along
a given submultiple, and (*b*) for a given carrier frequency, several
pitches (corresponding to different submultiples) may be perceived
simultaneously. In both Figs. 10 and 12, when the submultiple is
above the modulating frequency, the pitch is judged higher than that
expected on the basis of the submultiple hypothesis, but when the
submultiple is below the modulating frequency, the reverse is true.
Moreover, in Fig. 11, when the modulating frequency is changed but
the carrier frequency is held constant, pitch actually decreases before
it jumps to a higher value. It can be shown, as Schouten *et al.* (1962)
have done, that if one such effect occurs, the other is to be expected.

These authors refer to these effects collectively as the "second effect of pitch shift."

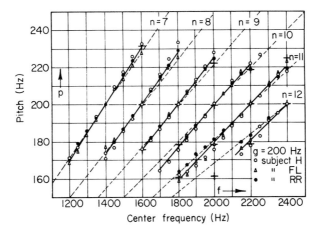

Figure 12 Pitch of a sinusoidally amplitude-modulated signal as a function of carrier center frequency f. Modulating frequency g was 200 Hz ($n = f/g$). Pitch matching was effected as for Figs. 10 and 11. Each subject contributed twelve judgments for each data point. (Schouten *et al.*, 1962. By permission from *Journal of the Acoustical Society of America*.)

De Boer (1956) proposed and Schouten *et al.* (1962) reviewed the concept of a pseudoperiod as an explanation of at least part of these data. They suggested that the pitch mechanism may measure the distance between those peaks in the carrier wave that are closest to (but not necessarily coincident with) the peaks in the waveform envelope. The reciprocal of this value then corresponds to periodicity pitch. Figure 13 illustrates the hypothesis. For example, if the carrier frequency is increased, the interval, I_1, becomes shorter and periodicity pitch increases, which is in line with the general features of the data shown in Figs. 10 and 12. If the pitch mechanism responds in this fashion, it is not difficult to conceive of the situation in which several pitches (defined for example by I_2 or I_3) are heard simultaneously. Although such a mechanism accounts for certain features of the data, it provides no explanation for the so called "second effect." Indeed, it can be shown in Fig. 10 that, because of envelope fluctuations, I_2 and I_3 are both shorter than would be expected on the basis of an unmodulated carrier frequency. This deviation from the "expected value" is not in accord with the "second effects."

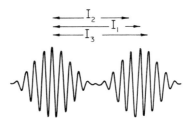

Figure 13   Waveform of an amplitude-modulated sinusoid. A pitch mechanism may operate on the basis of measuring the time interval between these peaks in the waveform that occur near the envelope maxima, such as I_1, I_2, and I_3. (Schouten *et al.*, 1962. By permission from *Journal of the Acoustical Society of America*.)

Additional data on the pseudoperiod were offered by Ritsma and Engel (1964), who worked with quasi-frequency modulated signals of the same type as used by Mathes and Miller (1947) (Section II, B, 1). Two subjects matched the pitch of these signals with that of a companion amplitude-modulated signal (that gave rise to a periodicity pitch). If the pitch of the FM signal is assumed to be determined by the pseudoperiod, then differential predictions may be made about how the perceived pitch varies with the ratio of carrier frequency to modulating frequency. Although the data are meager, they are in accord with the predictions.

These data demonstrate clearly that periodicity pitch is not determined simply by the periodicities in the envelope of the waveform. Rather it is determined by the envelope in conjunction with the fine structure of the waveform contained within the envelope. Sinusoidally amplitude-modulated signals of the type used in the de Boer and Schouten *et al.* studies provide a unique contribution to the question as to whether a difference tone is responsible for periodicity pitch. If the modulating frequency is kept constant and the carrier frequency is increased, within limits, periodicity pitch increases. The spacing of the spectral components is uniquely determined by the modulating frequency, and a difference tone in turn is determined by this spacing. Consequently if periodicity pitch changes when in fact the spacing of the spectral components does *not* change, we have compelling evidence that periodicity pitch is unrelated to difference tones.

Spectral Characteristics. Both the waveform envelope and the waveform fine structure are important in the perception of periodicity pitch, as are certain aspects of the signal spectrum. These critical spectral features include (a) the number and relative magnitude of the spectral components, (b) the spacing of these components, and (c) the region of the spectrum in which they are located.

Small (1955), manipulated certain temporal aspects of ac pulse trains (Fig. 7). The most reasonable interpretation of his data is that perceptual changes occurred by virtue of spectral changes that were, in turn, brought about by the temporal variation. For example, as the rise and decay time of the individual ac pulses making up the pulse train is increased, the perceptibility of the periodicity pitch declines. In a similar fashion, as the duty cycle of the pulse train increases, the audibility of periodicity pitch decreases. An increase in rise-decay time lessens the dispersion of energy among signal components; that is, the bandwidth of the signal is narrowed. An increase in duty cycle increases the amplitude of the carrier frequency or central component of the spectrum while the other components remain essentially unchanged. Under these conditions, signal threshold is probably determined to an increasing degree by the large central component. Thus, if the signal is maintained at a constant sensation level as duty cycle is varied (as it was here), then the levels of the other components are in effect lowered. Since the amplitude of a component usually becomes smaller as the frequency difference between component and carrier increases, the net result of this increase in duty cycle is to decrease the effective bandwidth of the signal. These results support the hypothesis that peridocity pitch should be more perceptible as the number of effective spectral components increases. Additional support comes from the observation that, with sinusoidal amplitude modulation, where there are only three spectral components, periodicity pitch is much less pronounced than for signals comprising a greater number of spectral components (Small, 1955; de Boer, 1956; Ritsma, 1963a). To have periodic variations in the envelope waveform, the signal needs a minimum of two components. It follows from this discussion that any periodicity pitch resulting from such two-component signals should be very faint indeed. And indeed, stimuli of this type led to the original controversy regarding "non-place" pitch (see Section I). We have gone full circle.

The use of sinusoidally amplitude-modulated signals provides certain advantages in the study of periodicity pitch. Foremost among these advantages is the simple nature of the spectrum and the ease with which it may be manipulated. Ritsma (1962) used such signals to try to delineate what he termed the existence region of tonal residue. Specifically, he manipulated the carrier and modulating frequencies and the depth of modulation (the markedness of waveform envelope variations). Spectrally, the modulating frequency determines the spacing between components, the carrier frequency fixes the location of the components, and the depth of modulation determines the amplitude of the side frequencies relative to the carrier (the deeper the modulation—the higher the modulation index—the greater the relative amplitude of the side bands). Ritsma investigated a number of carrier and modulating frequencies in which the ratio of carrier to modulating frequency formed an integer. His three subjects were considered to be perceiving a periodicity pitch when they could precisely match the pitch in question with a second stimulus. The second stimulus was similarly complex, but had a lower carrier frequency ($f_c = f_c - 4f_m$). Although matching to a pure-tone stimulus permits the traditional definition of pitch in terms of a sinusoid, quality differences between a pure tone and a periodicity pitch associated with complex stimuli create an appreciable amount of variability in the data. Therefore, Ritsma and others have chosen not to use pure tones as comparison stimuli.

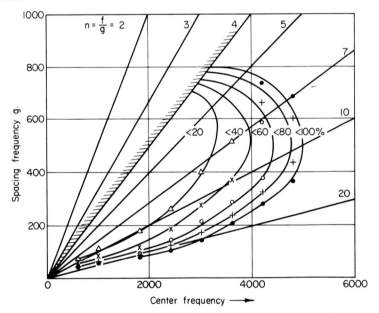

Figure 14 The frequency region within which periodicity pitch may be perceived using sinusoidal amplitude modulation. Modulating or spacing frequency g is shown on the ordinate, and carrier or center frequency f appears on the abscissca. The solid lines radiating from the origin are for reference purposes and represent constant values of the ratio f/g, M is the modulation index. (Ritsma, 1962. By permission from *Journal of the Acoustical Society of America*.)

Figure 14 shows, for one subject, the conditions under which periodicity pitch exists for a sinusoidally amplitude-modulated signal. The range of carrier and modulating frequencies for which periodicity pitch is perceived becomes larger as the depth of modulation increases. Further, for both the carrier and modulating frequencies, there are limits above which periodicity pitch is not perceived.

These data of Ritsma, obtained with three-component signals, bear out the earlier findings of Small (1955), who used signals with large numbers of components. Small found that periodicity pitch is less well heard (and therefore less precisely matched) when, with a modulating fundamental frequency of 100 Hz, carrier frequency is increased above 2000 Hz. Other pertinent observations were made but not reported at that time. Specifically, with that rate of modulation, effective signal components had to exist in the region below 2000 Hz in order for periodicity pitch to be perceived. Several techniques were used to control the location of spectral energy: (a) the components were moved upward by increasing the carrier frequency; (b) with the carrier frequency substantially above 2000 Hz, the rise-fall time was increased, thus lessening the energy spread down into the region below 2000 Hz; (c) components below 2000 Hz were rejected by a high-pass filter; and (d) components below 2000 Hz were masked by a low-pass thermal noise.

Ritsma (1963a) confirmed Small's observations of a critical region that must contain signal components. He used dc pulses at a repetition rate of 200 or 280 Hz, and with the spectrum limited by filters. The location of the components was determined by a frequency shifter that moved the components in frequency steps equal to the pulse repetition rate. The subject's task was to determine whether, following each shift, the pitch of the complex still corresponded to the repetition rate. Figure 15 shows his results for the highest pass band for which the criterion could be met. As the sensation level of the signal is increased, the center frequency of permissible pass bands increases, but the low-frequency skirt remains unchanged. Apparently, it is necessary to have approximately three spectral components below some critical frequency before periodicity pitch is audible. For the conditions Ritsma (1963a) employed, this critical frequency is about 3000 Hz and corresponds closely to the upper limit established for a three-component complex (Ritsma, 1962).

In summary, certain aspects of signal spectrum are important in determining the perceptibility of periodicity pitch. Generally, the greater number of spectral components contained in the signal, the more apparent is periodicity pitch. Further, periodicity pitch seems

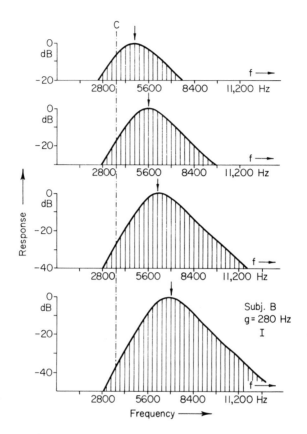

Figure 15 Spectral composition of a filtered pulse train shifted upward in frequency as far as possible with periodicity pitch still audible. Panels from top to bottom represent sensation levels of 25, 35, 45, and 55 dB, respectively. Components are spaced at 280-Hz intervals. The factor of principal importance seems to be the configuration of the low-frequency components. The vertical dashed line represents the upper limit of periodicity pitch for a three-component complex (see Fig. 14). (Ritsma, 1963a. By permission from *Journal of the Acoustical Society of America*.)

to exist only when signal components are located below some critical frequency. The relation between the spacing of the spectral components and the audibility of periodicity pitch is dependent upon the carrier frequency, but the pitch is best heard for spacings (modulation rates) below 700 Hz.

C. Relations between Place and Periodicity Pitch

One way to establish whether place pitch and periodicity pitch share a common mechanism is to ask whether both pitches are affected in a similar fashion by similar variables. This section reviews such experiments.

Pitch Shifts. The apparent change in the pitch of a pure tone as its level is changed is well known. Snow (1936), for example, reported that a 125-Hz tone may lower its pitch by as much as 25% with an extreme increase in level. Stevens (1935) reported data of a "typical" listener who showed shifts of similar magnitude at low frequencies, and in addition showed an upward shift in pitch with increased level at high frequencies. More recent data do not completely support these findings: Morgan *et al.* (1951) and Cohen (1961) noted very small shifts—less than two percent.

If this pitch shift with level is a characteristic of the pitch associated with a pure tone (i.e., a "place" pitch) then it would be interesting to see whether similar effects occur with periodicity pitch. Schouten (1940a) noted that, as intensity is raised, the pitch of the residue or periodicity pitch is unchanged while "the fundamental tone [of the complex exhibited] the well-known fall up to about half a tone." It is interesting to speculate whether Lewis and Cowan (1936), who reported that the pitch of complex musical tones (produced by violins and cellos) did not change as a function of level, were in fact listening to periodicity pitch. Tones produced by these instruments often have little energy at the fundamental frequency. Small and Campbell (1961a) used a variety of complex signals that produced periodicity pitch, and in addition used pure tones as control stimuli. They found no monotonic shift in pitch for the stimuli with envelope periodicity, but they found no pitch shifts with the pure tones either.

Békésy (1961), however, reported that the pitch associated with the envelope fluctuations of a sinusoidally amplitude-modulated signal decreases as depth of modulation increases (Fig. 16). To the extent that an increase in depth of modulation is similar to an increase in overall signal level, these data disagree with those reported by Schouten and by Small and Campbell. So it is difficult to offer a clear statement as to whether changes in sound level produce different shifts in periodicity pitch than in place (pure-tone) pitch.

Van den Brink (1965) reported an attempt to shift periodicity pitch by means of the presentation of an intense fatiguing stimulus. He found that shifts occur for both pure-tone and complex signals. However, he interpreted his data as supporting the hypothesis that periodicity pitch "is perceived at that place on the basilar membrane where its components are perceived." It is, however, a difficult experiment, and for a variety of reasons, not the least of which is the fact that data for only one subject were presented, his conclusion should be regarded as tentative.

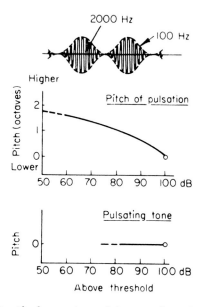

Figure 16 Pitch shift with changes in modulation index. The top drawing indicates that sinusoidal amplitude modulation was employed with a carrier of 2000 Hz and a modulating frequency of 100 Hz. The top graph shows that the pitch corresponding approximately to the modulating frequency falls as the modulation index is increased. The bottom graph indicates that, under the same conditions, the pitch associated with the carrier does not change. (Békésy, 1961. By permission from *Journal of the Acoustical Society of America.*)

Differential Thresholds for Frequency. Many data provide information on minimum perceptible frequency difference between two sinusoids (e.g., Shower and Biddulph, 1931; Harris, 1952). Generally these data indicate that the differential threshold is smaller for low frequencies than for high frequencies. If a moderately high-frequency sinusoid is interrupted periodically, a low-periodicity pitch is perceived. What is the minimum detectable change in interruption or modulation rate? And is the differential threshold small, as one would predict on the basis of the low pitch, or large, as one would predict from the high-frequency content of the signal?

Campbell (1963) presented data on this point, but unfortunately they do not allow any simple interpretation. Signals were sinusoids of 150 and 2200 Hz, and a pulsed signal derived from a band-pass filter—with a center frequency of 2200 Hz—that was excited by dc

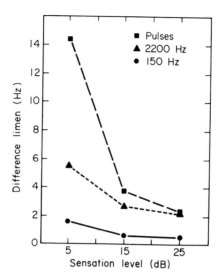

Figure 17   Differential thresholds for repetition rate (pulses) and frequency (sinusoids). The pulses consisted of a 2200-Hz sinusoid interrupted 150 times per sec. Each data point is based on 40 pitch matches for each of nine subjects. (Campbell, 1963. By permission from *Journal of the Acoustical Society of America*.)

pulses 150 times per sec. The subject's task was to match the pitch of a test signal with a comparison signal of the same type. The precision of matching is shown in Fig. 17. At very low sensation levels, the differential threshold for the pulses is higher than for either of the sinusoids. As sensation level is increased, the differential threshold for the pulses decreases and rapidly approaches the curve representing the 2200-Hz sinusoid.

In general, the differential threshold function for pulses resembles the function for the 2200-Hz tone more closely than it does the function for the 150-Hz signal. To the extent that this statement is true, one can argue that these data support the hypothesis that periodicity pitch is carried by high-frequency channels within the auditory system.

Ritsma (1963b) also reported data on the variability of pitch matching. In his case however, periodicity pitch was derived from a sinusoidally amplitude-modulated signal and was not matched by a similar

stimulus, but by one with a different center frequency. The results
are shown in Fig. 18 and suggest that the precision of matching is
similar for low periodicity pitch and low-frequency pure tones.
Higher-frequency pure tones, however, show less pitch-matching
variability than corresponding periodicity pitch. Therefore, the results of Ritsma and those of Campbell are not in complete accord.
However, the intensities under which the data were gathered were
not the same.

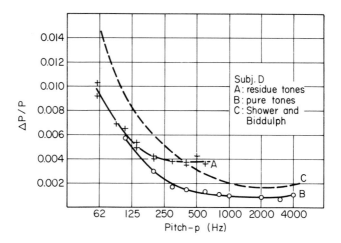

Figure 18 Differential thresholds for modulating frequency (residue tones) and simple
frequency (pure tones). The periodicity pitch was derived from a sinusoidally amplitude-modulated signal. Listening was done at 40 dB SL. The subject provided 80
matches for each data point. The pure-tone data of Shower and Biddulph are provided
for comparison. (Ritsma, 1963b. By permission from *International Audiology*.)

III. ELECTROPHYSIOLOGICAL DATA

Psychoacoustic data necessarily provide only indirect descriptions
of the mechanisms of pitch perception. A more direct approach involves the recording of electrical potentials from various parts of the
auditory nervous system. However, electrical potentials cannot be
considered the same as pitch, since the precise coding of pitch information within the nervous system is not clear.

A. Recordings from the Cochlea

Little work has been done on neuroelectric correlates of periodicity
pitch as recorded from the cochlea. A substantial amount of cochlear
research is pertinent to the problem of periodicity pitch.

Cochlear Microphonics. The cochlear microphonic mirrors the displacement pattern of the basilar membrane. That is, for high frequencies, a maximum potential is seen in the basal region; for low frequencies the maximum potential is found in the apex of the cochlea. Signals of intermediate frequency produce electrical maxima at intermediate cochlear positions. Davis and his co-workers have demonstrated these relations many times (for an early example, see Davis *et al.*, 1950). When 8000-Hz tone pips—the auditory neurophysiologist's term for an ac pulse train—are presented at a fairly rapid rate, the cochlear microphonic in the guinea pig shows a maximum in the region of the basal turn. When the same stimulus is presented to human subjects, they judge it to have a low pitch corresponding approximately to the repetition rate (Davis *et al.*, 1951). On the basis of the pitch, the electrical activity should be in the low-frequency or apical region of the cochlea. It appears then that this observation of Davis *et al.* supports the hypothesis that, for periodicity pitch at least, pitch information is not coded in terms of place, but perhaps in terms of rate of responding (volleying). It should be added, however, that Leibbrandt (1966), in a similar situation, failed to substantiate the Davis *et al.* results.

A related observation was reported by de Boer and Six (1960). They were concerned with the locus of a difference tone produced by the simultaneous presentation of two sinusoids. The distribution of cochlear microphonics along the length of a guinea pig's basilar membrane was investigated for each of the primaries and for the difference tone. At low to moderate sound levels, the distribution of potentials was identical for both the high-frequency primaries and for the low-frequency difference tone. With high sound levels, the distribution of potentials corresponding to the difference tone changed so that a larger relative voltage was seen in the apical region. In the former case, the authors suggested that the difference tone (as seen in the cochlear microphonic) arises from the same region as is excited by the primaries—perhaps due to nonlinearities associated with the "mechano-electrical conversion process." At high sound levels, distortion arises in the middle ear, and the distortion products have the same cochlear distribution as they would if they were simply the result of nonsimultaneous, independent sinusoidal signals.

Action Potentials. The role of cochlear microphonics in the production of a neural response is not settled. Some hold that it is the necessary and immediate precursor of the neural response (Davis, 1957); others suggest it is independent of and causally unrelated to neural activity and is simply a by-product of the movement of membranes that separate fluids of different electrical potential (Hallpike and Rawdon-Smith, 1937). In any case, the research that relates the microphonic to periodicity pitch is pertinent to the extent that neural excitation occurs at the position of maximum amplitude of the traveling wave. Still to be faced is the problem of the neural coding of pitch information at both peripheral and central levels. The place hypothesis stated in neural terms is simply that the locus of maximum neural activity is determined by signal frequency, and that pitch is a function of these loci. A commonly advanced alternative to a place theory suggests that pitch is coded in terms of temporal rather than frequency cues. It is clear that for any temporal analysis, relevant time relations found in the signal must be preserved in the nervous system. Among other things, this requirement calls for the nervous system to be able to respond at high rates and, more importantly, maintain synchrony with the signal waveform. Whether the nervous system is able to convey temporal information to higher neural centers with sufficient precision to account for periodicity pitch data has been questioned. However, techniques of computer averaging of neural responses make it possible to discern synchronous activity that, under other conditions of observation, might be obscured by nonsynchronous neural responses. Derbyshire and Davis (1935) recorded at the cochlea in cats, and found synchronous activity up to 2000 Hz in response to sinusoidal signals. With the aid of averaging techniques, Peake *et al.* (1962) were able to detect synchronized responses to bursts of noise for rates as high as 3000 bursts per sec. Moreover, they concluded that this upper limit "may represent a limitation of our method rather than a limit of synchronous firing."

B. Recordings from the Nervous System

Subcortical. A more straightforward method of ascertaining the upper limit of synchronous activity is to record directly from the nervous system rather than from the cochlea. Several authors (Galambos and Davis, 1943, 1948; Tasaki, 1954) have reported that, in mammals at least, although single neurons tend to discharge during a particular interval of the sinusoidal signal they do not respond to every cycle nor to every *n*th cycle. Rather, they respond in a probabilistic way, so the synchronous activities observable in whole-nerve responses may be due to a "statistical" synchrony rather than a "deterministic" synchrony.

Data from single neurons of the eighth nerve in the bullfrog (Frishkopf and Goldstein, 1963) and in the green frog (Sachs, 1964) are of interest with respect to synchrony, time coding, and pitch. In both experiments, two groups of neurons were found: one was characterized as responding most readily to low frequencies (about 300 Hz), possessing no spontaneous activity, and having evoked responses that could be inhibited by tones; the other as responding principally to high-frequency stimuli (about 1400 Hz), usually having spontaneous activity, and being impossible to inhibit. The frog's auditory system might have among its more important functions the capacity to respond to frog croaks—particularly those of its own species. The croak is impulsive in character (about 100 impulses per sec) with most of its energy in the frequency region to which the high-frequency fibers are maximally sensitive. Single neural units produce spikes that are time-locked to the impulsive aspects of the waveform of both actual and synthetic croaks, even when there is no signal energy at the neural discharge rate. Further, Capranica (1964) reported that, in order to elicit responsive vocal activity from a bullfrog, the initiating signal must have a periodicity of about 1/100 sec. In other words, for the bullfrog at least, envelope periodicity and timing cues play an important role in the functioning of the auditory system.

As responses are observed at successively higher neural centers, the upper limit at which synchrony may be maintained steadily decreases (Kemp et al., 1937). Within the auditory area of the cat's cerebral cortex, stimulus-locked activity of cortical origin may be found up to 200 noise bursts per sec (Goldstein et al., 1959). It is curious that these upper limits of synchronous activity are of the same magnitude as the upper limit of noise interruption for which Miller and Taylor's (1948) subjects were able to perform pitch matches.

Cortical. Several studies of the cortex deal explicitly with possible neural correlates of periodicity pitch. Small and Gross (1962) used a variety of impulsive signals to map the auditory cortex of the cat for evoked potentials. They reasoned that, if pitch is represented cortically by the locus of response, then stimuli differing in physical characteristics, but producing the same pitch sensation (in man), should produce similar spatial patterns of activity. They found that the topical distribution of evoked cortical activity corresponds not to "pitch sensation," but to a Fourier analysis of the signal. Those signals with similar spectra show similar patterns of activity. For example, an increase in spectral dispersion of signal energy results in an increase in the spread of evoked activity over the cortex. Thus, at least at the cortex of the cat, frequency, not pitch, is represented.

One of the interesting response characteristics of single auditory neural units is their tuning; that is, they show maximum sensitivity to a pure tone of a particular frequency (termed characteristic frequency) and decreasing sensitivity to frequencies increasingly remote from the optimal one. Such findings have been reported by large numbers of investigators (beginning with Galambos and Davis, 1943) for a wide variety of species, from moths (Suga, 1961) to monkeys (Katsuki *et al.*, 1961). It has been presumed that this tuning is related to the spatial pattern of excitation within the cochlea. Thus, if a unit responds to a high-frequency sinusoid, it is assumed that this unit, or at least its excitation, originates in the basal region of the cochlea. Glattke (1968) made use of this reasoning in an investigation of the neurophysiological correlates of periodicity pitch as recorded from single neural units in the cochlear nucleus of the cat. He divided those units he sampled into "low-frequency" and "high-frequency" categories depending upon whether their characteristic frequency was below or above 800 Hz. In the case of low-frequency units, stimuli were presented that possessed low-frequency periodicity in their waveform envelopes, but had spectra containing essentially no low-frequency energy. For each high-frequency unit, the stimuli consisted of a sinusoid corresponding to the unit's characteristic frequency, but interrupted at rates of 100 to 1000 times per sec. In addition, interrupted noise was used with both types of units. Tuning curves were obtained (as a function of repetition rate) for these modulated stimuli. The results indicated that, in order for units to respond, it is necessary that energy be located in the vicinity of the unit's characteristic frequency. Low-frequency units do not respond to low-frequency envelope periodicities corresponding to their characteristic frequency. However, the temporal patterns of the discharge of high-frequency units mirrors stimulus periodicity over a wide range of modulation rates. Thus, these results suggest that demodulation does not occur in the cochlea, a concept consonant with the hypothesis that, for these types of signals, the low-pitch information is coded in the temporal patterning of the responses of the high-frequency units.

Hind (1953) demonstrated that tuning within the auditory nervous system is not restricted to single neural units. With a gross electrode, he observed tuning in response to a sinusoid, presumably sampling a population of neurons on the cortex of the cat. Kiang and Goldstein (1959) expanded on Hind's observation of tuning; they used steady tones and repetitive bursts of tone and of noise (Fig. 19). Kiang and Goldstein, as well as Hind, applied bits of filter paper soaked in a three percent strychnine sulfate solution to the cat's cortex and by means of evoked activity determined the tuning function of the areas treated. Their results indicate that, although a particular spot responds preferentially to certain frequency sinusoids as compared to others, its threshold is independent of the burst rate of noise. Since, for a human observer, the pitch of an interrupted noise changes as a function of repetition rate — at least up to 200–300 interruptions per sec — this finding does not support the representation of periodicity pitch by the "tuning" mechanism. In general, the tuning curves reflect the spectral characteristics of their complex signals — a finding in agreement with Small and Gross (1962) and, at a subcortical level, with Glattke (1968). Thus, rather than being structured in terms of pitch, the auditory cortex possesses an organization based on frequency, both for the tuning of local areas, and for all spatial patterning.

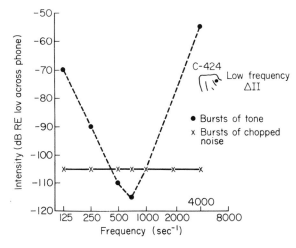

Figure 19 Lowest intensity at which responses evoked by auditory stimuli could be detected. Inset shows the position of the electrode and strychnine patch. Dashed curve depicts response thresholds to onsets of tonal stimuli vs. tone frequency in hertz. Solid curve indicates response thresholds to onsets of repeated bursts of noise vs. burst repetition rate. (Kiang and Goldstein, 1959. By permission from *Journal of the Acoustical Society of America.*)

Measurements at the cortex may be interpreted in several ways. First, one may question whether, in cats at least, frequency discrimination (and therefore pitch) is a cortical function. Thompson's (1960) data, for example, suggest that it is not. Second, the cortical activity reported here was in response to the onset of the stimulus, not to a steady-state situation. This response may not be related to subjective pitch, which tends to be a steady-state rather than an onset phenomenon (Doughty and Garner, 1948). Third, species differences should not be overlooked. These experiments, conducted with cats, used stimuli that evoke certain pitch characteristics in human observers. Whether cats or other nonhuman species perceive periodicity pitch remains to be determined.

An important question arises: Is periodicity pitch an effect found only in human observers, perhaps related to learning (Thurlow, 1963), or is it an experience that is basically physiologically determined and therefore common to many species? The only information on this point comes from informal and inconclusive observations on pigeons recounted by Licklider (1959). Their responses in a conditioning situation yield results similar to those obtained by electrophysiological methods, i.e., they respond to Fourier frequency, not to waveform periodicity.

In summary, the only electrophysiological or conditioning data that reflect periodicity perception is that obtained with the bullfrog. In that case, there is little evidence that pitch is necessarily involved; periodicity may manifest itself quite differently.

IV. COCHLEAR MODELS

A. Simple "Békésy" Models

Models, including models of the ear, provide a useful approach to the understanding of complex systems. For example, they allow the manipulation of system parameters in ways that might well be impossible in the actual system. There are several different classes of models, but those used most commonly in the study of the cochlea have been dimensional models of a hydromechanical variety. Békésy (1928) was one of the first to use such models to simulate the action of the cochlea. More recently, others have worked with models similar to those Békésy originated. A typical model consists of a rectangular piece of metal with a triangular section cut from its center. The missing section conforms to the width-length function of the basilar membrane. The "membrane" itself is formed by applying rubber cement to the opening in the metal. Because of the effect of surface tension, the cement forms a thicker film at the narrow end of the opening than at the wide end, and as a consequence, the film of rubber achieves an elastic gradient comparable to that of the basilar membrane. The frame is mounted in an uncoiled plastic "cochlea" and the "perilymphatic fluid" consists of a glycerin and water solution. Models are commonly twice the size of the actual cochlea.

In 1959 and 1962, Tonndorf reported observations of a model in which the inputs were amplitude-modulated signals. In essence, he found that the cochlear model detects any fluctuation in the signal waveform envelope. When fluctuation is periodic, a maximum appears in the displacement pattern of the "basilar membrane" at the place corresponding to the frequency of envelope periodicity. For example, if a 250 Hz sinusoid were amplitude-modulated with a 40 Hz sinusoid, maxima would occur in the displacement pattern at the positions corresponding to both 250 and 40 Hz. Remember that, in the same stimulus situation, human observers report pitches corresponding to both frequencies. If results obtained on a cochlear model reflect the situation as it exists in the human cochlea, then it would be unnecessary to call upon complex neural mechanisms to account for periodicity pitch. On the other hand, such envelope detection is a known property of nonlinear systems. The auditory system—in particular the cochlea—exhibits other attributes of nonlinearity under appropriately large input amplitudes (Tonndorf, 1958). It is difficult to know precisely the scaling factor between signal levels applied to cochlear models and those delivered to the actual ear. Therefore, the signal amplitude at which these effects are observed in cochlear models may in fact correspond to rather high levels in the real ear. If so, then nonlinear effects—including envelope detection—are to be expected.

B. Cochlear Model with Nerve Supply

In his chapter of this book, Békésy describes his investigations of responses of the skin to vibratory stimuli. He believes that, in many respects, the skin is a "primitive basilar membrane," and consequently that information gained there can furnish insight into the functioning of the auditory system. He has used two types of stimuli: a simple rigid frame, and a model of the cochlea. Generally results obtained with either vibrating system are similar except that, in the latter case, because of the relative complexity of the stimulus, subjects note a greater number of attributes in the evoked sensation.

I will limit this discussion to the results obtained with the model with nerve supply. This model takes the form of a fluid-filled cylinder with a portion of the otherwise rigid cylinder wall consisting of a narrow, flexible membrane whose long axis is parallel to that of the cylinder. The forearm (complete with nerve supply) is placed on the membrane whose mechanical characteristics are similar to those in earlier and less elaborate Békésy models. When the fluid within the cylinder is set into vibration, the membrane is displaced in the typical traveling wave fashion, and this vibratory motion is sensed by the skin. One of the most striking features of the response to such a stimulus is that, although a large area of the skin is set into motion, the spatial sensation is quite small and precisely localized. Békésy suggested that this restricted response results from mutual facilitation and inhibition within the peripheral nervous system, and refers to the effect as "funnelling." In the case of sinusoidal stimuli, the position of the sensation changes as a function of frequency, and is localized at the maximum of the envelope of the traveling wave (Békésy, 1955).

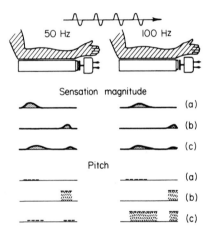

Figure 20 Sensation patterns obtained using pulsed sinusoids as the input to the cochlear model with nerve supply. The frequency of the uninterrupted sinusoid was either 50 Hz (left) or 100 Hz (right). The top drawings labeled *a*, *b*, and *c* show the distribution of sensation magnitude along the forearm when the attention is concentrated (*a*) near the elbow, (*b*) near the wrist, or (*c*) overall. The *a*, *b*, and *c* drawings at the bottom of the figure have the same meanings as in the top drawings, and depict the subjective attribute corresponding to rate of vibration for each of the sensation loci. The height of the dotted line is proportional to the perceived rate of vibration. (Békésy, 1961. By permission from *Journal of the Acoustical Society of America.*)

When complex stimuli with marked envelope periodicity are presented to this model, two local maxima appear — one at the locus corresponding to the rate of envelope variation, the other at the locus corresponding to the frequency of the waveform (Fig. 20). Similar results are obtained for dc and ac pulses as well as sinusoidal amplitude-modulated signals (Békésy, 1961).

These findings agree with those of Tonndorf (1959) who made optical rather than tactile observations. Such results suggest that periodicity pitch (and, perhaps, allied phenomena) may be accounted for on a simple physical basis utilizing a place principle of pitch perception.

C. Electrical Analogs of the Cochlea

A number of electrical analogs of the cochlea have been developed; most have grown out of computational models. The analog to be discussed here was developed in this fashion by Flanagan (1960, 1962). It is the only electrical model whose output has been observed with input signals that yield periodicity pitch in man.

Flanagan's goal was an analytical relation for estimating basilar membrane displacement at a given point from a knowledge of the sound pressure at the eardrum. The basic data from which he worked were Békésy's observations regarding the phase and amplitude of basilar membrane displacement as a function of frequency. His method was to approximate Békésy's data by a function whose Laplace transformation was the ratio of rational polynomials and was computationally tractable. It was then possible to construct electrical circuits whose transmission properties were identical to those of the developed functions.

A similar procedure was followed in deducing the transmission characteristics of the middle ear; in this case, he used Zwislocki's (1962) data. The results shown in Fig. 21 are typical of those obtained from such an electrical analog. In this figure, the input consists of short pulses (with a repetition rate of 200 Hz) that have been passed through a high-pass filter with a 4 kHz cutoff frequency. Under these conditions, there is no "displacement" of the "basilar membrane" in the region corresponding to 200 Hz. Yet, under these same stimulus conditions, a pitch may be perceived that corresponds to a frequency of 200 Hz. The results with this model, although at variance with the observations of Tonndorf and Békésy are in accord with the findings of psychoacoustic investigations. For example, the results of Small and Campbell (1961b) with masking and Small and Yelen (1962) with fatigue suggest very strongly that no effective stimulus is present in the apical region of the membrane under the described conditions.

200 Hz
HP 4 KC

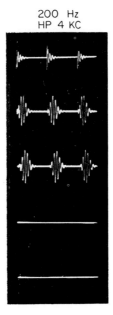

Figure 21 Response of an electrical analog of the cochlea to ac pulses. The input to the analog is shown at the top of the figure and consists of a train of short-duration dc pulses repeated 200 times per sec, high-pass filtered at 4 kHz. The response at the output of the middle ear and at the point on the basilar membrane responding maximally to 5000, 1000, and 200 Hz are shown. (Flanagan, 1962. From the *Bell System Technical Journal*. Copyright 1962, The American Telephone and Telegraph Company, reprinted by permission.)

V. NONPLACE HYPOTHESES

Several hypotheses have been advanced to account for periodicity pitch with a pitch mechanism that operates on something other than a place principle. These hypotheses vary in scope from those that purport to explain *all* of pitch perception to those whose horizons are restricted to the data of a particular periodicity pitch experiment. Central to all of these hypotheses is the notion that the important cue for periodicity pitch is in the time waveform of the signal, and that the essentials of this time information are preserved in the firing of the neurons associated with the auditory system.

A. Specific Proposals

Schouten's (1940b) original contention was that periodicity pitch, at least as perceived with amplitude-modulated signals, is mediated by synchronous firing in the auditory nerve. Further, this synchronous firing originates in that place in the peripheral auditory mechanism that responds to high frequencies. Figure 22, which schematizes Schouten's idea, depicts the situation existing when repetitive dc pulses are applied to a series of resonators. The resonators in this figure are drawn with equal Qs and have center frequencies spaced at 200-Hz intervals. Low-frequency components of the signal are resolved, but at higher frequencies, more than one component is found within a single resonator. Schouten suggested that these unresolved components beat together to produce a waveform that retains the original envelope periodicity; this periodicity then forms the basis for neural timing cues. Such a hypothesis is a reasonable first attempt to produce a model that accounts for the important features of periodicity pitch.

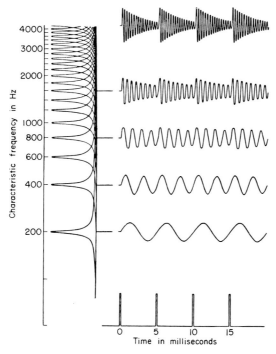

Figure 22 Response of a set of tuned resonators to a complex wave of 200 pulses per sec. This figure demonstrates how waveform periodicity may be maintained in the cochlea in the region that normally responds to high frequencies. The tuning of the resonators is such that only a single component passes through the low-frequency resonators but several appear at the output of the high-frequency resonators. These latter components beat together to produce an output whose envelope reflects the periodicity of the complex wave at the input. (Schouten, 1940b. By permission from *Proceedings Koninklijke Nederlandse Akademie van Wetenschappen.*)

Recall that de Boer (1956) and Schouten *et al.* (1962) found periodicity pitch to be determined not only by the waveform envelope, but also by the fine structure of the waveform. Consequently, Schouten's original hypothesis was modified (by the introduction of the concept of the pseudoperiod — see Fig. 13) to take this finding into account. The hypothesis was amended to state that the timing cues associated with the unresolved components (upper part of Fig. 22) are taken from the major positive peaks in the fine structure rather than from the envelope.

Goldstein (1957) and, in a slightly different sense, Huggins and Licklider (1951) attempted to provide an adequate mathematical description of the auditory signal. That is to say, the auditory system, for purposes of pitch perception, utilizes certain aspects of the signal and neglects certain other aspects. If the signal could be described in the same terms as the auditory system "sees" it, then such a description could be used to predict pitch perception for any type of signal. Goldstein (1957) developed a transform for obtaining a time-variant spectral representation of the signal (the work is an extension of that of Fano, 1950, and Booton, 1952). Goldstein called this representation the bifrequency transform and suggested its principal usefulness lies in its ability to represent both the characteristic of the waveform envelope and the spectral distribution of signal power for either random or nonrandom signals.

Huggins and Licklider (1951) were concerned about the lack of a sufficiently restricted response in the place domain. They tried, therefore, to derive a rational transform that would provide sharper spatial responses either on the basilar membrane or in the peripheral portion of the auditory nervous system. Their goal and Goldstein's were similar in that they were all attempting to specify the "effective" signal.

Those who want to build a comprehensive theory of pitch perception almost without exception come to the conclusion that pitch is based on two or more aspects of the signal. The theoretical differences arise from the relative importance ascribed to each signal aspect. Wever (1949), for example, hypothesized that volleying — i.e., synchrony of neural discharge with stimulus envelope periodicity — is of major importance over a wide range of stimulus frequencies. He suggested that the place principle plays a dominant role only above 5000 Hz. Békésy (1963), on the other hand, admitted to an inadequacy of the place principle only below 50 Hz. Licklider (1951, 1956, 1959, 1962) has proposed a theory of pitch perception that, in contrast to some, is explicit. Figure 23 schematizes his 1959 proposal. All signals undergo a spatial filtering action within the cochlea. Lick-lider conceived of a multitude of individual channels proceeding centrally from both cochleas. In the central processor, several im-portant transforms occur, one of which pertains directly to periodicity pitch, and has as its basis a neural network that produces a running autocorrelation function of the input from each "channel" of the cochlear output. One such network is shown in Fig. 24. Each channel feeds an autocorrelator whose action is described in the legend of the figure. Patterns of neural activity are formed with multiple loci spaced, in the Z dimension, by a distance related to the periodicty of the wave-form, while the position of the loci in the X dimension are determined by the spectrum of the signal. The autocorrelator thus acts as a periodicity-to-place transformer, and makes spatial patterns of neural activity change as a function of both the periodicity and spectrum of the signal. Licklider completed his model by hypothesizing an "each to every" matrix of interconnections between his H and J blocks. Pre-sumably through learning processes, certain sets of patterns in H come to be represented through appropriately modified interconnec-

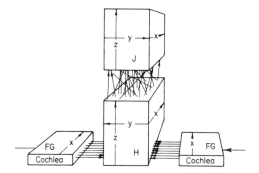

Figure 23   Schematic illustration of a hypothetical auditory system. Signals enter the cochleas where cochlear frequency analysis maps stimulus frequency into the spatial dimension X. The time-domain analyzer H preserves the order in X but adds an analysis in the Y dimension (based chiefly on interaural time differences) and an analysis in the Z dimension (based on periodicities in the waveform envelope received from FG). In the projection from H to J, each point in H is initially connected to every point in J (except that the ordering of the X dimension is largely preserved). Under the influence of acoustic stimulation, the H–J transformation organizes itself according to the rules imposed by the dynamics of the neural network. The patterns in J thereby acquire properties that are reflected in pitch perception. (Licklider, 1959. From *Psychology: a study of a science*, Vol. I, S. Koch (ed.). Copyright 1959 by McGraw-Hill. Used with permission of McGraw-Hill Book Company.)

tions between *H* and *J* as a single focus in *J*. This latter consideration is thought to be the basic condition for the emergence of pitch.

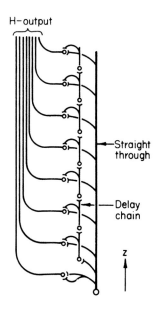

H–output

Straight
through

Delay
chain

z

Figure 24 Schematic illustration of a neural autocorrelator. The straight-through neuron is an ascending neuron oriented along the Z axis of the *H* block. Consider an example of the autocorrelator's operation. Following appropriate cochlear frequency analysis, certain groups of neurons in *H* receive inputs in the form of neural impulses synchronized to the envelope periodicity of the original signal. An impulse travels up the straight-through neuron, and a corresponding impulse travels up the delay chain with appropriate synaptic delays. Meanwhile, a second impulse enters "at the bottom" and follows the same pathways. At some point in the Z dimension, the straight-through second impulse will catch up with the delayed version of the first impulse. At this point, the *H* output fiber is excited by the coincidence of impinging impulses. Such a sequencing of events occurs continuously and, thereby, this mechanism provides a time-to-place conversion. (Licklider, 1959. From *Psychology: a study of a science.* Vol. 1, S. Koch (ed.). Copyright 1959 by McGraw-Hill. Used with permission of McGraw-Hill Book Company.)

Thurlow (1963), though, felt that there is no firm basis for postulating the existence of a precise time-analyzing mechanism. He argued that the data are more parsimoniously accounted for by a multicue mediation theory. In some respects, Thurlow's proposal simply emphasizes what Licklider termed the *H* to *J* transformation. Thurlow suggested that pitch arises on the basis of place information, the response to which is mediated by vocal activity. The vocal activity may be overt, subliminal, or involve only auditory imagery. For example, if a 2000 Hz carrier is amplitude-modulated by a 200 Hz sinusoid, components will be located at 1800, 2000, and 2200 Hz with corresponding maxima in the displacement pattern of the basilar membrane. The mediation hypothesis states that the subject "sings or hums," and produces physically or in his mind, a "comparison" signal whose fundamental frequency is adjusted so that its harmonics coincide with the components of the amplitude-modulated tone. The pitch perceived then corresponds to the fundamental of the implicit "comparison" signal. Such a theory, although elegant in the way it accounts for sometimes disconcerting individual differences, suffers from many of the shortcomings of the difference-tone hypothesis of periodicity pitch. For example, it does not predict the findings of de Boer (1956) and Schouten *et al.* (1962) that periodicity pitch may be manipulated independently of the frequency separation between components.

B. Origin of Timing Cues

There are several interesting but somewhat neglected aspects of time-based theories of pitch perception. One deals with the origin of the timing information; the other probes the related question of whether the time system that *may* exist for pitch, is in fact, the same as that utilized for binaural localization.

All impulsive signals apparently produce a traveling wave that progresses from the base to the apex of the cochlea, but shows a maximum determined by the signal's spectral characteristics (Tonndorf, 1960). Thus, timing cues may derive either from the basal turn (Davis, 1957) through which all signals must pass, or from the point of maximum stimulation. The psychoacoustic data, particularly those relating to the masking and fatiguing of periodicity pitch, point strongly toward the latter conclusion. And most theorists accept this point of view (Schouten, 1940b; Licklider, 1951).

It seems likely that with dc pulses (clicks), timing cues for localization derive from the region of the cochlear basal turn. However, Békésy (1933) and Schubert and Elpern (1959) suggested that, with appropriate noise masking, the origin of the time cues may be shifted apically. Further, if the signal consists of bursts of a sinusoid, time cues for lateralization seen to arise from that point on the basilar membrane that responds maximally (Harris, 1960). Thus, there is a basic similarity between the origin of "timing" for periodicity pitch and for binaural localization.

Nordmark (1963) attempted to provide further information regarding timing as related to pitch mechanisms and as related to localization. His conclusions support the hypothesis of a close relation, but the signals he used give rise to a pitch phenomenon other than periodicity pitch and consequently, the results are discussed in his chapter. Nieder and Creelman (1965) investigated what they call "central periodicity pitch." Their basic stimulus paradigm consisted of interrupted thermal noise delivered to one ear, and steady noise presented simultaneously to the other. Depending upon the parameters of the noise, the apparent position of the tonal sound image may be manipulated through intracranial space. One of their more important findings is that, in order for a central tonal image to be formed, the noise in the two ears must be significantly correlated. Although not a critical test of the hypothesis, their results suggest that (in this situation at least) periodicity pitch is centrally determined and they further imply that there is a communality of mechanisms relating pitch to localization.

REFERENCES

von Békésy, G. (1928). Zur Theorie des Hörens. *Phys. Z.*, **29**, 793–810. (English transl.: Vibratory patterns of the basiler membrane. *Experiments in hearing.* pp. 404–429. McGraw-Hill, New York, 1960.)

von Békésy, G. (1933). Über den Knall und die Theorie des Hörens. *Phys. Z.*, **34**, 577–582. (English transl.: Clicks and the theory of hearing. *Experiments in hearing.* McGraw-Hill, New York, 1960.)

von Békésy, G. (1934). Über die nichtlinearen Verzerrugen des Ohres. *Annln Phys.*, **20**, ser. 5, 809–827. (English transl.: Nonlinear distortion in the ear. *Experiments in hearing.* pp. 332–344, McGraw-Hill, New York, 1960.)

von Békésy, G. (1955). Human skin perception of traveling waves similar to those on the cochlea. *J. Acoust. Soc. Am.*, **27**, 830–841.

von Békésy, G. (1961). Concerning the fundamental component of periodic pulse patterns and modulated vibrations observed on the cochlear model with nerve supply. *J. Acoust. Soc. Am.*, **33**, 888–896.

von Békésy, G. (1963). Hearing theories and complex sounds. *J. Acoust. Soc. Am.*, **35**, 588–601.

de Boer, E. (1956). On the "residue" in hearing. Unpublished doctoral dissertation, University of Amsterdam.

de Boer, E. and Six, P. D. (1960). The cochlear difference tone. *Acta Oto-Lar.*, **51**, 84–88.

Booton, R. C., Jr. (1952). An optimization theory for time-varying linear systems with nonstationary statistical inputs. *Proc. Inst. Radio Engrs.*, **40**, 977–981.

van den Brink, G. (1965). Pitch shift of the residue by masking. *Int. Audiol.*, **4**, 183–186.

Campbell, R. A. (1963). Frequency discrimination of pulsed tones. *J. Acoust. Soc. Am.*, **35**, 1193–1200.

Capranica, R. R. (1964). Evoked vocal response of the bullfrog. *J. Acoust. Soc. Am.*, **36**, 2007 (A).

Cohen, A. (1961). Further investigation of the effects of intensity upon the pitch of pure tones. *J. Acoust. Soc. Am.*, **33**, 1363–1376.

Davis, H. (1957). Biophysics and physiology of the inner ear. *Physiol. Rev.*, **37**, 1–49.

Davis, H., Fernández, C., and McAuliffe, D. R. (1950). The excitatory process in the cochlea. *Proc. Natn. Acad. Sci. U. S. A.*, **36**, 580–587.

Davis, H., Silverman, S. R., and McAuliffe, D. R. (1951). Some observations on pitch and frequency. *J. Acoust. Soc. Am.*, **23**, 40–44.

Dennert, H. (1887). Akustisch-physiologische Untersuchungen mit Demonstration. *Arch. Ohrenheilk.*, **24**, 171–184.

Derbyshire, A. J. and Davis, H. (1935). The action potentials of the auditory nerve. *Am. J. Physiol.*, **113**, 476–504.

Doughty, J. M. and Garner, W. R. (1948). Pitch characteristics of short tones. II. Pitch as a function of tonal duration. *J. Exp. Psychol.*, **38**, 478–494.

Fano, R. M. (1950). Short-time autocorrelation functions and power spectra. *J. Acoust. Soc. Am.*, **22**, 546–550.

Flanagan, J. L. (1960). Models for approximating basilar membrane displacement. *Bell Syst. Tech. J.*, **39**, 1163–1191.

Flanagan, J. L. (1962). Models for approximating basilar membrane displacement – Part II. *Bell Syst. Tech. J.*, **41**, 959–1009.

Flanagan, J. L. and Guttman, N. (1960a). On the pitch of periodic pulses. *J. Acoust. Soc. Am.*, **32**, 1308–1319.

Flanagan, J. L. and Guttman, N. (1960b). Pitch of periodic pulses without fundamental component. *J. Acoust. Soc. Am.*, **32**, 1319–1328.

Fletcher, H. (1934). Loudness, pitch and the timbre of musical tones and their relation to the intensity, the frequency and the overtone structure. *J. Acoust. Soc. Am.*, **6**, 59–69.

Frishkopf, L. S. and Goldstein, M. H., Jr. (1963). Responses to acoustic stimuli from single units in the eighth nerve of the bullfrog. *J. Acoust. Soc. Am.*, **35**, 1219–1228.

Galambos, R. and Davis, H. (1943). The response of single auditory-nerve fibers to acoustic stimulation. *J. Neurophysiol.*, **6**, 39–57.

Galambos, R. and Davis, H. (1948). Action potentials from single auditory-nerve fibers? *Science*, **108**, 513 (L).

Glattke, T. J. (1968). Unit responses of the cat cochlear nucleus to amplitude-modulated stimuli. Unpublished doctoral dissertation, University of Iowa.

Goldstein, M. H., Jr. (1957). Neurophysiological representation of complex auditory stimuli. *M. I. T. Res. Lab. Electron. Tech. Rep.* **323**.

Goldstein, M. H., Jr., Kiang, N. Y-s., and Brown, R. M. (1959). Responses of the auditory cortex to repetitive acoustic stimuli. *J. Acoust. Soc. Am.*, **31**, 356–364.

Gray, A. A. (1900). On a modification of the Helmholtz theory of hearing. *J. Anat. Physiol., Lond.*, **34**, 324–350.

Guttman, N. and Flanagan, J. L. (1964). Pitch of high-pass-filtered pulse trains. *J. Acoust. Soc. Am.*, **36**, 757–765.

Hallpike, C. S., and Rawdon-Smith, A. F. (1937). The Wever and Bray phenomenon. *Ann. Otol. Rhinol. Lar.*, **46**, 976–990.

Harris, G. G. (1960). Binaural interactions of impulsive stimuli and pure tones. *J. Acoust. Soc. Am.*, **32**, 685–692.

Harris, J. D. (1952). Pitch discrimination. *J. Acoust. Soc. Am.*, **24**, 750–755.

Harris, J. D. and Rawnsley, A. 1. (1953). Patterns of cochlear adaptation at three frequency regions. *J. Acoust. Soc. Am.*, **25**, 760–764.

von Helmholtz, H. (1863). *Die Lehre von den Tonempfindungen als physiologische Grundlage für die Theorie der Musik.* Braunschweig: Friedrich Vieweg und Sohn. (English transl.: *On the sensations of tone.* [2nd English ed. of the 4th German ed.] Longmans, Green, London. 1885.)

Hind, J. E. (1953). An electrophysiological determination of tonotopic organization in auditory cortex of cat. *J. Neurophysiol.*, **16**, 475–489.

Hoogland, G. A. (1953). The missing fundamental: a place theory of frequency analysis in hearing. Unpublished doctoral dissertation, University of Utrecht.

Huggins, W. H. and Licklider, J. C. R. (1951). Place mechanisms of auditory frequency analysis. *J. Acoust. Soc. Am.*, **23**, 290–299.

Jones, A. T. (1935). The discovery of difference tones. *Am. Phys. Teacher*, **3**, 49–51.

Katsuki, Y., Kanno, Y., Suga, N., and Mannen, M. (1961). Primary auditory neurons of monkey. *Jap. J. Physiol.*, **11**, 678–683.

Kemp, E. H., Coppée, G. E., and Robinson, E. H. (1937). Electric responses of the brain stem to unilateral auditory stimulation. *Am. J. Physiol.*, **120**, 304–315.

Kiang, N. Y-s. and Goldstein, M. H., Jr. (1959). Tonotopic organization of the cat auditory cortex for some complex stimuli. *J. Acoust. Soc. Am.*, **31**, 786–790.

König, R. (1876). Ueber den Zusammenklang zweier Töne. *Annln Phys.*, **157**, *ser. 2*, 177–237. (English transl.: On the simultaneous sounding of two notes. *Lond. Edinb. Dubl. Phil. Mag.*, **1**, *ser. 5*, 417–446, 511–525, 1876.)

Leibbrandt, C. C. (1966). Periodicity analysis in the guinea pig cochlea. *Acta Oto-Lar.*, **61**, 413–422.

Lewis, D. and Cowan, M. (1936). The influence of intensity on the pitch of violin and cello tones. *J. Acoust. Soc. Am.*, **8**, 20–22.

Licklider, J. C. R. (1951). A duplex theory of pitch perception. *Experientia*, **7**.

Licklider, J. C. R. (1954). "Periodicity" pitch and "place" pitch. *J. Acoust. Soc. Am.*, **26**, 945 (A).

Licklider, J. C. R. (1955). Influence of phase coherence upon the pitch of complex, periodic sounds. *J. Acoust. Soc. Am.*, **27**, 996 (A).

Licklider, J. C. R. (1956). Auditory frequency analysis. In C. Cherry (Ed.) *Information theory.* Butterworths *and* Academic Press, London *and* New York.

Licklider, J. C. R. (1959). Three auditory theories. In S. Koch (Ed.) *Psychology: a study of a science.* Vol. 1. McGraw-Hill, New York.

Licklider, J. C. R. (1962). Periodicity pitch and related auditory process models. *Int. Audiol.*, **1**, 11–36.

Mathes, R. C. and Miller, R. L. (1947). Phase effects in monaural perception. *J. Acoust. Soc. Am.*, **19**, 780–797.

Miller, G. A. and Taylor, W. G. (1948). The perception of repeated bursts of noise. *J. Acoust. Soc. Am.*, **20**, 171–182.

Moe, C. R. (1942). An experimental study of subjective tones produced within the human ear. *J. Acoust. Soc. Am.*, **14**, 159–166.

Morgan, C. T., Garner, W. R., and Galambos, R. (1951). Pitch and intensity. *J. Acoust. Soc. Am.*, **23**, 658–663.

Müller, J. (1826). *Zur vergleichenden Physiologie des Gesichtssinnes des Monschen und der Thiere Nebst einem Versuch über die Bewegungen der Augen und über den menschlichen Blick.* C. Cnobloch, Leipzig.

Munson, W. A. and Gardner, M. B. (1950). Loudness patterns—a new approach. *J. Acoust. Soc. Am.*, **22**, 177–190.

Nieder, P. C. and Creelman, C. D. (1965). Central periodicity pitch. *J. Acoust. Soc. Am.*, **37**, 136–138.

Nordmark, J. (1963). Some analogies between pitch and laterization phenomena. *J. Acoust. Soc. Am.*, **35**, 1544–1547.

Ohm, G. S. (1943). Über die Definition des Tones, nebst daran geknüpfter Theorie der Sirene und ähnlicher tonbildender Vorrichtungen. *Annln Phys.*, **59**, *ser. 2*, 513–565.

Peake, W. T., Kiang, N. Y-s., and Goldstein, M. H., Jr. (1962). Rate functions for auditory nerve responses to bursts of noise: Effect of changes in stimulus parameters. *J. Acoust. Soc. Am.*, **34**, 571–575.

Plomp, R. (1965). Detectability threshold for combination tones. *J. Acoust. Soc. Am.*, **37**, 1110–1123.

Ritsma, R. J. (1962). Existence region of the tonal residue. I. *J. Acoust. Soc. Am.*, **34**, 1224–1229.

Ritsma, R. J. (1963a). Existence region of the tonal residue. II. *J. Acoust. Soc. Am.*, **35**, 1241–1245.

Ritsma, R. J. (1963b). On pitch discrimination of residue tones. *Int. Audiol.*, **2**, 34–37.

Ritsma, R. J. and Engel, F. L. (1964). Pitch of frequency-modulated signals. *J. Acoust. Soc. Am.*, **36**, 1637–1644.

Sachs, M. B. (1964). Responses to acoustic stimuli from single units in the eighth nerve of the green frog. *J. Acoust. Soc. Am.*, **36**, 1956–1958 (L).

Schaefer, K. L. and Abraham, O. (1901a). Studien über Unterbrechungstöne (I). *Pflügers Arch. Ges. Physiol.*, **83**, 207–211.

Schaefer, K. L. and Abraham, O. (1901b). Studien über Unterbrechungstöne (II). *Pflügers Arch. Ges. Physiol.*, **85**, 536–542.

Schaefer, K. L. and Abraham, O. (1902). Studien über Unterbrechungstöne (III). *Pflügers Arch. Ges. Physiol.*, **88**, 475–491.

Schouten, J. F. (1938). The perception of subjective tones. *Proc. K. Ned. Akad. Wet.*, **41**, 1086–1093.

Schouten, J. F. (1940a). The residue, a new component in subjective sound analysis. *Proc. K. Ned. Akad. Wet.*, **43**, 356–365.

Schouten, J. F. (1940b). The residue and the mechanism of hearing. *Proc. K. Ned. Akad. Wet.*, **43**, 991–999.

Schouten, J. F., Ritsma, R. J., and Lopes Cardozo, B. (1962). Pitch of the residue. *J. Acoust. Soc. Am.*, **34**, 1418–1424.

Schubert, E. D. and Elpern, B. S. (1959). Psychophysical estimate of the velocity of the traveling wave. *J. Acoust. Soc. Am.*, **31**, 990–994.

Seebeck, A. (1841). Beobachtungen über einige Bedingungen der Entstehung von Tönen. *Annln Phys.*, **53**, *ser. 2*, 417–436.

Shower, E. G. and Biddulph, R. (1931). Differential pitch sensitivity of the ear. *J. Acoust. Soc. Am.*, **3**, 275–287.

Small, A. M. (1955). Some parameters influencing the pitch of amplitude modulated signals. *J. Acoust. Soc. Am.*, **27**, 751–760.

Small, A. M. and Campbell, R. A. (1961a). Pitch shifts of periodic stimuli with changes in sound level. *J. Acoust. Soc. Am.*, **33**, 1022–1027.

Small, A. M. and Campbell, R. A. (1961b). Masking of pulsed tones by bands of noise. *J. Acoust. Soc. Am.*, **33**, 1570–1576.

Small, A. M. and Gross, N. B. (1962). Response of the cerebral cortex of the cat to repetitive acoustic stimuli. *J. Comp. Physiol. Psychol.*, **55**, 445–448.

Small, A. M. and Yelen, R. D. (1962). Fatigue as an indicator of pitch channels. *J. Acoust. Soc. Am.*, **34**, 1987 (A).

Smith, R. (1749). *Harmonics, or the philosophy of musical sounds.* Printed by J. Bentham and sold by W. Thurlbourn, Cambridge.

Snow, W. B. (1936). Change of pitch with loudness at low frequencies. *J. Acoust. Soc. Am.*, **8**, 14–19.

Stevens, S. S. (1935). The relation of pitch to intensity. *J. Acoust. Soc. Am.*, **6**, 150–154.

Stumpf, C. (1926). *Die Sprachlaute experimentell-phonetische untersuchungen nebst einem anhang über instrumentalklänge.* J. Springer, Berlin.

Suga, N. (1961). Functional organization of two tympanic neurons in noctuid moths. *Jap. J. Physiol.*, **11**, 666–677.

Tasaki, I. (1954). Nerve impulses in individual auditory nerve fibers of guinea pig. *J. Neurophysiol.*, **17**, 97–122.

Thompson, R. F. (1960). Function of auditory cortex of cat in frequency discrimination. *J. Neurophysiol.*, **23**, 321–334.

Thurlow, W. R. (1963). Perception of low auditory pitch. *Psychol. Rev.*, **70**, 461–470.

Thurlow, W. R. and Small, A. M. (1955). Pitch perception for certain periodic auditory stimuli. *J. Acoust. Soc. Am.*, **27**, 132–137.

Tonndorf, J. (1958). Harmonic distortion in cochlear models. *J. Acoust. Soc. Am.*, **30**, 929–937.

Tonndorf, J. (1959). Beats in cochlear models. *J. Acoust. Soc. Am.*, **31**, 608–619.

Tonndorf, J. (1960). Response of cochlear models to aperiodic signals and to random noises. *J. Acoust. Soc. Am.*, **32**, 1344–1355.

Tonndorf, J. (1962). Time/frequency analysis along the partition of cochlear models: a modified place concept. *J. Acoust. Soc. Am.*, **34**, 1337–1350.

Wever, E. G. (1949). *Theory of hearing.* Wiley, New York.

Wien, M. (1905). Ein Bedenken gegen die Helmholtzsche Resonanztheorie des Hörens. In *Festschrift Adolph Wüllner.* pp. 28–35. B. G. Teubner, Leipzig.

Young, T. (1800). Outlines of experiments and inquiries respecting sound and light. *Phil. Trans. R. Soc. Pt. 1*, **1**, 106–150.

Zwislocki, J. (1962). Analysis of the middle-ear function. Part I. *J. Acoust. Soc. Am.*, **34**, 1514–1523.

Chapter Two

Time and Frequency Analysis

FOREWORD

Almost no one questions that high-frequency tones are analyzed differently than low-frequency tones. The best-accepted theoretical writers talk of a temporal analysis for long-period signals and a place analysis for short-period signals. Where long and short meet may vary somewhat according to the writer, but the jumping-off places range from, perhaps, 150 to as much as 1500 Hz, depending upon the experiment and upon the experimenter. For some kinds of studies, the *temporal* analysis appears to be more precise and more useful to the auditory system. Jan Nordmark takes the extreme point of view that such an analysis is best, not just for low frequencies, but throughout the audible range. This viewpoint has led him to raise some problems that established theories overlook, and to perform some experiments that are intriguing in their concept and important in their results.

Time and Frequency Analysis

Jan O. Nordmark*

I. INTRODUCTION

A comprehensive theory of auditory analysis did not exist before Helmholtz. It is doubtful if one has existed since. For more than sixty years his theory dominated the field of hearing. When it finally became possible to observe the cochlear partition in motion, Helmholtz's basic assumptions were proved untenable, but there were still too many unexplained aspects of the analytical process to allow the formulation of an alternative theory. Simple and all-embracing theories, appropriate though they might have been for a scientifically more innocent age, are nowadays not considered very meaningful. The most we can expect, it is sometimes argued, is a partial reduction in conceptual complexity — a reduction that can only be achieved through concentration on limited areas of auditory experience.

Still, Helmholtz's attempt at a complete solution to the analytical problem is worth reconsidering. Although the newer theories may not have the specific aim of solving the problems he attacked, an examination of Helmholtz's approach can suggest further refinements of these theories.

A. Helmholtz's Theory of Auditory Analysis

The second chapter of *Sensations of Tone* (Helmholtz, 1863) contains a summary of what Helmholtz considered to be the main problems of auditory analysis. He started by pointing out that we have no

---

*Mathema AB, Stockholm, Sweden.

difficulty in following the individual instruments in a concert, or in directing our attention at will to the words of one speaker to the exclusion of others. It follows, first, that many different trains of sound waves can be propagated without mutual disturbance, and second, that the ear can analyze a sound complex into its constituent elements.

It is easy, he wrote, to understand how the eye, in surveying a surface of water, can separate the different wave systems from each other by noticing which waves are connected. But the ear is incapable of such spatial analysis; the mass of air that sets the tympanic membrane in motion must be considered as if it were a single point in the surrounding medium. The ear is in the situation the eye would be in if it were required to analyze a composite wave by looking at the up-and-down movement of a single point on the water surface through a long, narrow tube.

How then does the ear perform the analysis? For his explanation, Helmholtz used two earlier theoretical concepts. One was Ohm's law of hearing, which states that the ear separates a complex sound into sinusoidal components corresponding to those in a mathematical analysis, and that all tones that can be discriminated have their origins in physical sinusoids. Helmholtz made the important addition to this law that apparent exceptions—such as the difference tone—can be explained by assuming that new sinusoids, not present in the physical stimulus, are introduced by nonlinearity in the ear. The other concept was Müller's doctrine of specific nerve energies, which states that the sensation a stimulus gives rise to depends on the kind of nerve fiber that is stimulated; he suggested five specific nerve energies—one for each of the senses. Helmholtz extended this concept by assuming that every discriminable pitch corresponds to one particular nerve or small group of nerves. The further assumption of a connection between these nerves and the cochlear segments resonating to specific tones enabled Helmholtz to formulate a theory of pitch.

This description was not enough, Helmholtz realized, for a complete solution to the problem of sound analysis. For instance, we still do not understand why complex sounds generally are heard as unanalyzed wholes.

B. Modern Views on Auditory Analysis

After some time it became obvious that Helmholtz's system was less consistent than had been originally thought. The greatest difficulty concerned the selectivity of the resonators, which depends on their damping—that is, on the degree to which their motion is retarded by frictional forces. The selectivity and damping of a resonator are inversely related, so to explain the fine frequency discrimination of the human ear, one must assume high selectivity and low damping of the cochlear resonators. On the other hand, low damping implies that tones presented even for a short interval have a long persistence. From studies of musical trills, Helmholtz had to conclude that the resonators must have considerable damping. The selectivity was not as great as he wished—even a pure tone should excite several resonators.

No attempts were made to resolve these inconsistencies until Gray (1900) suggested that only the nerve fiber associated with the maximally stimulated segment of the basilar membrane gives rise to a sensation of pitch; impulses from the other nerves are suppressed. This principle has influenced most subsequent writers on auditory theory.

When Békésy (1960, pp. 429–446) measured basilar membrane vibrations, a solution to the selectivity problem became even more essential. He found that there is a mechanical analysis in the cochlea, so that sinusoids are distributed along the basilar membrane according to their frequency, but also that each stimulating sinusoid displaces a large part of the membrane.

Hypotheses to explain the fine pitch discrimination of the ear fall into two classes. One type assumes that pitch in the low and middle ranges of the tonal spectrum is determined by the frequency of the neural impulses rather than by position on the membrane. The evidence supporting this view comes mainly from experiments indicating that a periodicity in the waveform of the sound may give rise to a pitch, even when no corresponding frequency component is present. The other type of theory assumes that the preliminary mechanical analysis at the basilar membrane is supplemented by a neural sharpening process that limits the pitch information to a small group of nerves. Inhibitory phenomena such as these theories require are important in the vertebrate retina, and a detailed theory exists for the interactions in the eye of the horshoe crab, Limulus (Hartline et al., 1961). Békésy (1960, p. 553) used a mechanical model of the cochlea to demonstrate a similar kind of sharpening performed by the nerves of the skin. In spite of a very broad amplitude distribution along the forearm (representing the membrane), only a small section seems to vibrate.

A similar mechanism can be invoked to explain why short tones have a well-defined pitch. Since the spectrum for short tones is broad, an inhibition even greater than that for long-duration pure tones is required. Békésy showed that only two periods of a sinusoid are necessary to give a localized impression on the skin; in fact, continuous tones are less sharply localized. According to the skin model, then, nearly instantaneous frequency analysis should be possible in hearing.

However, the analysis requires more time than the stimulus duration; also it must include the time taken to complete the inhibition. Békésy's experiment offers no way of estimating this time, but the Hartline *et al.* (1961) work in the Limulus eye showed it to be appreciable. So a simultaneous second tone, or one presented before the inhibitory process is finished could disturb the analysis.

The duration of the inhibitory effect must also be considered. Békésy (1960, p. 632) noted that it takes more than 30 msec to establish a new inhibition or to break up an old one. This finding is in accord with physiological experiments on the inhibition produced by single impulses (Lloyd, 1961).

The time course of inhibition constitutes a problem for the neural-sharpening model, particularly when it comes to explaining pitch discrimination for sounds of rapidly changing frequency. Lewis *et al.* (1940) showed that the accuracy of estimating the extent of a frequency change improves as the modulation time increases from 25 to 100 msec, at which point it is almost as good as for a relatively slow change. Interestingly, upward and downward glides are discriminated equally well. These findings present a theoretical problem of the first magnitude. It is a particularly intriguing one because none of the familiar theories of hearing appears to be able to handle it with any degree of success. The place theory must account for the smooth and continuous pitch sensation that occurs even when the inhibitory processes cannot possibly have time to be both established and broken up along the basilar membrane. The frequency theory is no better. If pitch is determined by the frequency of nerve impulses over some given time, the sensation resulting from this kind of stimulus obviously could not be one of a gliding pitch. Two theories representing a special form of frequency theory assume a correlational analysis (Licklider, 1959; Schief, 1963). But neither is well equipped to handle rapidly changing frequency. Schief's aim was to account for the sharpness of frequency discrimination with short-duration stimuli. He postulated a bank of coincidence filters in tandem, but they were to be actuated after about two periods of a sinusoid, so they could not respond at all to a continuously changing frequency.

II. HYPOTHESIS ON COMPLEX-SOUND ANALYSIS

Auditory theory has devoted far less attention to the analysis of complex sounds than the problem requires; we know very little about the capabilities of our analytical mechanism. Not until 1964 did Plomp measure the number of distinguishable partials of multitone signals. Contrary to what Helmholtz and his followers assumed, only the first six or seven partials can be distinguished. Plomp interpreted these results to indicate that the individual partials of a complex sound are heard only if their frequency separations exceed critical bandwidths. He stated that it is very difficult to imagine how the nervous system could discriminate the partials if they are not presented separately to the haircells. Plomp regarded a mechanical analyzing system with bandwidths corresponding with the critical bands to be much more acceptable. Thurlow and Bernstein (1957) on the other hand, found that two simultaneous tones around 1000 Hz do not have to differ by more than 50 Hz before two distinct pitches can be perceived—an amount that is considerably less than the critical bandwidth at that frequency. As the limit for two-tone discrimination is of the same order when the tones are led to different ears, the determining factor may not necessarily be a mechanical one.

A. Place Theories

Again the analytical ability poses problems for both place and frequency theories. Separate maxima on the basilar membrane do not exist until the frequency separation exceeds one octave (Zwislocki, 1948); the place theory obviously requires that this unimodal amplitude distribution be transformed into a bimodal neural distribution. Békésy (1960, p. 417) suggested that the discrimination may be achieved through a mechanism similar to that involved with the Mach bands in vision. Mach bands appear to be concentric light and dark rings, but they result from changes in the *rate of change* of lightness rather than from the lightness itself. The auditory effect could be that of Fig. 1. But this example from Békésy is scarcely representative of complex sounds in general. It is not clear how a curve compounded from more than two closely spaced sinusoids is analyzed, or indeed that, even in principle, it could be uniquely decomposed. Also if a sharpening of this kind occurs in the cochlea, it must be different in some respect from the sharpening mechanism of the skin model, where it is not possible to obtain a frequency discrimination for two beating tones (Békésy, 1960, p. 576).

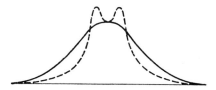

Figure 1 A form of amplitude distribution on the basilar membrane (solid line) and its expected sensory effect (broken line). (From *Experiments in Hearing*, by G. von Békésy. Copyright 1960 by McGraw-Hill. Used with permission of McGraw-Hill Book Company.)

According to the place theory, pitch changes should occur when there is activity on portions of the basilar membrane that are far removed from the pitch-determining position. Huggins and Licklider's (1951) work can serve as an illustration. They computed the displacement curve produced by mixing a sinusoid at 1600 Hz with one at 200 Hz. The higher-frequency tone was 30 dB less intense than the lower one, making its displacement maximum fall far below the displacement amplitude of the 200-Hz-tone curve at the same point. To account for the fact that both tones can be heard, the authors suggested a contrast phenomenon similar to the Mach bands. Figure 2 shows the displacement curve and its first and second derivative. Huggins and Licklider said that the negative second derivative has maxima in approximately the same position as the maxima of curve A and curve B, which represent the two components. This small change in position, however, is still enough to result in clearly audible pitch changes. Yet such changes have not been reported for mixtures of two tones. The sharpening concept is thus incomplete in its explanation of how the ear performs its analysis of closely spaced tones. In a mechanical system with incomplete resolution, analysis based on the transformation of frequency into position suffers from the further disadvantage that a one-to-one correspondence between frequency and position cannot be expected for complex waveforms. The addition of noise to a tone, for instance, should produce a shift in the position of the maximum, and consequently, a shift in pitch in the direction of the frequencies contained in the noise band.

There is conflicting evidence whether such pitch shifts occur. Békésy (1963b) reported that noise with high-frequency cutoffs between 75 and 600 Hz, at a level 30 dB above threshold, always lowers the pitch of a 40 dB SL, 600-Hz tone. The shifts range from about

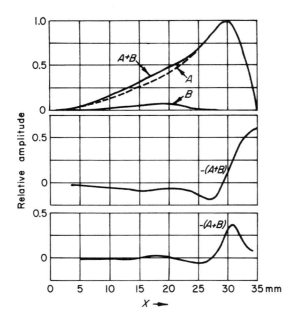

Figure 2 Effects of differentiation and double differentiation upon the maximum displacement curve of the cochlear partition under simultaneous stimulation by two tones. (Huggins and Licklider, 1951. By permission from *Journal of the Acoustical Society of America*.)

eight to eighteen percent, with the larger shifts occuring for lower cutoffs, in agreement with observations on the skin model. Similarly, with high-frequency noise, the pitch shifts increase as the cutoff frequency increases from 600 to 9600 Hz.

Egan and Meyer (1950) and Webster and Schubert (1954), on the other hand, found that the pitch shifts away from a masking noise toward a region of better hearing, although the upward shift is more noticeable than the downward one. These results were confirmed in a later study by Webster and Muerdter (1965), who measured pitch shifts in a 600-Hz tone in the presence of noise bands at various frequencies. Only when the noise bands were well above the tone did they find small shifts in the direction that Békésy did. As Békésy's experiment was explicitly performed as a test of the place theory, the failure of others to substantiate his findings regarding both the magnitude and the direction of the pitch shifts ought to have aroused greater interest than it apparently did.

B. Frequency Theories

Presumably the problem of frequency analysis of complex tones would be easier to handle if it could be assumed that the information contained in the basilar membrane movement is preserved not only in a *spatial* pattern of nerve activity, but in a *temporal* one as well. Localization studies with low-frequency tones definitely show that the temporal pattern is preserved. It is difficult, however, to find evidence of temporal patterns for high-frequency tones. For this reason, it is commonly believed that a limit exists for a neural frequency representation of pitch.

The agreement on where to put this limit is less apparent. Frequencies almost everywhere between 50 and 5000 Hz have been suggested. A limit of 400 Hz could be taken for instance, because the refractory period of the nerve prevents any fiber from responding to each acoustic peak at higher frequencies (Davis, 1951). But the individual nerve fibers may take turns in responding to the sound waves, and the synchronous activity extends to 2000 to 3000 Hz (Davis, 1961), so that the limit is sometimes considered to lie in this range. Or, it could be argued that this limit (as well as the even lower limits of frequency representation found in more central parts of the auditory neural chain) is too low due to imperfections in our methods of physiological measurement, and that synchronism is present, but masked, up to the point where the same pitch sensation arises for all frequencies (Chocholle, 1957). Some support for this view can be found in the fact that new refinements in the processing of neuro-electric data tend to push the limit of synchronous activity to ever higher frequencies.

More commonly, the absence of a binaural phase effect above a certain frequency has been considered to show a definite limit for the transmission of temporal information in any form to higher neural centers. From such reasoning, the limit above which a place principle must operate has been variously put at 4000 Hz (Wever, 1949), 3000 Hz (Békésy, 1955), and, far more often than any other, close to 1500 Hz.

In my view, the real problem for the frequency theories is not the limit on frequency representation, but the limited resolution on the basilar membrane — the same problem that confronts the place theory. Schouten (1940) stated that for complex sounds, the number of discriminable pure-tones is determined by the efficiency of the spatial analysis, and that as soon as the excitation curves overlap, beats or beat tones (residues) arise. The experiments of Thurlow and Bernstein (1957), however, must be interpreted as showing that overlapping tones can be discriminated. The tones cannot be separately represented by frequency of nerve impulses except where no overlap occurs. For the middle of three adjacent tones, no separate representation at all is possible. The temporal pattern of activity in the auditory nerve must represent the composite motion of the basilar membrane. If pitch were simply proportional to the number of nerve impulses, it would be constantly too high in a mixture of closely spaced tones. Békésy (1963a) made the related objection that an increase in the firing rate of a nerve should produce not only an increase in loudness, but, if pitch is assumed to be connected with the firing rate, a rise in pitch as well. The greatest problem of the pure periodicity theory, he said, is to explain how pitch and loudness are separated in the auditory nervous system.

Both place and periodicity theories therefore have to assume that the mechanical analysis on the basilar membrane is followed by a further analysis. Is this analysis based on the temporal or on the spatial pattern of nerve activity, or on both?

III. ANALYSIS OF TEMPORAL PATTERNS

Inherent in the theories considered so far is the assumption that frequency analysis is completed before the pitch-sensing mechanism in the brain is reached. Only the so-called telephone theory of hearing (Rutherford, 1886) called for prominent central analysis, an idea that had little influence. Instead of solving the problem of analysis, the theory relegated it to an area inaccessible to experimental study. At the time, the opposite view was far more widely accepted: analysis is completed in the cochlea, and the function of the auditory nerves is merely to conduct a signal from the resonating element to a corresponding place in the projection area of the brain, where somehow a pitch sensation arises. Today, a certain amount of processing in the nervous system is assumed, but place theorists (Békésy, 1963a) still maintain the idea of a separate nerve element for every pitch. The doctrine of specific nerve energies therefore remains a cornerstone of the theory. The problematic nature of Helmholtz's enormous extension of Müller's doctrine has carried little weight in discussions of pitch. Indeed, Ranke (1955) stated that analysis according to a frequency principle is contrary to the universally valid law of specific nerve energy.

It is interesting, therefore, that the basic doctrine has been called into question (Weddell, 1955; Pfaffman, 1962). Anatomical and physiological evidence from the cutaneous and gustatory senses show that the end organs, although differentially sensitive, do not fall into rigidly specific categories. Qualitative discrimination appears to depend on the pattern of activity in a group of nerves rather than on the activity in any one nerve fiber. We must assume that the pattern is interpreted by the brain and that, in this sense, central analysis occurs.

Nor is it necessary to postulate "some mystical property of the brain" (Boring, 1942) to argue that the auditory information reaching it is probably subjected to further processing. In the following paragraphs, some experiments are discussed that show the presence in the nervous system of an analyzing mechanism that operates on the temporal patterns of activity. Most of the experiments used pulses rather than sinusoidal stimuli because, with suitable filtering, a separation can easily be made of factors that have to do with the spectrum of the signal, and thus with position on the basilar membrane, and of those that have to do with the temporal pattern of basilar membrane motion.

A. Perception of Time Difference between Two Pulse Trains

In 1955, Thurlow and Small observed that, if a train of sound pulses of low repetition rate is added to a second pulse train of nearly identical rate, a tone can be heard whose pitch glides downward as the time difference between the two pulse trains increases. In Fig. 3, letters a_1, a_2, a_3 represent pulses of one train; b_1, b_2, b_3 represent those of the other. If, for example, the interval $a_1 b_1$ is 2 msec, the pitch is close to that of a pure tone whose period is 2 msec.

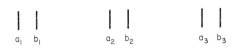

Figure 3 Schematic diagram of two pulse trains.

The stimulus has no obvious spectral characteristics that could explain this phenomenon in place-theory terms. The close correspondence between time separation and pitch, on the other hand, suggests that a time mechanism is operating. In a later paper, however, Thurlow (1958) noted evidence that argues against this interpretation. Reversing the polarity of one of the pulse trains produces a change of pitch. If, for example, the pulse rate of each train is near 100 per sec, and the pulse separation *ab* is 3 msec, the two-phase tonal complex has two pitches — one higher than for the single-phase condition, and one lower. Assuming that neural firings take place at some amplitude level on the upward deflection of the basilar membrane, an impulse of pressure rarefaction (which initially produces an outward movement of the eardrum and an upward movement of the basilar membrane) should have a shorter latency than a condensation pulse (which initially causes downward movement of the membrane). If a time-analyzing system were operating, such changes of latency should show up as shifts in pitch. These shifts would be in different directions, depending on whether the condensation pulse precedes or follows the rarefaction pulse; but the pitches are the same in both conditions.

It can nevertheless be shown that these observations are compatible with the time-mechanism hypothesis. If the objections were valid, we would expect a shift in *position* when the stimulus configuration for the case where the pulse trains are led to separate ears is changed from rarefaction-condensation to condensation-rarefaction. Matching the image positions produced by the two configurations, however, shows that the pulse separations are the same (Nordmark, 1963). This finding is also true when the pulse separation is zero; that is, the image, though more diffuse, is still centered when the polarity of one click is reversed.

In order to understand why we hear two pitches but only one sound image, we should consider some experiments made by Flanagan (1962). They were an attempt to relate psychoacoustic phenomena to a computational model for the mechanical operation of the ear. According to this model, the displacement response to 1200 and 600 Hz, respectively, will have the form shown in Fig. 4. The curves suggest that a time difference of about one-half cycle on the displacement waveform should exist between the neural firings of a rarefaction pulse and those of a simultaneous condensation pulse. It can be assumed that simultaneous neural firings at the two ears produce a fused image. If a rarefaction pulse were led to one ear and a condensation pulse to the other, the listener should consequently be able to fuse the sound image by making the condensation pulse lag or lead in time so as to bring its positive displacement peak into coincidence with one of the rarefaction peaks. For unmasked pulses, where the greatest neural response is likely to originate near the central portion of the basilar membrane, the lag or lead would have to be about 250 to 500 μsec.

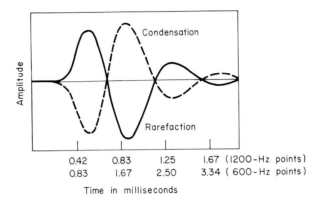

Figure 4   Apical displacement of the basilar membrane for rarefaction and condensation pressure impulses at the eardrum. (Flanagan, 1962. From the *Bell System Technical Journal*. Copyright, 1962, by the American Telephone and Telegraph Co., reprinted by permission.)

The results confirm these predictions. Further experiments by Cummings *et al.* (1961), as well as those mentioned earlier, show that the centered image is different from these fusions. It looks as if the position of the image is determined by a point halfway between the neural firings corresponding to the fusions. The resolution of closely spaced pulses therefore appears to be less sharp for the binaural mechanism than for the monaural one.

The curve in Fig. 4 also implies that if the dominant response were made to originate at points that are maximally displaced by lower frequencies, the lag or lead would have to be greater. Flanagan tested these predictions by selectively masking the membrane response with filtered random noise and recording the time shift necessary for making the condensation pulse fuse with the principal or the secondary positive excursion of the rarefaction waveform. The results indicate that the time difference increases as the cutoff frequency of the filtered noise is lowered. As the maximally responding unmasked place on the membrane should be just below the cutoff frequency f_c of the filter, the difference ought to be about $\pm 1/2\ f_c$. The data agree reasonably well with this prediction.

If the pitch of the time separation tone is dependent on the time interval between neural impulses, one would expect to find pitch changes of the same order as the interaural lag or lead in the lateralization experiments. Nordmark (1963) asked his subjects to offset the upward and downward shift in pitch that occurred when the polarity pattern was changed from single-phase to two-phase clicks. The shifts to lower and higher pitch were found to be approximately equal, and to increase as the frequency composition of the pulses was altered so as to make the maximal neural response come from increasingly apical parts of the basilar membrane.

The time needed to compensate for the pitch shifts can be compared with that required to obtain a fused image in Flanagan's experiment. As shown in Fig. 5, the agreement is so close that a similarity in the underlying mechanisms appears likely.

This interpretation is further strengthened when the possibility of explaining the time-separation tone in terms of the place theory is considered. Pollack (1961) stated that the Thurlow and Small findings

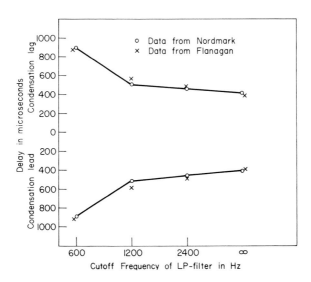

Figure 5 Effects of the frequency content on pitch shift for antiphasic pulses compared with the fusion shifts found by Flanagan. (Nordmark, 1963. By permission from *Journal of the Acoustical Society of America*.)

are entirely reasonable in terms of a Fourier spectral analysis. But Small and McClellan's (1963) series of spectral measurements for various delays at a given repetition rate do not bear out this view. The place theory predicts that the pitch should correspond to the frequency component with the maximum amplitude. Yet spectra were found with *no* component corresponding to the pitch heard. Nor is it likely that the auditory system responds to the maximum in the spectral *envelope;* one spectrum showed a minimum rather than a maximum at the expected position. Furthermore, the low-frequency portion of the spectrum may be eliminated entirely by filtering or masking without destroying the time-separation tone. Thurlow (1958) suggested that the *spacing* of envelope maxima may be a cue for pitch, but this hypothesis receives no support from these measurements.

Some further evidence can be adduced to show that the explanation for these phenomena is to be found in temporal rather than spectral factors. The shift in polarity of one of the pulse trains reverses the position of maxima and minima in the spectrum. The *spacing* of maxima in the envelope, however, is the same. The pitch shift therefore cannot be explained in spectral terms, whereas as we have seen, it is unquestionably similar to time phenomena. As one of the pulse trains is lowered in intensity, the spectrum changes gradually until it is practically identical with that of one train presented alone. In all these transformations the only invariant feature is the time difference between the pulse trains. For these reasons it is natural to assume that the time relations are directly perceived.

B. Time-Separation Tones from Sinusoidal Stimuli

These phenomena are not limited to pulse signals, however, and can be shown to be present for pure tones as well. If, for instance, a 1200-Hz tone of moderate intensity is mixed with a 2399-Hz tone, preferably at a slightly lower intensity, a tone can be heard whose pitch once per sec glides upward about a musical third above the higher frequency. This gliding tone is much easier to hear than the higher stationary tone. Changing the higher tone to 2401 Hz reverses the direction, but not the compass or frequency level of the glide. Similar glides can be obtained if the lower tone is changed to 800 Hz.

Figure 6 shows a schematic diagram of the first configuration, when the tones are in an approximate-octave relation. Since only pressure rarefaction leads to neural firings, the probable explanation is that the pitch is produced by neural pulses from the portion of the basilar membrane where the high-frequency and the attenuated low-frequency tones overlap. A completely analogous localization phenomenon can be obtained by leading, for instance, a 120- or 80-Hz tone to one ear and a 240-Hz tone at a slightly lower intensity to the other. The image then moves once per sec from a central position out toward one ear. The movement takes place during exactly the same part of the cycle as the pitch glide. The results cannot be explained by assuming that a harmonic of the low-frequency tone is introduced by nonlinear distortion. They seem to offer the strongest and simplest possible proof of a time mechanism operating in pitch perception. The place theory is unable to explain the gliding pitch and, in fact, requires quite different pitch changes (Békésy, 1960, p. 587).

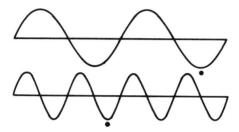

Figure 6 Schematic diagram of pure tones in an octave relationship.

C. Temporal Inhibition

An interesting aspect of the mistuned consonance phenomena is that some form of temporal inhibition must be assumed to take place in the nervous system. There are many other facts that show that not every constant time relation between neural pulses gives rise to a tone or to a localized image. For single-phase pulses, the neural pulses corresponding to the oscillatory motion of the membrane are apparently not separately resolved. As they can be resolved under certain circumstances, we can assume that inhibition normally prevents the appearance of a multiplicity of pitches or images. Not even every distance between separate events in the stimulus can be perceived. No pitch, for instance, can be heard that would correspond to the distance b_1-a_2 in Fig. 3. The well known fact that only one image is produced by two binaurally presented pure tones is a related example.

In other cases the inhibition is less complete. If a third pulse train (labeled c in Fig. 7) is added to the a and b trains with equal separation between the trains, the pitch corresponding to the distance a–c is weaker than if the b train is absent, but it can be heard. A fourth train (d in the figure) almost completely abolishes the a–c pitch, however, whereas the a–d can be heard clearly, and the a–b, (b–c, c–d) pitch very clearly. The inhibition is not complete and appears to be mutual. A clear mutual inhibition effect can be observed when the c and d trains are arranged so that all the intervals between the pulse trains are different from each other.

Figure 7   Schematic diagram of four pulse trains.

The gradual lessening of one inhibition and the emergence of an inhibition in the opposite direction can be found in the localization of pure tones as the frequency goes higher. Hartley (1919) suggested that the progressive decrease in definiteness of the sound image is connected with the appearance of a second image, at first confined to a small part of the cycle and gradually extending over the remainder. The second image would correspond to the time separation between b_1 and a_2 in Fig. 3. Viewed in this light, the absence of a binaural phase effect for high frequencies could indicate some form of inhibition rather than a limit for the transmission of temporal information. This interpretation is supported by an experiment in which two tones whose frequencies are close to 1000 Hz are led to both ears. Two separate images arise if the phase relations between each pair of frequencies can be independently regulated. In this case, the rate of transmission must be higher than what has been thought possible – probably due to the absence of inhibition between the tones.

There are other ways to remove the inhibition. If the b train in Fig. 3 is further separated from the a train, so that the distance a_1–b_1 is longer than the distance b_1–a_2, again only the shorter time interval gives rise to a corresponding pitch sensation. The longer, it must be assumed, is in some way prevented from doing so. If, at this point, the pulse trains are triggered from a random noise source, we get a stimulus that can be described as two identical aperiodic pulse trains separated by a constant time delay. In this case, the time-separation tone will correspond to the constant separation a_1–b_1 rather than to the shorter, but varying, separation b_1-a_2; the former inhibition is broken. Analogous results can be obtained by leading the trains to separate ears. The sound image normally corresponds to the shorter distance, but in the aperiodic configuration, it is determined by the longer. By slowly increasing the degree of randomness, the point where tones or images corresponding to both the shorter and the longer distance are present, that is, when the inhibition is beginning to weaken, can be determined. The degree of randomness required for disinhibition is the same both for tones and for localized images.

Some other aspects of these findings are worth noting. Periodicity is apparently not necessary for this pitch phenomenon, as long as a constant time relation is present in the stimulus. Nor does a slight inconstancy immediately abolish the phenomenon; it only gradually weakens it.

D. Paired Aperiodic Sounds

The time-separation tone can also be heard when random noise is substituted for pulse trains. When, for instance, low-pass-filtered noise delayed 2 msec is added to the same noise undelayed, one can hear a clear tone around 500 Hz. Reversing the polarity of either noise produces pitch shifts of a magnitude that depends on the cutoff of the low-pass filter, exactly as in the case of periodic pulse trains. Leading the two noise signals to separate ears produces a spreading out of the sound image rather than a shift in position. With no time separation, a phase reversal in either ear spreads the image symmetrically (Licklider, 1948). Again, the symmetry is probably due to the limited resolving power of the binaural system.

Coherence, then, is important in overcoming the disturbing influence of other activity on the basilar membrane. In another example, if random pulses are added to two random pulse trains separated by a constant time difference, the masking of the tone will be slight even if the number of random pulses is several times that in the connected pulse trains. No regularity is apparent in oscilloscope tracings, yet one pitch stands out clearly. Similar phenomena can be demonstrated if two nonidentical random pulse trains are led to separate ears together with one random train that is led to both ears, but with a delay in one channel. Although transient images appear continually, one image corresponding to the constant delay stands out from the background.

From these experiments, it appears that an important factor in determining the degree to which the time interval between pulses in a group of nerves will contribute to a sensation of pitch is its rate of occurrence in relation to other intervals. If it is frequent in comparison with some other interval, it will be masked only if the total number of other intervals is many times larger. If it occurs exactly as often as some other interval, there will be inhibition that, for obscure reasons, will vary from small to complete depending on the configuration. Obviously, in these examples, the word *interval* does not necessarily mean the smallest distance in time between neural pulses; it may equally well mean the distance between pulses separated by other pulses.

E. Paired Sounds with Varying Delays

In a further experiment the accuracy of pitch and lateralization discrimination was compared for pulse intervals of various degrees of randomness. The interval between two identical pulse trains was made to vary in such a manner that a normal interval-distribution curve was formed. The just discriminable time difference for pitch when the trains were led to one ear, and for lateralization when they were led to separate ears, was plotted against the degree of randomness expressed as the standard deviation for the pulse interval distribution. The straight line in Fig. 8 was drawn on the assumption that the relation is linear. However, the reasonably close fit to this line of the values of two observers was unexpected, and more data are needed before a simple relation can be accepted. Nevertheless, the similarity between the mechanisms underlying pitch and lateralization seems to be established beyond doubt.

IV. RELATION BETWEEN FREQUENCY AND PITCH

These experiments can be interpreted to indicate that a physiological mechanism exists that can determine the magnitude of the time interval between neural pulses, and can convert it into a pitch. Although time interval and frequency are reciprocal terms, this hypothesis is not necessarily identical to the frequency or periodicity theory. Measuring time intervals is, in principle, a different activity from counting the number of events during some period. A differentiation between these concepts is seldom made, but at times the implication seems to be that periodicity means rate or number of pulses per unit time (Flanagan and Guttman, 1960; Békésy, 1963b). Pitch hypotheses involving delay-line mechanisms, on the other hand, imply

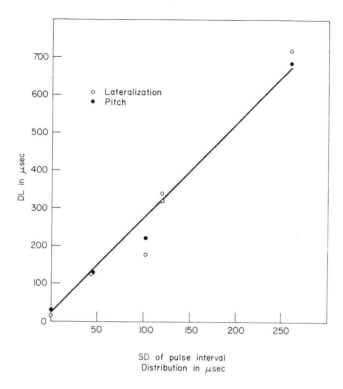

Figure 8   Effects of degree of randomness (SD) on just discriminable time difference for pitch and for lateralization.

the time-interval concept. A pitch extractor that might use such a mechanism was postulated by Schouten *et al.* (1962) to explain certain pitch phenomena where the periodicity concept is insufficient. De Boer (1956), in discussing these phenomena, also suggested the possibility of time-interval measurement.

In this connection, Kneser (1948) pointed out that, depending on the method of measurement, frequency can be defined in two different ways. One he calls *phase frequency,* which is the inverse of the time interval between two points of equal phase in a recurring phenomenon. The phase frequency can be defined with arbitrary accuracy by only one time interval. The *group frequency,* on the contrary, physically the value of the resonator that reacts most strongly to the input wave, cannot be measured with an accuracy better than that given by the uncertainty relation.

In auditory theory, the second definition of frequency is almost universally implied, if not stated; but the phase-frequency or time-interval concept has many advantages. One possible application concerns the pitch sensation resulting from sounds of rapidly changing frequency. Strictly speaking, group frequency, in contrast to phase frequency, is not defined other than for periodic waves, but the concept can be extended to include changing frequency as well (Carson and Fry, 1937). Nevertheless, a considerable simplification of the problem results from assuming that the gliding pitch corresponds to a measurement of changing time intervals. For this kind of stimulus, no two intervals are exactly alike, and all contribute equally to the pitch sensation. Under certain circumstances, therefore, two neural pulses are enough to give rise to a tonal impression.

The fact that tones of short durations may have a well-defined pitch can also be interpreted in this light. As early as 1880, Kohlrausch made some ingenious but forgotten experiments on the pitch resulting from two sound pulses. For pulse separations within a tonal range from 80 to 240 Hz, the average accuracy of discrimination was slightly better than 1.5 percent. If we compute the "uncertainty product" from this figure and the duration for the different pulse-pairs, we get even lower values than 0.05, which was obtained by Lopes Cardozo (1962) for a 1000-Hz tone. It is doubtful, however, if the uncertainty relation has any real meaning in hearing. Although attempts have been made to show its existence in pitch discrimination by Gabor (1947), by Liang Chih-an and Chistovich (1960), and by Lopes Cardozo (1962), a numerically satisfying agreement with the theoretical results can be found only in Liang Chih-an and Chistovitch's experiments, and then only for very short durations.

A reduction of the frequency-difference limen in proportion to increasing duration would be incompatible with the time-interval conception of pitch. With the exception noted, no such proportionality is evident from the experiments on this question. The improvement in discrimination with longer durations can more likely be ascribed to the decreasing effect of neural noise with repetition of temporal information. It is significant that Tobias and Zerlin (1959) found a decrease with longer duration in the interaural time-difference threshold for wide-band noise. The curve describing the relation between threshold and duration is very similar in shape and magnitude to the pitch discrimination curves for tones around 1000 Hz, replotted in terms of least discriminable time difference versus duration, from Békésy (1960, p. 221), Oetinger (1959) and Liang Chih-an and Chistovich

(1960). The smallest interaural threshold is about 6 μsec; the pitch thresholds range between 3 and 7 μsec.

Pitch discrimination curves that use frequency instead of duration as the parameter can also serve to illustrate the difference between the two definitions of frequency. The DL for pitch is usually represented as the least discriminable number of cycles per second. Investigations such as that of Harris (1952) show that, with this form of representation, the DL decreases with frequency. If Harris's data are replotted as least discriminable changes in time interval, we get a different result. On a double logarithmic scale, pitch discrimination is seen to improve linearly with frequency up to about 2000 Hz. A similar relation was obtained in my own experiments (Nordmark, 1968); an excellent fit to a straight line is evident both in my data (Fig. 9) and in the replotting of other data from pitch discrimination experiments.

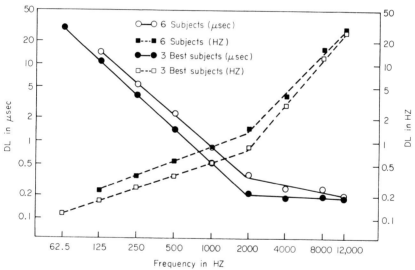

Figure 9 DL's for pure tones as a function of frequency plotted both as least discriminate change in frequency and as least discriminable change in time interval (Nordmark, 1968). (By permission from *Journal of the Acoustical Society of America*.)

In itself, the linear relation does not prove that the DL for pitch should be expressed as the least discriminable change in time interval (period); the double logarithmic representation also gives a straight line when the DL is measured in cycles per second. There are reasons, however, for believing that the time-interval representation is the appropriate one. For one thing, it is difficult to see why pitch discrimination should improve as the frequency goes down. A much

more important reason comes from measurements of frequency discrimination down to 1 Hz effected through the use of trains of short
pulses instead of pure tones. The resulting curve has no discontinuity
at the point where the sensation of pitch disappears. In the very low-
frequency region, the discrimination task is experienced as an estima-
tion of differences in duration. The differentiation between three
pulses with a frequency of 2.00 Hz and three others with a frequency
of 2.02 cannot be based on the number of impulses per unit time or on
the place of maximum stimulation on the basilar membrane, for the
simple reason that the stimuli are identical in both respects. The continuity of this part of the curve with that in the tonal region indicates
that, up to about 2000 Hz, pitch is based on perception of time interval.

Although some kind of time mechanism is often assumed for the
low-frequency range, an acceptance of the form of representation
shown in Fig. 9 leads to some interesting consequences. The main
argument in favor of a place mechanism in the high-frequency range
has been that any other mechanism has seemed physiologically unrealizable. But a time-differentiating mechanism with a precision of
the order of a few μsecs also seems unrealizable considering the
variability in firing times of individual neurons, yet we have to accept
that it exists from what we know of binaural hearing. If a similar
mechanism is assumed for pitch, the place theory becomes redundant,
since only a negligible increase in precision is required for higher
frequencies. It is difficult to imagine what evolutionary advantage
could have accrued from substituting an entirely different form of
frequency measurement for the rest of the auditory range. Piéron
(1952) pointed out how highly improbable the coexistence of two
completely heterogenous mechanisms in pitch must be. A coexistence,
peaceful or otherwise, becomes even more improbable when the
time-interval rather than the frequency form of pitch perception is
assumed. Figure 9 therefore brings out more clearly the fundamental
dichotomy between the explanatory concepts of time and place—a
dichotomy that is obscured in the duality theories.

We thus have some grounds for believing that a mechanism for
time-interval measurement (related to that operating for the binaural
system) underlies pure-tone, periodicity, and time-separation pitch.
What the hypothesis does and does not say, however, must be clearly
understood. It does not imply that pitch is necessarily uniquely determined by the temporal pattern of the basilar membrane motion.
We may, for instance, very well imagine that central effects can influence pitch perception to a limited extent, or even give rise to some
pitch phenomena.

V. PERCEPTION OF COMPLEX SOUNDS

The discussion up to this point has suggested some basic principles that should be of value in understanding auditory analysis. Analysis is commonly considered the fundamental problem of hearing. The term may be slightly misleading, however. Largely through the influence of Helmholtz, it has come primarily to mean the analysis of complex tones rather than the separation and identification of different sound sources. Helmholtz took great pains to show why it should be more difficult to hear out the partials of one tone than to distinguish complex tones in a mixture of sounds. There are many circumstances, he wrote, which assist us in separating the musical tones arising from different sources and also in keeping together the partial tones of each separate source. Thus, when one musical tone is heard for some time before being joined by a second, we know immediately what we have to deduct from the compound effect. Even when the instruments start together, dynamic factors, such as the rapid dying away of the piano tone, or the slow build-up of intensity in brass instruments, help us in hearing them as separate. The rules of counterpoint emphasize the independence of the parts and the stepwise progression of their melodic lines; distinction is made easy. In short, Helmholtz attributed our ability to separate simultaneous sounds to what in Gestalt terminology would be the law of common fate. The difficulty felt in analyzing a single complex tone into its constituent elements, on the other hand, also exists for other senses and can be overcome with practice.

For Helmholtz, therefore, the basic problem was to answer the question of how we can analyze a single complex tone rather than of how we analyze the composite tone produced by several musical instruments acting at the same time. Auditory theory seems to agree with this view even though the resonance concept has been long abandoned. The traditional view, however, needs reexamining in the light of newer knowledge. The ability to analyze a complex tone into its partials is, as Plomp showed, considerably more limited than Helmholtz imagined. The ability to "hear out" one tone in a mixture, on the other hand, though fully as great as he assumed in both the scientific and the musical part of his book, is not primarily dependent on the factors he enumerated. For example, if we eliminate all dynamic factors in the presentation of a mixture of complex tones with different sound qualities, such as amplitude-modulated tones, square waves, and filtered pulse trains, they still retain enough of their quality to allow identification. It is far from easy to understand how.

Since tone quality depends on the formant structure — that is, on the dominant regions in the amplitude spectrum of the tone — the addition of a second complex tone may change the envelope of the spectrum, and we should expect some change in the sound quality. This kind of change seldom occurs, however. Broadbent and Ladefoged (1957) showed that when the formants of two vowels spoken simultaneously overlap — even when the formants of one vowel are separated by one or more formants of the other vowel — we hear the two vowels as if they were completely separate. The simple place theory cannot account for the fact that listeners group the appropriate formants together and identify the vowels correctly, when they might equally well couple any other pairs of regions stimulated on the basilar membrane, which would result in the perception of different vowel qualities. Presumably, the authors argued, the related formants must resemble one another in some respect. The resemblance is probably associated with the modulation of the stimulus, which suggests that the key to the fusion of sounds is the waveform envelope of the sounds. Synthetically produced speech, they noted, fuses when the formants have the same fundamental, or envelope, frequency, but not otherwise.

A further reason for directing our attention to tone mixtures rather than to single complex tones is the surprising number of closely spaced instrumental tones that musical practice has shown can be distinguished, or at least in some way separately perceived. Again, traditional theory can offer no ready explanation. If the position of fundamentals on the basilar membrane determines pitch, they are in many cases too closely spaced to have clearly separate maxima. Whatever definition is given the critical band, it cannot indicate a limit for hearing out the pitch of complex tones in a mixture.

If instead we assume that the periodicity of the harmonics contributes to the impression of fundamental pitch, we are in a somewhat better position to answer these questions. The problem is that we still cannot explain how the harmonics can determine tone quality. The overlap in membrane position among the harmonics must be so extensive that it is difficult to understand how they can contribute to tone quality at all, and even less how they can be combined in groups.

One way out of these difficulties is to abandon the assumption that analysis presupposes separate representation of the auditory information in the nervous system. This assumption underlies all auditory theory — place theory in its different forms as well as the residue concept. The neural response to a mixture of sounds must, however, be exceedingly complicated; the basilar membrane cannot perform more than a very incomplete analysis, and the waveforms will intermingle. The neural analysis that must complement the preliminary mechanical analysis on the basilar membrane is, in all probability, related to the time-interval-measuring mechanism discussed in the preceding sections. Such a mechanism is eminently suitable for complex sound analysis: it is instantaneous, extremely accurate, it works in a statistical manner giving prominence to the regularities of an interval distribution, and it functions even when other temporal information is present in the same group of nerves. The mechanisms of temporal coherence and inhibition will also doubtless be of great importance for an understanding of complex sound perception. We can, at least in principle, deduce how the harmonics of a complex tone can be fused, if we assume that simultaneous temporal intervals from different regions of the membrane are grouped perceptually. We must furthermore assume that the neural information originating from a restricted area will often be scrambled, and that only the whole pattern over a much larger area will allow a meaningful interpretation.

The picture of the ear emerging from these considerations is that of a temporal pattern analyzer. Once this notion is accepted, I am convinced that phenomena of auditory analysis will turn out to be considerably easier to explain than is at present thought possible.

REFERENCES

von Békésy, G. (1955). Beitrag zur Frage der Frequenzanalyse in der Schnecke. *Arch. Ohr.-, Nas.- u. KehlkHeilk.*, **167**, 238–255.

von Békésy, G. (1960). *Experiments in hearing.* McGraw-Hill, New York.

von Békésy, G. (1962). Can we feel the nervous discharges of the end organs during vibratory stimulation of the skin? *J. Acoust Soc. Am.*, **34**, 850–856.

von Békésy, G. (1963a). Hearing theories and complex sounds. *J. Acoust. Soc. Am.*, **35**, 588–601.

von Békésy, G. (1963b). Three experiments concerned with pitch perception. *J. Acoust. Soc. Am.*, **35**, 602–606.

de Boer, E. (1956). On the "residue" in hearing. Unpublished doctoral dissertation, University of Amsterdam.

Boring, E. G. (1942). *Sensation and perception in the history of experimental psychology.* Appleton-Century-Crofts, New York.

Broadbent, D. E. and Ladefoged, P. (1957). On the fusion of sounds reaching different sense organs. *J. Acoust. Soc. Am.*, **29**, 708–710.

Carson, J. R. and Fry, T. C. (1937). Variable frequency electric circuit theory with application to the theory of frequency-modulation. *Bell Syst. Tech. J.*, **16**, 513–540.

Chocholle, R. (1957). Comments in D. Albe-Fessard and P. Buser. Activités de projection et d'association du néocortex cérébral des mammifères. *J. Physiol., Paris*, **49**, 1065–1068.

Cummings, F. T., Hall, J. L., II, and Peake, W. T. (1961). Lateralization of antiphasic clicks. *M. I. T. Res. Lab. Electron. Q. Prog. Rep.*, **62**, 239–243.

Davis, H. (1951). Psychophysiology of hearing and deafness. In S. S. Stevens (Ed.) *Handbook of experimental psychology.* pp. 1116–1142. Wiley, New York.

Davis, H. (1961). Peripheral coding of auditory information. In W. A. Rosenblith (Ed.) *Sensory communication.* pp. 119–141. M. I. T. Press *and* Wiley, New York.

Egan, J. P. and Meyer, D. R. (1950). Changes in pitch of tones of low frequency as a function of the pattern of excitation produced by a band of noise. *J. Acoust. Soc. Am.*, **22**, 827–833.

Flanagan, J. L. (1962). Models for approximating basilar membrane displacement—Part II. *Bell Syst. Tech. J.*, **41**, 959–1009.

Flanagan, J. L. and Guttman, N. (1960). On the pitch of periodic pulses. *J. Acoust. Soc. Am.*, **32**, 1308–1319.

Gabor, D. (1947). Acoustical quanta and the theory of hearing. *Nature, Lond.*, **159**, 591–594.

Gray, A. A. (1900). On a modification of the Helmholtz theory of hearing. *J. Anat. Physiol., Lond.*, **34**, 324–350.

Harris, J. D. (1952). Pitch discrimination. *J. Acoust. Soc. Am.*, **24**, 750–755.

Hartley, R. V. L. (1919). The function of phase difference in the binaural location of pure tones. *Phys. Rev.*, **13**, *ser. 2*, 373–385.

Hartline, H. K., Ratliff, F., and Miller, W. H. (1961). Inhibitory interaction in the retina and its significance in vision. In E. Florey (Ed.) *Nervous inhibition.* pp. 241–284. Macmillan (Pergamon), New York.

von Helmholtz, H. (1865). *Die Lehre von den Tonempfindungen als physiologische Grundlage für die Theorie der Musik.* Friedrich Vieweg und Sohn, Braunschweig.

Huggins, W. H. and Licklider, J. C. R. (1951). Place mechanisms of auditory frequency analysis. *J. Acoust. Soc. Am.*, **23**, 290–299.

Kneser, H. O. (1948). Bemerkungen über Definition und Messung der Frequenz. *Arch. Elekt. Übertr.*, **2**, 167–169.

Kohlrausch, W. (1880). Über Töne, die durch eine begrenzte Anzahl von Impulsen erzeugt werden. *Poggendorff's Annln. Phys. Chem.*, **10**, *ser. 3*, 1–13.

Lewis, D., Cowan, M., and Fairbanks, G. (1940). Pitch and frequency modulation. *J. Exp. Psychol.*, **27**, 23–36.

Liang, C-a. and Chistovich, L. A. (1960). Frequency-difference limens as a function of tonal duration. *Soviet Phys. Acoust.*, **6**, 75–80.

Licklider, J. C. R. (1948). The influence of interaural phase relations upon the masking of speech by white noise. *J. Acoust. Soc. Am.*, **20**, 150–159.

Licklider, J. C. R. (1959). Three auditory theories. In S. Koch (Ed.) *Psychology: a study of a science.* Vol. 1. Pp. 41–144. McGraw-Hill, New York.

Lloyd, D. P. C. (1961). A study of some twentieth century thoughts on inhibition in the spinal cord. In E. Florey (Ed.) *Nervous inhibition.* Pp. 13–31. Macmillan (Pergamon), New York.

Lopes Cardozo, B. (1962). Frequency discrimination of the human ear. *Proc. IV Int. Congr. Acoust.*, paper H16. Harlang and Toksvig, Copenhagen.

Nordmark, J. O. (1963). Some analogies between pitch and lateralization phenomena. *J. Acoust. Soc. Am.*, **35**, 1544–1547.

Nordmark, J. O. (1968). Mechanisms of frequency discrimination. *J. Acoust. Soc. Am.*, **44**, 1533–1540.

Oetinger, R. (1959). Die Grenzen der Hörbarkeit von Frequenz- und Tonzahländerungen bei Tonimpulsen. *Acustica*, **9**, 430–434.

Pfaffmann, C. (1962). Sensory processes and their relation to behavior: studies on the sense of taste as a model S-R system. In S. Koch (Ed.) *Psychology: a study of a science.* Vol. 4. pp. 380–416. McGraw-Hill, New York.

Piéron, H. (1952). *The sensations: their functions, processes and mechanisms.* Yale Univ. Press, New Haven, Connecticut.

Pollack, I. (1961). Hearing. In P. R. Farnsworth (Ed.) *Annual review of psychology.* Vol. 12. pp. 335–362. Annual Reviews, Palo Alto.

Ranke, O. F. (1955). Die Fortentwicklung der Hörtheorie und ihre klinische Bedeutung. *Arch. Ohr.-, Nas.- u. KehlkHeilk.*, **167**, 1–15.

Rutherford, W. (1886). A new theory of hearing. *J. Anat. Physiol., Lond.*, **21**, 166–168.

Schief, R. (1963). Koinzidenz-Filter als Modell für das menschliche Tonhöhenunterscheidungsvermögen. *Kybernetik*, **2**, 8–15.

Schouten, J. F. (1940). The residue and the mechanism of hearing. *Proc. K. Ned. Akad. Wet.*, **43**, 991–999.

Schouten, J. F., Ritsma, R. J., and Lopes Cardozo, B. (1962). Pitch of the residue. *J. Acoust. Soc. Am.*, **34**, 1418–1424.

Small, A. M. and McClellan, M. E. (1963). Pitch associated with time delay between two pulse trains. *J. Acoust. Soc. Am.*, **35**, 1246–1255.

Thurlow, W. R. (1958). Some theoretical implications of the pitch of double-pulse trains. *Am. J. Psychol.*, **71**, 448–450.

Thurlow, W. R. and Bernstein, S. (1957). Simultaneous two-tone pitch discrimination. *J. Acoust. Soc. Am.*, **29**, 515–519.

Thurlow, W. R. and Small, A. McCollum (1955). Pitch perception for certain periodic auditory stimuli. *J. Acoust. Soc. Am.*, **27**, 132–137.

Tobias, J. V. and Zerlin, S. (1959). Lateralization threshold as a function of stimulus duration. *J. Acoust. Soc. Am.*, **31**, 1591–1594.

Webster, J. C. and Muerdter, D. R. (1965). Pitch shifts due to low-pass and high-pass noise bands. *J. Acoust. Soc. Am.*, **37**, 382–383. (L)

Webster, J. C. and Schubert, E. D. (1954). Pitch shifts accompanying certain auditory threshold shifts. *J. Acoust. Soc. Am.*, **26**, 754–758.

Weddell, G. (1955). Somesthesis and the chemical senses. In C. P. Stone (Ed.) *Annual review of psychology.* Vol. 6. pp. 119–136. Annual Reviews, Palo Alto.

Wever, E. G. (1949). *Theory of hearing.* Wiley, New York.

Zwislocki, J. (1948). Theorie der Schneckenmechanik. *Acta Oto-Lar., Suppl.* **72.**

Chapter Three

Masking

FOREWORD

One of the older problems of psychoacoustics is to determine how the presence of one signal affects the presence of another. Monographs, texts, and reference books all detail the nature of masking, of its mechanisms, and of its effects. But the advent of new measuring techniques led to new insights into the masking process. Experiments devised to test procedures for data collection turned out additionally to raise problems for people who thought they already knew everything about the ways in which tones interfere with each other. Questions about the statistical nature of the signals were never included in the basic masking studies because it was assumed that whatever variations occurred would either average out, or be too small to be consequential. The mode of presentation seemed unlikely to be very important to understanding masking because the listening problems inherent in near-threshold hearing are solved by the high levels used for masking work. Pedestal experiments would never have been considered by most investigators because pedestals, in some funny way, seem to give the subject too much information, because they are not in the tradition of masking studies (rather, they look something like DL measurements), and because they are not amenable to the simple programing procedures that can be replicated in every laboratory. Lloyd Jeffress has brought his background in the study of binaural masking to bear upon the new problems of monaural masking.

Masking

Lloyd A. Jeffress[*]

I. INTRODUCTION

A. Historical

Masking is the obscuring of one sound by another. As Licklider (1951) pointed out, it is the opposite of analysis; when we fail to hear the signal in the noise, it is because the analysis was inadequate or because we were not listening. Analysis implies some sort of filter system and most of our theories of hearing have been filter theories from the time of Helmholtz. We should, therefore, expect that a study of the phenomena of masking would bring us closer to an understanding of the basic problem of how we hear.

Much of the early work was conducted by the Bell Telephone Laboratories and is summarized in Fletcher's (1929) book, *Speech and Hearing*. Much earlier, Mayer (1894) found that a tone could be rendered inaudible by another tone of lower frequency, but not readily by one of higher frequency. Figure 1, which summarizes a series of experiments done at the Bell Telephone Laboratories by Wegel and Lane (1924), support Mayer's observation. The figure also shows that frequencies near the signal, whether above it or below, are more effective than frequencies farther removed.

Wegel and Lane's curves are characterized by notches occuring at frequencies near the signal. These notches result from beats between

---

[*]Applied Research Laboratories and Department of Psychology, University of Texas, Austin, Texas.

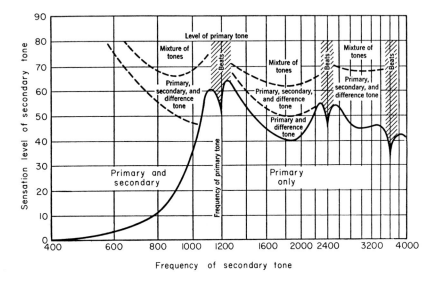

Figure 1 The various sensations produced by a two-component tone. The primary component is a sinusoid of 1200 Hz, 80 dB above threshold. The secondary component is a sinusoid of the frequency and sensation level indicated by the coordinates. When the secondary component falls below the solid curve it is masked. When the secondary component is above its masked threshold, however, the auditory sensation may be quite complex, as indicated by the descriptions in the several regions of the graph. (From Licklider, 1951, after Fletcher, 1929, from Wegel and Lane, 1924. By permission from John Wiley and Sons, Inc.; from *Speech and Hearing* by Harvey Fletcher, copyright, 1929, by D. Van Nostrand Company, by permission of Van Nostrand Reinhold Company; and from Bell Telephone Laboratories.)

the masker and the signal — fluctuations of level that render the signal more conspicuous and easier to detect. When these beats are avoided by employing a narrow band of noise rather than a tone as the masker (Egan and Hake, 1950) or by using a signal duration too short to permit a full cycle of beating to occur, the notches are eliminated and the curves show a peak rather than a notch at the signal frequency (Fig. 2).

B. White Noise

Probably the most commonly used masking stimulus is *white noise*, noise with a uniform power spectrum from one extreme of its frequency range to the other. The power is usually measured for a bandwidth of 1 Hz and, when expressed in decibels relative to 0.0002 μbar, is called the *pressure spectrum level* or the *spectral level* (L_{ps})

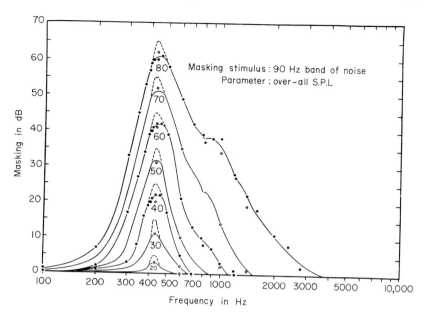

Figure 2 Masking audiograms of a narrow band of noise (90 Hz wide, centered at 410 Hz) presented at various over-all sound-pressure levels (decibels re 0.0002 dyne/cm²). The pressure spectrum level of the noise may be obtained by subtracting 19.5 dB from the corresponding number under the curve. The peak of each masking curve is extended by 4.2 dB in order to represent better the amount of excitation near the frequency of the masking stimulus. (Egan and Hake, 1950. By permission from *Journal of the Acoustical Society of America.*)

of the noise. A white noise therefore has the same spectral level at all its frequencies. A series of measurements of the instantaneous voltage associated with a band of white noise, whether wide or narrow, would show a mean of zero and a normal distribution. Because of this normal or Gaussian distribution, the noise is often referred to as Gaussian, and because it is often developed from thermal agitation in a resistor, it is also referred to as *thermal* noise.

C. Critical Bands

Fletcher (1940) proposed the *critical band* concept to account for many of the phenomena of masking. He suggested that different frequencies produce their maximal effects at different locations along the basilar membrane, and that each of these locations responds to a

limited range of frequencies. The frequency range to which a particular segment (or filter) responds is its critical band. Masking occurs,
according to Fletcher, when the noise preempts a filter (or its output
channels) that would otherwise respond to the signal, and only those
frequencies of the noise that fall within the bandwidth of the filter
are effective in masking the particular signal. The signal is just
detectable, according to Fletcher, when its energy equals the energy
of the part of the noise that affects the filter. Fletcher (1929, p. 167)
says, "When the ear is stimulated by a sound, particular nerve fibers
terminating in the basilar membrane are caused to discharge their unit
loads. Such nerve fibers then can no longer be used to carry any other
message to the brain by being stimulated by any other source of sound.
Masking experiments appropriately chosen, then, should enable us
to determine what portions of the membrane are being stimulated
by an external sound."

D. Noise Level and Masking

Hawkins and Stevens (1950) studied the masking of tones of different frequencies by a wide band of white noise. Their results are presented in Fig. 3. The abscissa is noise level, and the ordinate is the
amount of masking, expressed as the amount of signal required for
detection over that required in the absence of external noise. Had
Hawkins and Stevens used the spectral level of the masking noise as
their abscissa, they would have obtained six parallel lines — one for
each frequency — instead of their single line. Instead, the abscissa is
the "effective level" of the noise — the overall level within a specified
band around the signal frequency. The effective level is numerically
equal to the spectral level plus $10 \log W$, where W is the bandwidth in
cycles per second. For each frequency, they chose W so as to make the
line for that frequency pass through a point where the masking in dB
equalled the effective level in dB. That the line is straight over most
of its course and also passes through other points where the amount of
masking and the effective level are equal indicated a linear relation
between masking and noise level. Watson (1963) obtained a similar
function (Fig. 4) for masking in cats by choosing an appropriate bandwidth. The bandwidth, W, chosen in this way has been referred to by
some experimenters as the "critical bandwidth"; others prefer to call
it the "critical ratio" and reserve the term "critical band" for the
bandwidth arrived at by band-narrowing experiments.

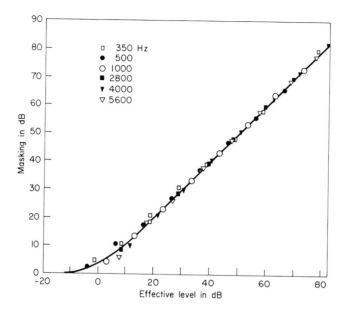

Figure 3 The relation between the masking produced by a white noise and the effective level of the noise. The effective level is the amount of noise power in a narrow frequency band, the "critical band" (see text), centered about the frequency of the masked sinusoid. It is expressed in decibels relative to the absolute threshold (in power units) at that frequency. When the intensity is given in terms of effective level, the function shown in the graph is essentially independent of the frequency of the masked sinusoid. (Hawkins and Stevens, 1950.)

II. VARIETIES OF MASKING

A. Masking, Difference Limens, and Absolute Thresholds

G. A. Miller (1947) pointed out that the difference limen and the masked threshold are essentially the same thing. The increment needed to produce a just noticeable difference in loudness may be expressed as Δp (where the original stimulus was p) or as a number of decibels. For example, we can equally well say that $p = 0.002$ μbar and $\Delta p/p = 0.15$, or that the SPL of the noise is 20 dB and the masked threshold is 21.2 dB (i.e., there is 1.2 dB of masking).

Diercks and Jeffress (1962) went a step further and argued that the

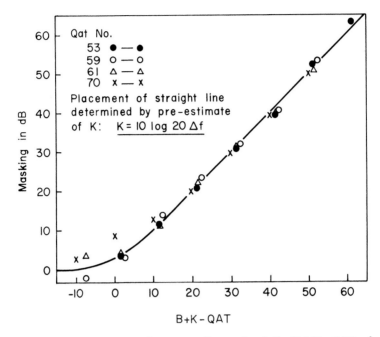

Figure 4 A function relating masking M to effective level, $Z = B + K - QAT$, where B is the spectrum level of a band of noise broader than the estimated critical bandwidth K, and QAT is the quiet absolute threshold. The function is estimated from the relation $K = 20 \, \Delta f$; the points represent data from each of four cats. (Watson, 1963. By permission from *Journal of the Acoustical Society of America*.)

absolute threshold is itself really a masked threshold. By comparing binaural thresholds for an antiphasic (reversed in phase at one ear compared with the other) tone with thresholds for diotic (same in both ears) stimulation, they concluded that noise, which is always present in one cochlea, is partially correlated with noise in the other. They pointed out that the amount of masking is commensurate with the amount of noise measured physically in the external meatus by Shaw and Piercy (1962).

B. Remote Masking

In addition to the masking by noise within the same critical band as the signal, there can be masking by frequencies well outside of the band, even above it. This phenomenon was discovered by Bilger and Hirsh (1956) and called "remote masking." It occurs only at high noise

levels, 60 to 80 dB Lps, and exhibits itself as an elevation of threshold
for frequencies below those of the band of noise. Thus a band of noise
from 2450 to 3120 Hz at a spectral level of about 70 dB will elevate
the threshold for tones from 100 to 1000 Hz by about 20 dB. Deatherage *et al.* (1957) demonstrated a similar phenomenon in the guinea
pig. The action potentials and cochlear microphonics recorded from
the third turn of the cochlea in response to 500 Hz tone bursts were
masked by an intense high-frequency noise. At the same time a
random, low-frequency, cochlear-microphonic potential appeared.
The authors explained their finding as being the result of nonlinear
distortion that generates out of the high-frequency noise a low-
frequency disturbance, fluctuating in frequency and amplitude. Hirsh
and Burgeat (1958) confirmed this hypothesis.

They measured binaural masking level differences (comparisons
between various binaural conditions and simple monaural masking)
by reversing the phase of a low-frequency tone that was masked remotely by a high-frequency noise. The results were similar to those
obtained with low-frequency noise, suggesting that the masking was
due to low frequencies actually existing in the cochlea. Cox (1958)
showed that low frequencies are indeed generated from a limited
(clipped) high-frequency band of noise.

C. Backward and Forward Masking

Backward masking is the masking of a signal by a noise that occurs
later; forward masking is the reverse, the noise being terminated
before the signal is begun. Both phenomena have other names; backward masking has been called precedent masking, and forward masking has been called residual masking, poststimulatory threshold shift,
and adaptation. Lüscher and Zwislocki (1949) reviewed earlier experiments and offered data on the spread of adaptation (forward masking)
as a function of level, time, and frequency. Masking as a function of
frequency is similar to simultaneous masking: a tone is masked by an
earlier tone when the frequencies are close together or when the
earlier tone is lower in frequency. There is little forward masking
when the masker has a higher frequency than the signal. The masking
effect of an earlier sound falls off rapidly with the size of the interval
between, and the slope of this drop is a function of the level of the
masking sound. For an 80-dB, 400-msec, 3000-Hz masker, the masking
is 40 dB when the signal follows in 20 msec. The value falls to zero

when the interval is increased to 200 msec. The drop, when expressed in decibels of masking, is approximately linear with time.

Pickett (1959) and Elliott (1962) summarized earlier work on backward masking, much of it done in the Soviet Union, and presented the results of several experiments in which the masker was a burst of white noise and the signal, a 1000-Hz tone of short duration. The dependence of masking on the level of the masker is linear, but the linear relation between interval and masking found by Lüscher and by Zwislocki for forward masking does not hold for backward masking. The masking decreases much more rapidly as the interval between signal and masker is increased. Elliott, in one case for example, found about 60 dB of masking when the noise began 1 msec after the termination of the signal, but only about 20 dB when the interval was increased to 10 msec. Virtually no masking was found for intervals longer than about 25 msec.

Both forward and backward masking are the results of time-dependent properties of the neural mechanism of hearing. Forward masking suggests that recently stimulated cells are not as sensitive as rested cells, a not very surprising fact. Backward masking, however, is the interference of a later noise with some process initiated by the signal but not completed before the onset of the noise. The intervals are too long to explain in terms of energy integration at the cochlea and suggest instead some kind of interaction at higher centers, where the later activity produced by the more intense stimulus can overtake and obscure the effects of the earlier stimulus. The effect is large; a short tone terminating 1 msec before the onset of the noise may experience 60 dB of masking, but the same tonal pulse, starting 1 msec after the termination of the noise, experiences only about 30 dB.

D. Masking of Speech

Although speech is probably our most important signal, it is an awkward one to use, and has not been employed much in masking experiments. Where it has been used, the purpose has often been to study the nature of speech itself, or the nature of the masker — room reverberation, street noise, etc. Licklider (1948) used speech in a study of binaural phenomena, and Pollack and Pickett (1958), in their study of the masking of speech by speech, were primarily concerned with binaural effects. Swets (1964) devoted four chapters to the masking of speech, but his major concern was with speech as a signal in the theory of signal detectability (TSD).

III. MASKING AND THE THEORY OF
SIGNAL DETECTABILITY

A. Noise and Noise-Plus-Signal Distributions

The theory of signal detectability covers the detection of a great variety of signals. Let us look at it here only as it applies to the detection of a (usually) tonal signal in a background of (usually) Gaussian noise. The two probability density curves (for noise and for noise plus signal) of TSD are usually exhibited along an unspecified abscissa, representing whatever it is about the stimulus that the subject is responding to. In this section an attempt will be made to specify the abscissa, that is, to determine just what aspect of the stimulus causes the subject to vote more frequently for the interval containing the signal.

Narrow-Band Noise. The concept of critical bands is one of the important ideas to grow out of the experimental work on masking. The picture of the cochlea as a series of narrow-band filters helps in understanding not only many phenomena of masking, but also a number of other functions of the ear. Figure 5, from Licklider (1951), shows estimates of critical bandwidths based on data from studies of masking, of pitch discrimination, of pitch scaling, and of speech intelligibility. Data for pitch discrimination, pitch scaling, and speech intelligibility do not yield critical bandwidths directly. They were adjusted along the ordinate to conform with the masking data at one frequency to show the *form* of the function, not its magnitude. The functions agree surprisingly well considering the diversity of the sources.

Figure 5 shows that the bandwidth associated with, say, 500 Hz is about 50 Hz. Thus, in a masking experiment where the noise level is not excessively high, only the noise frequencies from about 475 to 525 Hz (the critical band) play an important role in the masking of a 500-Hz tonal signal. The idea of the critical band as a filter (resembling an electrical filter) is only an analogy that is imperfect in many respects. The bandwidth of an electrical filter is the same over a wide range of measured levels; the ear's is not. Also, the bandwidth of a filter is either its width at the half-power (3-dB down) points or its equivalent rectangular width; and both of these measures lose some of their meaning (especially their predictive value) when the filter response is as unsymmetrical as the ear's. An ear's filter skirt is considerably steeper on the high-frequency side than on the low — that is, low frequencies mask higher frequencies more effectively than the reverse. (Many masking studies show the shape in reverse because the masker is kept at a constant frequency and the signal is varied, thus making each measurement in a number of critical bands.)

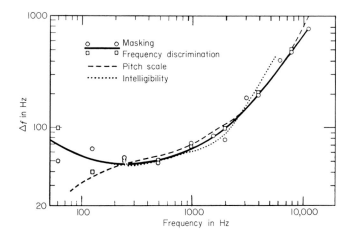

Figure 5   Four functions relating Δf to f. The critical band function (circles and solid curve) shows the width of the band of noise that contributes to the masking of a sinusoid at the center of the band. In the frequency-discrimination curve (squares and solid curve), Δf is 20 times the jnd. The curve based on the pitch scale gives the width in frequency of intervals that are 50 mels wide in pitch. The curve based on intelligibility data shows the widths of frequency bands that contribute equally—2 percent of the total—to the intelligibility of speech. The similarity of the curves suggests that they have a common basis in the auditory mechanism. (Licklider, 1951. By permission from John Wiley and Sons, Inc.)

Figure 6 shows a 50-Hz narrow band of noise centered at 500 Hz. The upper picture is an oscilloscope photograph of the noise, and the lower is a simultaneous photograph of the same stretch of noise with a 500-Hz tone added. The signal has the same rms voltage as the noise. Both functions closely resemble sine waves that are slowly fluctuating both in amplitude and in frequency or phase; the axis crossings are not quite evenly spaced. These functions might be sinusoids with a basic frequency of 500 Hz, randomly modulated in amplitude and in phase. The fluctuations of phase are equivalent to fluctuations in frequency, 360° per sec being 1 Hz. Because the filter is so narrow, the amplitude and phase modulation rates are slow compared with the frequency of the sinusoid.

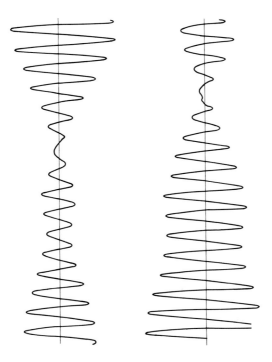

Figure 6 Narrow-band noise (bandwidth 50 Hz, center frequency 500 Hz) (upper trace). Narrow-band noise plus signal (lower trace).

The instantaneous displacement (voltage or pressure) for the narrow band of noise can be written

$$y(t) = a(t) \sin [2\pi f t + \varphi(t)] \tag{3.1}$$

where f is the center frequency (500 Hz in the example), $a(t)$ is the amplitude (frequently called the envelope), and $\varphi(t)$ is the phase angle between the noise and some reference zero. Both $a(t)$ and $\varphi(t)$ are slowly varying, random functions of time. The amplitude, $a(t)$, is always positive in sign and varies from zero upward. If the noise is Gaussian, the instantaneous voltage, $y(t)$, will be normally distributed around zero as its mean, and the standard deviation of the distribution of instantaneous voltages, σ, will be identical with the rms voltage of the band of noise (the square-root of the mean of the squared voltages).

If for a Gaussian noise the voltages are normally distributed, then the amplitudes cannot be. Their distribution must be skewed since they are bounded on one side by zero and can reach toward infinity on the other. The literature of both acoustics and physics is often confusing because of the widespread, careless use of the word "amplitude" when voltage or displacement is meant. The amplitude of a pure sinusoid is a constant, it is the voltage or displacement or pressure that varies sinusoidally. In the case of a narrow band of noise the amplitude, $a(t)$, fluctuates but remains positive in sign; it is the voltage that shows a Gaussian distribution.

Rayleigh's Distribution. In 1894, Rayleigh (1945, pp. 35–42) discussed the distribution function associated with the amplitudes of Eq. (3.1). He considered a narrow band of noise, obtained by combining n sinusoids of equal amplitude and of random phases, and derived the expression for the distribution function when n is allowed to become infinite. He found the function to be

$$f(a) = \left[a/\sigma^2 \right] \exp\left[-a^2/2\sigma^2 \right] \tag{3.2}$$

where σ is the standard deviation of $y(t)$ of Eq. (3.1) and hence is the rms voltage of the band of noise. The probability that a, the amplitude in this expression, will exceed some magnitude, a_i, is given by

$$P(a > a_i) = \int_{a_i}^{\infty} f(a)\, da = \exp\left[-a_i^2/2\sigma^2 \right] \tag{3.3}$$

The probability-density function of Eq. (3.2) is graphed in the left-hand curve of Fig. 7.

The density function of Eq. (3.2) can be obtained from a bivariate normal distribution function of x and y, where the means of x and y are equal to zero, where σ_x and $\sigma_y = \sigma$, and where the correlation between x and y is zero. The radius*, from the center (origin) to any point (x, y), is the quantity, a.

---

*The expression of Eq. (3.2) can be obtained from the density functions for a bivariate normal distribution where x and y are independent and have the same standard deviation; i.e., σ_x and $\sigma_y = \sigma$. The joint density function is simply the product of the two independent density functions:

$$f(x, y) = \left[1/ (\sigma \sqrt{2\pi}) \right] \exp\left[-x^2/2\sigma^2 \right] \left[1/ (\sigma \sqrt{2\pi}) \right] \exp\left[-y^2/2\sigma^2 \right]$$

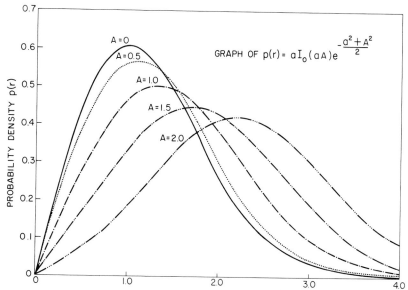

Figure 7 Distribution curves for narrow-band noise and noise plus signal. The parameter A is the amplitude of the signal relative to the rms noise voltage. The curve for A = 0.0 is for noise alone — the Rayleigh distribution. (Jeffress, 1964. By permission from *Journal of the Acoustical Society of America.*)

$$= \left[1/2\pi\sigma^2\right] \exp\left[-(x^2 + y^2)/2\sigma^2\right]$$

And letting $\rho^2 = x^2 + y^2$,

$$f(x, y) = \left[1/2\pi\sigma^2\right] \exp\left[-\rho^2/2\sigma^2\right]$$

the joint probability associated with a particular point (x, y). (The equation is not, of course, the density function for ρ, since there is an infinity of combinations of x and y that will yield the same value of ρ.) To find the density function for ρ, first determine the probability, $P(\rho)$. The increment involved is a ring of radius ρ, and of width $d\rho$. Therefore, multiply the expression by $2\pi\rho \, d\rho$ and integrate:

$$P(\rho) = \int_0^\rho \left[2\pi\rho/2\pi\sigma^2\right] \exp\left[-\rho^2/2\sigma^2\right] d\rho = 1 - \exp\left[-\rho^2/2\sigma^2\right]$$

Differentiating this expression yields

$$f(\rho) = \left[\rho/\sigma^2\right] \exp\left[-\rho^2/2\sigma^2\right]$$

which is Rayleigh's distribution.

Deriviations and tables associated with the circular-normal distribution are to be found in the *Handbook of Probability and Statistics with Tables*, by Burington and May (1953).

Narrow-Band Noise Plus Signal. A signal of frequency, f, added to the noise of Eq. (3.1), produces the function pictured in the lower part of Fig. 6. It too may be thought of as a sinusoid, modulated in amplitude and phase, and can be described by

$$y(t) = r(t) \sin [2\pi ft + \theta(t)] \qquad (3.4)$$

where $r(t)$ is the new amplitude—the vector sum of the random variable, $a(t)$, and the constant signal amplitude, A. The new phase angle, $\theta(t)$, is the angle between the resultant and the reference zero.

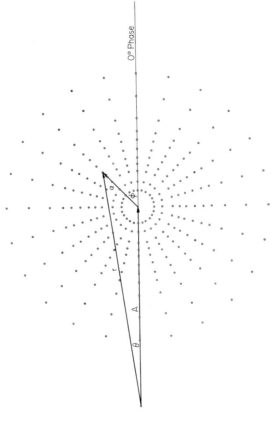

Figure 8 Adding a signal to noise. The vector A represents the signal and the vector a represents one possible value for the noise. The momentary phase angle between the signal and the narrow-band noise is φ, and between the signal and the signal-plus-noise vector, r, is θ. The dots indicate equi-probable locations of the terminus of the noise vector.

Distribution for Noise Plus Signal. From the distribution function for narrow-band noise, we can try to determine the function for noise plus signal. The amplitude function of the noise is the Rayleigh, or circular-normal, distribution. The phase function is rectangular: all angles are equally likely. Let us select a number, say ten, of equally likely values of the noise amplitude. These would be the mid-decile values, i.e., the values for $P = 0.05, 0.15, 0.25$, and so on. The corresponding values of a, computed from Eq. (3.3) are 0.32, 0.57, 0.76, and so on. Let us also select a number of equally likely phase angles — every 15° will serve. All the combinations of amplitude and phase produce 240 values of $a(t)$, all equally likely. These values are shown as dots in Fig. 8.

Figure 8 also shows the result of adding a signal of amplitude A, in phase with the reference zero. The signal vector is shown for A equal to four times the standard deviation (the rms voltage) of the noise and pointing along the x axis (0° phase). One of the 240 noise vectors is shown and the resultant drawn in. The resultant SN vector, has a length, r, and makes an angle, θ, with the x axis.[*]

---

[*]The rationale for resorting to vector triangles is not always obvious to nonengineers, and for their benefit some trigonometry is provided.

Treat the nearly sinusoidal narrow band of noise as if it were a sinusoid of the same frequency as the signal, but differing in phase, at the moment by the angle φ. The amplitude of the noise is a and of the signal, b. Now, adding two sinusoids of the same frequency but different phase yields another sinusoid of the same frequency, but usually different both in phase and in amplitude from the other two. Call the new amplitude c, and the new phase angle θ. Then

$$c \sin (2\pi ft + \theta) = a \sin (2\pi ft + \varphi) + b \sin 2\pi ft$$

This expression holds for all values of t, and hence for $t = 0$; therefore

$$c \sin \theta = a \sin \varphi$$

The expression also holds for the value of t that makes $2\pi ft = \pi/2$; hence

$$c \sin (\pi/2 + \theta) = a \sin (\pi/2 + \varphi) + b \sin (\pi/2)$$

but

$$\sin (A + \pi/2) = \cos A$$

and

$$\sin \pi/2 = 1$$

hence

$$c \cos \theta = a \cos \varphi + b$$

Repeating this process for each of the dots in Fig. 8 and measuring the length of the *SN* vector for each triangle produces a set of data from which to construct a frequency polygon. The polygon approximates the distribution function for noise plus signal for the case where $A = 4\rho$.*

Fortunately, solving vector triangles graphically is unnecessary. Rice (1954, pp. 236–241) derived the expression for the probability density corresponding to this frequency polygon. In our notation, with a for noise amplitude, A for signal amplitude, and σ for the rms noise voltage, the function is

$$f(a,A) = (a/\sigma^2) \, I_0(aA/\sigma^2) \, \exp \, [-(a^2 + A^2)/2\sigma^2] \qquad (3.5)$$

where I_0 is a Bessel function for which tables are readily available.†

Squaring the two expressions gives

$$c^2 \sin^2\theta = a^2 \sin^2\varphi$$

and

$$c^2 \cos^2\theta = a^2 \cos^2\varphi + 2ab \cos \varphi + b^2$$

Adding and combining terms leads to

$$c^2 (\sin^2\theta + \cos^2\theta) = a^2 (\sin^2\varphi + \cos^2\varphi) + 2 \, ab \cos \varphi + b^2$$

and from $\sin^2 A + \cos^2 A = 1$, to

$$c^2 = a^2 + b^2 + 2ab \cos \varphi$$

This statement is the familiar law of cosines with the sign changed because φ, as we have measured it, is the supplement of the included angle and $\cos \varphi = -\cos(\pi-\varphi)$.

So the new sinusoid can be found by simply solving a triangle involving the two original amplitudes and the phase angle. Such a triangle is shown in Fig. 8.

---

*This approach avoids several assumptions about which there have been arguments. It is unnecessary to assume Fourier-series, band-limited noise, or to assume the applicability of sampling theory, or to use likelihood ratios, even though these things are needed to obtain the analytical expressions. But the receiver operating characteristic (ROC) curves (see Section I) can be found by the brute-force method of combining the frequency polygon for noise plus signal with the one for noise alone. The only necessary assumption is that the noise *voltage* be normally distributed.

---

†Tables of e^{-x} and I_0 (x) (x) are to be found in the *Handbook of Chemistry and Physics*, by Weast *et al.* (1965).

When $A = 0.00$, the Bessel function, I_0, is unity, and Eq. (3.5) reduces to Eq. (3.2), the expression for noise alone. The right-hand curves of Fig. 7 represent the function $f(a, A)$ with $\sigma = 1.00$ for various values of the signal amplitude A. The curves for noise and for small values of A are decidedly skewed. The curves for large values of A approach the normal distribution, with a standard deviation equal to σ, the rms noise voltage. To turn the probability density functions of Fig. 7 into receiver operating characteristic (ROC) curves, it is necessary to accumulate the probabilities under the curves. The probabilities for noise are given by Eq. (3.3) and can be readily determined from tables of the exponential. The corresponding expression for SN is

$$P(r > a_i) = \int_{a_i}^{\infty} f(a, A) \, da \qquad (3.6)$$

The expression in Eq. (3.6) is not integrable, but it can be evaluated numerically. Marcum (1950) did so, and prepared a set of tables of the integral (with $\sigma = 1.00$) for values of a_i ranging in steps of 0.1 units from 0.1 to 20.0, and for A, in steps of 0.05 units, from 0.00 (the Rayleigh distribution) to 24.90. The probabilities are given to six decimal places. Using Marcum's table instead of our graphically derived frequency polygon, we can determine $P(a > a_i)$ and $P(r > a_i)$ for various values of the criterion, a_i, and of the signal amplitude, A. These probabilities correspond to $P(y \mid N)$ (the probability of a "yes, the signal was present" response to the noise alone) and $P(y \mid SN)$ (the probability of a "yes" response to the noise plus the signal), and can be used in plotting a family of ROC curves. The result is shown in Fig. 9.[*]

ROC Curves for Amplitude Distribution. The curves of Fig. 9 are slightly different in shape from the familiar ones of TSD, but they are to be found in the TSD literature. Peterson *et al.* (1954, p. 193) presented the family, and showed that it represents the behavior of the ideal detector for the case where the signal is completely specified except for phase. The more familiar curves are derived from overlapping normal curves of equal variance, and represent the behavior of the ideal detector when the signal is completely specified, including phase.

---

[*]Figure 9 is taken from Jeffress (1964), who also presented a condensed version of Marcum's table containing probabilities to three decimal places for values of a_i from 0.2 to 4.0 by steps of 0.2 units, and for values of A, from 0.0 (noise alone) to 5.0, by steps of 0.5 units.

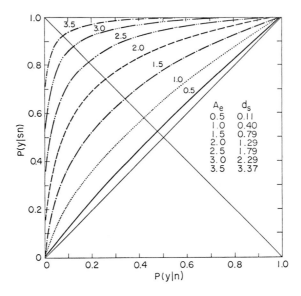

A_e	d_s
0.5	0.11
1.0	0.40
1.5	0.79
2.0	1.29
2.5	1.79
3.0	2.29
3.5	3.37

Figure 9 ROC curves derived from the distribution functions for noise and noise plus signal. The parameter is the same as that of Fig. 7. (Jeffress, 1964. By permission from *Journal of the Acoustical Society of America.*)

Watson *et al.* (1964), with a rating-scale device (with which the subject indicated his assurance that a signal was present in the stimulus interval), plotted 36 points on an ROC curve. On normal-normal probability paper, the points could be fitted only fairly well by straight lines having slopes less than unity. The authors commented, "It could be further conjectured that the functions that generate these ROC curves are somewhat more peaked than normal distributions . . . ." Jeffress (1964) later found that the ROC curves of Fig. 9 fitted the rating-scale data better than ROC curves derived from normal distributions did.* Similarly, Marill (1956) showed that ogives derived from Eq. (3.6) (Marcum's table), where $P(c)$, the probability of a correct response, is plotted against signal level, fitted his subjects' data better than ogives derived from normal curves.

These results indicate that the subject, in detecting a tonal signal in a background of Gaussian noise, responds to the *amplitude* of the stimulus, and does not use phase information. The abscissa for the

---

*It has been known for some time (e.g., Egan *et al.* 1959) that rating-scale data plotted on normal-normal probability paper yield lines having slopes almost always less than unity, and therefore violate the equal-variance assumption. Several *ad hoc* explanations of the unequal variance have been offered, none very satisfactory.

family of probability-density curves is the ratio of voltages (*SN* amplitude divided by rms noise voltage), and supports the observation by Tanner and Birdsall (1958) that d', their measure of detectability, is a voltage-like quantity, at least for audition.

"Pedestal" Experiments. Gaston (personal communication, 1964) pointed out that, since the curves of Fig. 9 became more nearly normal as *A* is increased, using one of the curves (say, for *A* = 2.0) for "noise" and another for *SN* should yield ROC curves like those for the normal, equal-variance assumption. An ROC plot on normal-normal probability paper for $A = 2.0$ (*N*) and $A = 3.0$ (*SN*) yields a line that is substantially straight and has a slope almost equal to unity.

"Pedestal" experiments use a "noise" made from a noise mixed with a sinusoid of the signal frequency. The "signal" is an increase in the level of the sinusoid and can be thought of as standing on the "pedestal." The experiment suggested by Gaston is therefore a pedestal experiment. So far no one has determined an ROC curve using a pedestal, but several experiments have determined the shape of the psychometric function relating signal level to detection percentage. Green (1960) pointed out that for a two-alternative, forced-choice experiment without a pedestal, the psychometric function does not fit the function for the ideal observer (phase known); when a pedestal is used, the fit is good. That the psychometric function for pedestal experiments fits the function for the ideal detector (phase known) better than data taken without a pedestal can be (and has been) interpreted as indicating that the human observer can use phase information when it is made available. Pfafflin and Mathews (1962), in discussing a series of pedestal experiments, pointed out that accounting for the observer's use of phase requires the assumption of some sort of correlation detector, whereas the assumption of a simple envelope detector will successfully predict the outcome of experiments both with and without a pedestal — even with a pedestal to which the signal is added in quadrature phase. For convenience, their mathematical treatment is based on an energy (square-law) detector, but (as they pointed out) a simple amplitude detector (rectifier) would yield almost the same functions and be more realistic neurophysiologically. Their approach to the detection problem is considerably different from mine, but the functions at which they arrive are substantially the same.*

---

*Green (personal communication, 1965) pointed out that increasing the size of the pedestal to where it, rather than the noise, is the dominant factor in masking, brings us under the jurisdiction of Weber's law. We discriminate changes in the level of a tone,

Meaning of d' for Rayleigh-Type Distributions. Tables of d' (Elliott, 1959) yield the values of d' associated with various combinations of $P(y|N)$ and $P(y|SN)$. The d' associated with the probabilities taken from any one of the ROC curves of Fig. 9 is different for each point on the curve. To circumvent this difficulty, Clarke *et al.* (1959), and Egan *et al.* (1961), employed the value of d' for the point where the ROC curve passes through the negative diagonal. Egan called this value d_s. Green (1964) showed that for two-alternative, forced-choice data, $P(c)$ is equal to the area under the ROC curve, no matter what shape the underlying probability-density functions may take. He therefore suggested using $P(c)$ as the measure of detection, which would still be a problem with data from a yes-no experiment. Without the shape of the ROC curves, we cannot know what curve the data point belongs to, and cannot discover the appropriate $P(c)$, nor for that matter, the appropriate d_s. Quite possibly some of the variability of yes-no data stems from the fact that points on the same curve yield different d' values because of the shape of the curve. The moral is that the first step in dealing with a new stimulus situation should be either to determine an ROC curve for it or to employ the two-alternative, forced-choice procedure and use $P(c)$.

For the Rayleigh-type distributions, $P(c)$ can be obtained from Marill's (1956) expression for $P(c)$ for two-alternative, forced-choice data,

$$P(c) = 1 - \tfrac{1}{2} \exp \left[-E/2N_0 \right]$$

where E is the signal energy and N_0 is the spectral level of the noise. The z-score corresponding to this $P(c)$ plotted as a function of $\sqrt{2E/N_0}$ gives a (very nearly) straight line with a slope of one. The line bends to the origin for small values of $\sqrt{2E/N_0}$. The straight portion, if extended, would intersect the ordinate at -0.707 (Jeffress, 1964). The

and $\Delta I/I$ should be nearly constant. Nothing in the foregoing approach would predict this fact. If the noise is just noise ($A = 0.0$) and the signal has $A = 2.0$, d_s should be about 1.3 (Jeffress, 1964). With a pedestal of $A = 2.0$ and a signal of $A = 4.0$, d_s should be the same (as it should be for a pedestal of $A = 10.0$ and a signal of $A = 12.0$). As Green pointed out, such an occurrence would obviously be in violation of Weber's law. It is like expecting a voltmeter to have the same accuracy in millivolts on the 100-V scale as on the 1-V scale. Green showed that Weber's law goes back into operation either by assuming a "self-noise" that is proportional to the stimulus, or by assuming that, like the voltmeter's the detector's error is proportional to the stimulus. The idea appears more reasonable physiologically — the firing rate of the "amplitude" fibers of the VIIIth nerve is a quasi-logarithmic function of amplitude.

z-score is numerically equal, or very nearly equal, to the d_s (the d' associated with the negative diagonal) for these distributions.

B. Energy, Bandwidth, and Duration

Energy vs. Amplitude as Stimulus. The literature of TSD has sometimes confused readers about whether subjects respond to the energy of the signal or to its amplitude. All of the evidence I have presented points to the latter, to the envelope of the waveform as the aspect of the stimulus to which subjects respond. The shape of ROC curves, the shape of the psychometric function relating detection to signal level (both with and without a pedestal), and the paramater of the family of distribution functions involved, all indicate that the ear acts as an envelope (amplitude) detector. The methods are sensitive enough to discover other bases for detection (such as interaural time difference under some binaural conditions) when they are operative. The sensitivity is also shown by the fact that the present data deny the use of phase information by the subject when phase information is not accessible to him.

Duration and Bandwidth. Peterson *et al.* (1954), in their derivation of the probability density functions of Fig. 7, used the parameter $\sqrt{2E/N_0}$ in the same way that we used A/σ.

For the same curve, the two quantities are equal: $A/\sigma = \sqrt{2E/N_0}$. Let us see what is implied by this relation. Our quantity, A, is the signal amplitude, and is therefore equal to $\sqrt{2}$ times the rms signal voltage, S. Our σ is the rms noise voltage of the band of noise. If for arithmetical convenience we make the conventional assumption of a unit resistive load, the noise power is σ^2 and is equal to the per-cycle noise power, N_0, times the bandwidth, W. The signal power is S^2, and the signal energy, E, is S^2 times the duration, T. Squaring both sides of the original equality, $A/\sigma = \sqrt{2E/N_0}$, gives $A^2/\sigma^2 = 2E/N_0$, and substituting for A, σ, and E, leads to $2S^2/WN_0 = 2S^2T/N_0$. Cancelling leaves the relation $1/W = T$. Since the curves of Peterson *et al.* were derived for the ideal detector for the case where signal phase is unknown, the relation shows the ideal observer (phase unknown) to be an envelope detector with a filter having a bandwidth equal to the reciprocal of the signal duration. Peterson *et al.* drew the same conclusion but used a somewhat different line of reasoning.

Signal Duration and Masking. There have been several studies of the effect of signal duration on masking. Probably the earliest was an experiment by Garner and Miller (1947), who found a linear relation between the masked threshold expressed in decibels of masking and the logarithm of signal duration (for durations between 12.5 and 200 msec at four signal frequencies). Increasing the duration by a factor of 2 increased detection by 3 dB. Other investigators (Hamilton, 1957; Blodgett et al., 1958) found similar relations, but with changes in the slope of the function at different durations. All found that the slope increases for short signals (where T is less than the reciprocal of the critical bandwidth). Durations longer than about 200 to 500 msec are apparently not so efficient as shorter ones and the line relating masking and duration levels off. Green et al. (1957), in an experiment where the signal energy was kept constant by increasing the power in proportion to the decrease in duration, found that the detection index, d', remained constant through a range of durations that varied from subject to subject. All had constant values of d' from 20 to 150 msec, but some subjects extended this range to about 10 msec at one end, some to nearly 300 msec at the other.

Studies of the effect of duration suggest that the ear integrates energy. The durations involved, however, are too long to make it reasonable that there is actual accumulation of energy before stimulation occurs. More likely, the integration is neural, and rather than accumulating energy, the mechanism accumulates neural events associated with envelope (amplitude) peaks. Elliott (1963) found that subjects with substantial high-frequency hearing loss, presumably neural, when tested at frequencies where the loss is serious, show less temporal integration than normal subjects. They require nearly as strong a signal at long durations as they do at short. It is difficult to see how this fact could be explained in terms of energy integration.

Bandwidth and Masking. Since the original experiments by Fletcher (1940), there have been several experiments attempting to discover the bandwidth and shape of the ear's filter system. Schafer et al. (1950) investigated the masking effects of narrow bands of noise obtained *a la* Rayleigh by combining a number of sinusoids of equal amplitudes and random phase. They determined the equivalent rectangular bandwidths at three frequencies — 200, 800, and 3200 Hz — to be 65, 65, and 240 Hz respectively. If the ear's filters are taken as single-tuned circuits, the corresponding Qs are 9.3, 37, and 39 respectively. The shapes of the masking functions obtained by Schafer et al. resemble curves for single-tuned circuits.

Swets et al. (1962) also studied the relation between masking and the bandwidth of the masking noise, using filters ranging from much wider to much narrower than the values usually assumed for the critical band. They made critical bandwidth estimates at 1000 Hz for various assumptions about the response characteristics: if the ear's filter is single-tuned, the band should be 41 Hz; if rectangular, 95 Hz; if Gaussian (3-dB-down points), 79 Hz; Gaussian (1-σ points), 95 Hz. They concluded, "We would suggest a consideration . . . of the possibility that the parameters of the mechanism of frequency selectivity vary from one task to another under intelligent control. If they do, then, of course, we cannot speak of, or measure, *the* critical band." The validity of their statement is supported by many experiments employing other than tonal signals and yielding bandwidths considerably wider than those mentioned.

Duration, Bandwidth, and Masking. The reciprocal relation between bandwidth and duration indicated by the equivalence of A/σ and $\sqrt{2E/N_0}$ has interesting implications for hearing. The most obvious is that the subject employs a bandwidth appropriate to the duration (or expected duration) of the signal. Something of the sort is implied in the quoted statement by Swets *et al.* (1962). It seems also to be implied in Békésy's (1959) concept of neural funneling, and in Marill's reference to the bandwidths employed by his subjects. Jeffress (1964) specifically considered a bandwidth that might be narrowed for long signals and widened for short, and examined Hamilton's (1957) data accordingly. Hamilton varied both the duration of the signal and the bandwidth of the noise. The interactions of bandwidth and duration were in the direction predicted, but were not clear-cut enough to be completely convincing. Hamilton's and Greenwood's (1961) estimates of critical bandwidth are considerably wider than most of those discussed here.

C. Signal Uncertainty

Frequency Uncertainty and Masking. In the physical domain, if we were looking for a signal of known frequency and duration (but unknown phase) in Gaussian noise, we would use a filter having a bandwidth equal to the reciprocal of the duration and a center frequency equal to that of the signal. If the signal might be either of two frequencies, we would select two appropriate filters and combine their outputs by means of an OR gate, unless the frequencies were close enough together so that one filter would suffice. An alternative to employing n filters for n different frequencies would be a single filter wide enough to encompass the range of frequencies involved. This method would be less efficient since the wider filter would not exclude the short, signal-like bursts of noise that would be rejected by the optimal filters.

The question of interest here is, does the ear do anything of the sort. Marill (1956) found that when two signals are presented simultaneously, if their frequencies lie close together (within one filter) they are detected more readily than either is alone; but if they are well separated, they are detected no better than one alone. This result is in agreement with the multifilter hypothesis. If the signals affect the same filter, they are occurring in a single band of noise and should increase the signal-to-noise ratio; if they occupy different filters, each will have its own band of noise and no improvement should occur.

The problem becomes more complicated when the signals are employed singly and the subject does not know which of two (or of several) to expect. A still different situation arises when the subject expects one frequency and gets another. Both situations have been studied. Greenberg (personal communication, 1964) found that when a subject is expecting a signal of 1100 Hz but is given one of some other frequency without knowing that this change can occur, his detection drops sharply. The curve of detection vs signal frequency resembles the masking curves of Schafer *et al.* (1950), which suggests that the subject is employing a single filter and disregarding signals that lie outside of its band.

If the subject knows that two possible signals are equally likely to occur, what happens? One possibility, suggested by Tanner *et al.* (1956), is that the subject scans the filter back and forth between the frequencies involved, and frequently misses the signal because he is looking in the other place. Green (1958) examined this idea and rejected it because it predicts too low a detection score. He suggested instead a multifilter model in which the outputs of the separate filters are added. Creelman (1960) made the further suggestion that the detector decides on the basis of the maximal output of the filters taken separately. Some of the experimental data appear to agree with one hypothesis and some with another. Creelman found that some of his data even suggest that the subject widens his filter to encompass the range of frequencies involved.

As Swets (1963) pointed out, there is no doubt that the subject is somehow selecting what to listen for—that there is some sort of control of the peripheral apparatus by the central nervous system. The question appears to be, what sort. At this point it might be wise to invoke the Huggins and Licklider (1951) principle of diversity, which says that if there are two ways of doing something, the nervous system probably uses both.

Let us examine the possibility that the outputs of the filters are combined by way of an OR gate. In a yes-no experiment, if the criterion were maintained at a constant level, $P(y \mid SN)$ would remain unaltered, but $P(y \mid N)$ would be doubled; a signal-like noise occurring in either filter would appear in the output of the gate, and receive a "yes" vote. (The gate responds to A or B or both.) If the ROC curves of Fig. 9 are appropriate here (and they should be), they can be used to predict almost any degree of drop in detection in a two-frequency experiment, depending upon the choice of criterion and of signal level. For example, consider a d_s of 2.0 for a single frequency, and assume that $P(y \mid SN) = 0.57$. The corresponding value of $P(y \mid N)$ will be 0.05. Doubling this value requires a new ROC curve, the one for $d_s = 1.7$. If instead of 0.57, the initial detection is $P(y \mid SN) = 0.80$, then $P(y \mid N) = 0.12$. Doubling this probability calls for the curve for $d_s = 1.55$, a considerably greater drop in detection efficiency. The former corresponds to about a 1 dB change of level, the latter to about 1.5 dB (Jeffress, 1964, p. 771). For a low signal level (hence a low value of d_s), the effect of doubling $P(y \mid N)$ is much greater and may amount to 3 or 4 dB. This increase of the effect of frequency uncertainty at low signal levels has been noted by Creelman (1960) and by Swets (1963).

When a two-alternative, forced-choice procedure is used, the subject is forced to remain near the negative diagonal of the ROC curve, and the OR gate becomes the equivalent of Creelman's model; the subject responds to the interval containing the larger stimulus. He may therefore respond correctly for the wrong reason: the interval containing the signal also contains a strong burst of noise from the other filter. Data taken with uncertain signal frequency are variable.

Other Uncertainties. In addition to the deliberately introduced frequency uncertainty, another form of uncertainty develops when the signal level is so low that the subject seldom hears the signal clearly. Then he may become uncertain about the frequency, the duration, and the time of onset of the signal. The frequency uncertainty probably is not as great as in the two-frequency experiments, and the subject might, if he has the machinery for it, widen his filter band slightly to take care of the uncertainties.

Marill (1956) in his work at very low signal levels, avoided this "forgetting" of the frequency and duration of the signal by presenting a sample of the signal without noise in advance of each stimulus trial. By rewriting his expression for $P(c)$ in a two-alternative, forced-choice experiment in terms of signal voltage and bandwidth instead of E/N_0, he obtained $P(c) = 1 - \frac{1}{2} \exp[-S^2/WN_0]$, where W is bandwidth. He found that his subjects maintained the same bandwidth at all signal levels.

Gaston (1964), in an experiment devised to determine the relation between d_s and signal voltage at low levels, found that his subjects responded as though they were employing a wider band at low levels than at high. He did not use a cueing signal in the initial study; but in a replication of it, Gaston and Jeffress (unpublished experiment, 1964) did use a cueing signal sufficient to be heard clearly above the noise, and found some improvement of detection at low levels. Their findings, however, did not quite reach the constancy of bandwidth reported by Marill. Greenberg (1962) has studied the effect of a variety of cueing signals. He found that such a signal is most effective when it precedes the stimulus interval by about one-half sec. His signal was at the same level as the signal to be detected and did not get as large an effect as Gaston and Jeffress did with a larger cueing signal.

It is, of course, equally possible to describe these results in terms of the efficiency measure, η, of TSD. Instead of thinking of the response to signal uncertainty as an increase of bandwidth, we may think of a decrease of efficiency. The two quantities η and W are reciprocally related.

REFERENCES

von Békésy, G. (1959). Neural funneling along the skin and between the inner and outer hair cells of the cochlea. *J. Acoust. Soc. Am.*, **31**, 1236–1249.

Bilger, R. C. and Hirsh, I. J. (1956). Masking of tones by bands of noise. *J. Acoust. Soc. Soc. Am.*, **28**, 623–630.

Blodgett, H. C., Jeffress, L. A., and Taylor, R. W. (1958). Relation of masked threshold to signal-duration for various interaural phase-combinations. *Am. J. Psychol.*, **71**, 283–290.

Burington, R. S. and May, D. C., Jr. (1953). *Handbook of probability and statistics with tables.* Handbook Publisher, Sandusky, Ohio.

Clarke, F. R., Birdsall, T. G., and Tanner, W. P., Jr. (1959). Two types of ROC curves and definitions of parameters. *J. Acoust. Soc. Am.*, **31**, 629–630 (L).

Cox, J. R., Jr. (1958). Spectrum of noise passed through a symmetrical limiter. *J. Acoust. Soc. Am.*, **30**, 696 (A).

Creelman, C. D. (1960). Detection of signals of uncertain frequency. *J. Acoust. Soc. Am.*, **32**, 805–810.

Deatherage, B. H., Davis, H., and Eldredge, D. H. (1957). Physiological evidence for the masking of low frequencies by high. *J. Acoust. Soc. Am.*, **29**, 132–137.

Diercks, K. J. and Jeffress, L. A (1962). Interaural phase and the absolute threshold for tone. *J. Acoust. Soc. Am.*, **34**, 981–984.

Egan, J. P. and Hake, H. W. (1950). On the masking pattern of a simple auditory stimulus. *J. Acoust. Soc. Am.*, **22**, 622–630.

Egan, J. P., Schulman, A. I., and Greenberg, G. Z. (1959). Operating characteristics determined by binary decisions and by ratings. *J. Acoust. Soc. Am.*, **31**, 768–773.

Egan, J. P., Greenberg, G. Z., and Schulman, A. I. (1961). Operating characteristics, signal detectability, and the method of free response. *J. Acoust. Soc. Am.*, **33**, 993–1007.

Elliott, L. L. (1962). Backward masking: monotic and dichotic conditions. *J. Acoust. Soc. Am.*, **34**, 1108–1115.

Elliott, L. L. (1963). Tonal thresholds for short-duration stimuli as related to subject hearing level. *J. Acoust. Soc. Am.*, **35**, 578–580.

Elliott, P. B. (1959). Tables of d'. *Tech. Rep. No. 97, Electron. Def. Group, University of Michigan.*

Fletcher, H. (1929). *Speech and hearing.* Van Nostrand, New York.

Fletcher, H. (1940). Auditory patterns. *Rev. Mod. Phys.*, **12**, 47–65.

Garner, W. R. and Miller, G. A. (1947). The masked threshold of pure tones as a function of duration. *J. Exp. Psychol.*, **37**, 293–303.

Green, D. M. (1958). Detection of multiple component signals in noise. *J. Acoust. Soc. Am.*, **30**, 904–911.

Green, D. M. (1960). Auditory detection of a noise signal. *J. Acoust. Soc. Am.*, **32**, 121–131.

Green, D. M. (1964). General prediction relating yes-no and forced-choice results. *J. Acoust. Soc. Am.*, **36**, 1042 (A).

Green, D. M., Birdsall, T. G., and Tanner, W. P., Jr. (1957). Signal detection as a function of signal intensity and duration. *J. Acoust. Soc. Am.*, **29**, 523–531.

Greenberg, G. Z. (1962). Cueing signals and frequency uncertainty in auditory detection. *U. S. A. F. Tech. Rep. AF* 19(628)–266.

Hamilton, P. M. (1957). Noise masked thresholds as a function of tonal duration and masking noise band width. *J. Acoust. Soc. Am.*, **29**, 506–511.

Hawkins, J. E., Jr. and Stevens, S. S. (1950). The masking of pure tones and of speech by white noise. *J. Acoust. Soc. Am.*, **22**, 6–13.

Hirsh, I. J. and Burgeat, M. (1958). Binaural effects in remote masking. *J. Acoust. Soc. Am.*, **30**, 827–832.

Huggins, W. H. and Licklider, J. C. R. (1951). Place mechanisms of auditory frequency analysis. *J. Acoust. Soc. Am.*, **23**, 290–299.

Jeffress, L. A. (1964). Stimulus-oriented approach to detection. *J. Acoust. Soc. Am.*, **36**, 766–774.

Licklider, J. C. R. (1948). The influence of interaural phase relations upon the masking of speech by white noise. *J. Acoust. Soc. Am.*, **20**, 150–159.

Licklider, J. C. R. (1951). Basic correlates of the auditory stimulus. In S. S. Stevens (Ed.) *Handbook of experimental psychology.* Wiley, New York.

Lüscher, E. and Zwislocki, J. (1949). Adaptation of the ear to sound stimuli. *J. Acoust. Soc. Am.*, **21**, 135–139.

Marcum, J. I. (1950). *Table of Q functions.* Rand Corporation, RM-339. ASTIA Doc. No. AD 116551. Santa Monica, California.

Marill, T. (1956). Detection theory and psychophysics. *M. I. T. Res. Lab. Electron. Tech. Rep.* **319**.

Mayer, A. M. (1894). Researches in acoustics. *Lond. Edinb. Dubl. Phil. Mag.*, **37**, *ser.* 5, 259–288.

Miller, G. A. (1947). Sensitivity to changes in the intensity of white noise and its relation to masking and loudness. *J. Acoust. Soc. Am.*, **19**, 609–619.

Peterson, W. W., Birdsall, T. G., and Fox, W. C. (1954). The theory of signal detectability. *Inst. Radio Engrs. Trans. Prof. Grp. Inf. Theory*, **4**, 171–212.

Pfafflin, S. M. and Mathews, M. V. (1962). Energy-detection model for monaural auditory detection. *J. Acoust. Soc. Am.*, **34**, 1842–1853.

Pickett, J. M. (1959). Backward masking. *J. Acoust. Soc. Am.*, **31**, 1613–1615.

Pollack, I. and Pickett, J. M. (1958). Stereophonic listening and speech intelligibility against voice babble. *J. Acoust. Soc. Am.*, **30**, 131–133.

Lord Rayleigh (J. W. Strutt) (1945). *The theory of sound.* 2 vols. (1st American ed. of the 2nd English ed. of 1894, bound as one volume) Dover, New York.

Rice, S. O. (1954). Mathematical analysis of random noise. In N. Wax (Ed.) *Selected papers on noise and stochastic processes.* pp. 133–294. Dover, New York.

Schafer, T. H., Gales, R. S., Shewmaker, C. A., and Thompson, P. O. (1950). The frequency selectivity of the ear as determined by masking experiments. *J. Acoust. Soc. Am.*, **22**, 490–497.

Shaw, E. A. G. and Piercy, J. E. (1962). Physiological noise in relation to audiometry. *J. Acoust. Soc. Am.*, **34**, 745 (A).

Swets, J. A. (1963). Central factors in auditory frequency selectivity. *Psychol. Bull.*, **60**, 429–440.

Swets, J. A. (Ed.) (1964). *Signal detection and recognition by human observers.* Wiley, New York.

Swets, J. A., Green, D. M., and Tanner, W. P., Jr. (1962). On the width of critical bands. *J. Acoust. Soc. Am.*, **34**, 108–113.

Tanner, W. P., Jr. and Birdsall, T. G. (1958). Definitions of d' and η as psychophysical measures. *J. Acoust. Soc. Am.*, **30**, 922–928.

Tanner, W. P., Jr., Swets, J. A., and Green, D. M. (1956). Some general properties of the hearing mechanism. *Tech. Rep. No. 30, Electron. Def. Group., University of Michigan.*

Watson, C. S. (1963). Masking of tones by noise for the cat. *J. Acoust. Soc. Am.*, **35**, 167–172.

Watson, C. S., Rilling, M. E., and Bourbon, W. T. (1964). Receiver-operating characteristics determined by a mechanical analog to the rating scale. *J. Acoust. Soc. Am.*, **36**, 283–288.

Weast, R. C., Selby, S. M., and Hodgman, C. D. (1965). *Handbook of chemistry and physics.* Chemical Rubber Co., Cleveland, Ohio.

Wegel, R. L. and Lane, C. E. (1924). The auditory masking of one pure tone by another and its probable relation to the dynamics of the inner ear. *Phys. Rev.*, **23**, *ser.* 2, 266–285.

Chapter Four

Fatigue and Adaptation

FOREWORD

Although the standard references on hearing mention adaptation and fatigue, most of the data postdate those books. The physiology of adaptation is quite different from the physiology of fatigue, although at one time the two processes were looked at as essentially similar. Now the similarities appear to be superficial, for the relation between the two is limited to the fact that both phenomena lead to threshold displacement and a concomitant loudness change. Donald Elliott and Winifred Fraser have brought together many of the studies pertinent to an understanding of how the auditory system handles continuous signals at various levels of intensity, and of what can be deduced regarding the construction of the system from the examination of fatigued and adapted ears, not only psychophysically, but anatomically and physiologically.

Fatigue and Adaptation

Donald N. Elliott* and Winifred (Riach) Fraser*

I. INTRODUCTION

One of the common functional characteristics of all sensory systems is a reduction in sensitivity following exposure to any stimulus of significant duration and intensity. For some systems (e.g., gustatory, olfactory), the sensation may disappear completely; for others (e.g., the auditory), there is merely a reduction in apparent magnitude or an increase in the threshold. In all cases, such changes are temporary so long as the stimulation does not exceed critical limits, which is the case in everyday life for most receptor systems. The ear, however, is often exposed to stimuli such as gunshots or to long periods of high-intensity noise; as a result, its sensitivity may be permanently impaired. Often, such damage accrues slowly from repeated exposure that individually cause only temporary sensitivity shifts. An interest in learning the safe limits of auditory exposure and an interest in discovering how the ear operates at various levels of stimulation have led to the investigation of the effects of various types of sensitivity-reducing stimuli upon auditory function.

In such studies, two psychophysical measures have been commonly employed: loudness decrements (obtained *during* the sensitivity-reducing stimulation) and shifts in the threshold (obtained *after* the stimulation). Clearly, both are indices of a reduction in the ear's sensitivity, but different terms are generally used for the two measures −presumably on the grounds that they reflect different types of

*Department of Psychology, Wayne State University, Detroit, Michigan.

change in the auditory system. The loudness decrement is termed *auditory adaptation* or *perstimulatory fatigue;* the temporary threshold shift (TTS) has been referred to as *auditory fatigue* (or more properly, *poststimulatory auditory fatigue*). Besides the difference in the time at which the data are obtained, and the difference in the type of measure involved, adaptation studies generally use weak to moderate levels of stimulation. Fatigue studies, on the other hand, tend to be concerned with the effects of moderate to quite intense levels of stimulation.

Although there is a good deal of evidence that *adaptation* and *fatigue* do reflect differing physiological changes, it is also true that these differences are often not complete. This overlap becomes evident when the various physiological changes that underlie decrements in the ear's sensitivity are considered. They include neural changes, hair-cell changes, endolymphatic changes, and some others.

A. Neural Changes

When a continuing auditory stimulus is presented, neural response rates rapidly decrease until, after about three minutes, a stable level is reached. Since this reduction in neural responsiveness occurs even for stimulus intensities too weak to cause a reduction in the cochlear microphonic (CM), it clearly indicates neural adaptation. Following cessation of the stimulus, neural discharge rates rapidly increase and reach their original level within about one minute (Derbyshire and Davis, 1935).

B. Hair-cell Changes

When a continuing stimulus of moderate to high intensity is presented, a decrement in the CM occurs, in the form of a shift in the linear portion of the input-output curve and of a reduction in the level of the maximum CM, with some sharpening of the peak of the input-output curve (Wever and Smith, 1944; Wever and Lawrence, 1955; Shimizu *et al.*, 1957; and Gisselsson and Sørenson, 1959). These changes are quite similar to those found when overstimulation has resulted in permanent injury (Davis *et al.*, 1953), and probably reflect alterations of the hair cells and their "moorings."

C. Endolymphatic Changes

Continued stimulation produces a reduction in the available oxygen in the endolymph. When stimulation ceases, the normal oxygen level is rapidly restored; often, in fact, the recovery process overshoots and temporary hyperoxia occurs (Misrahy *et al.*, 1958a,b,c). In addition to the change in oxygen content, the endolymphatic dc potential also decreases (Békésy, 1951; Tonndorf and Brogan, 1952); quite possibly —though not necessarily—these changes are interrelated (Misrahy *et al.*, 1958b). Since both the CM and the action potential (AP) are largely, if not completely, oxygen dependent, and since the CM is directly related to the size of the endolymphatic resting potential, these endolymphatic changes will likely lead to a reduction in both the CM and the AP (it appears that the AP is more sensitive to oxygen reduction than is the CM; see Misrahy *et al.*, 1958c). Perhaps, with continuing stimulation, metabolic waste products accumulate and interfere with receptor and nerve cell responses (Butler *et al.*, 1962).

D. Other Changes

Probably, in addition to the changes within the cochlear duct, other cochlear changes occur that may also be related to reduction in the ear's sensitivity. Thus, Békésy (1951) and Tonndorf and Brogan (1952) found that stimulation causes a reduction in the potential difference typically found between the scala vestibuli and scala tympani. This reduction may reflect a decrease in the impedance of Reissner's membrane—and the basilar membrane; if so, the ionic transfer between the endolymph and perilymph could increase and interfere with normal functioning (Shimizu *et al.*, 1957; Butler *et al.*, 1962).

In summary, then, stimulation results in reversible neural changes that indicate neural adaptation, reduction in hair-cell response, and in all probability, a variety of cochlear environmental changes that interfere with both hair-cell and nerve-cell functioning. Since auditory sensitivity—whether measured by loudness balancing or by determining thresholds—reflects the level of neural activity, one must consider a broad range of partially interdependent changes in the ear in attempting to understand the source of the reduction in sensitivity.

Although it appears reasonable to assume that *adaptation* and *fatigue* reflect different changes in the auditory system, the fact that both are measured in sensitivity decrement leads logically to the question of whether this differentiation is meaningful. In this connection, there are certain psychophysical data that suggest that the two phenomena reflect physiological changes of different natures.

First, *adaptation* to low or moderate stimulus levels is usually completely developed within three minutes; recovery is usually complete within one to two minutes. These intervals are similar to those observed electrophysiologically for neural adaptation (Derbyshire and Davis, 1935), which suggests that *adaptation* (as defined by loudness balance tests) results from neural adaptation (Hood, 1950). On the other hand, TTS may continue to increase for much longer periods of time; the rate and extent of the changes are generally proportional to the intensity and duration of the fatiguing stimulus. Further, recovery time is proportional to the size of the initial TTS and may require several hours or even days before it is complete. Quite clearly, then, the differences in times of development and recovery alone lead to the conclusion that the different measures reflect different physiological processes. In addition, other differences can be observed. In *adaptation*, changes in loudness are small near threshold but increase at higher and higher intensities (Hood, 1950; Egan, 1955); the result is, inferentially, a lower-than-normal loudness growth function. On the other hand, *fatigue* enhances loudness growth and intensity discrimination—both indices of hair-cell dysfunction (Davis *et al.*, 1950; and Békésy, 1960). Fatigue studies have disclosed other hearing changes that also suggest hair-cell dysfunction: pitch shifts (Rüedi and Furrer, 1946; Davis *et al.*, 1950), changes in the extent of temporal integration of short pulses (Jerger, 1955), susceptibility to fatiguing effects (Huizing, 1948), and level of overload onset (Lawrence and Yantis, 1957). Since such hair-cell changes occur only with moderate and stronger stimulation, TTS may be most useful in indexing changes to relatively severe levels of stimulation.

However, *adaptation* and *fatigue* are not always clearly distinguishable, particularly when the TTS is determined during the first minute or so after moderate stimulation ceases. Further, even though the slope of the loudness function may increase when the ear is fatigued and decrease when *adaptation* occurs, one also finds that, near threshold, both conditions lead to a reduction in normal loudness (Davis *et al.*, 1950; Hood, 1950). In addition, a TTS may be found for the *adapted* ear just as it is for the fatigued ear (Selters, 1964). It is not surprising, of course, that such overlapping changes occur since both processes reflect an ultimate reduction in neural responses. So, if one measures either the TTS or the loudness decrement during the first minute or so after the moderate to strong stimulation ceases, one observes the cumulative effects of both adaptation *and* fatigue, and it is extremely difficult to distinguish between them psychophysically. For extremes of stimulation (either very weak or very intense), of course, one may be able to observe, respectively, adaptation *or* fatigue. Thus, for weak levels of stimulation, the evidence points only to neural adaptation. But for more intense levels of stimulation, neural adaptation disappears after a minute or so of recovery, leaving only fatigue effects. However, the question continues to plague investigators as to whether, when the ear is stimulated, for example with a 60- or 80-dB tone, the changes observed during stimulation or immediately after its cessation are primarily indicative of adaptation or of fatigue. Consequently, although the terms are well established, we are using them with the realization that they often do not refer to completely independent physiological processes.

II. POSTSTIMULATORY AUDITORY FATIGUE

The most common index of auditory fatigue is the TTS. Usually, it is measured by first determining the normal threshold, then exposing the ear to fatiguing stimulation, and finally finding the postexposure thresholds. The difference between the pre and postexposure thresholds defines the severity of the fatigue. In such studies, five primary factors influence the size of the TTS: (a) the time between cessation of the fatiguing exposure and the postexposure threshold determination—we call this period the recovery interval (RI); (b) the intensity of the fatiguing exposure (I); (c) the duration of the fatiguing exposure (D); (d) the frequency of the fatiguing exposure (F_e); and (e) the frequency of the threshold-test signal (F_t).

Each of these factors will be considered in some detail, but since they interact, a summary of their relations will be useful. Generally, as the D and I of the fatiguing stimulus increase, the TTS becomes larger. At low to moderate intensities, TTS is symmetrically distributed about F_e, and is limited to the immediate neighborhood. However, as I increases, three changes occur (Hood, 1950): the TTS increases; the frequency range over which fatigue effects are manifest increases, with the increase almost entirely above F_e; and the frequency of the maximum TTS shifts one-half octave or more above F_e. In addition to this upward shift in the maximum TTS, one finds greater susceptibility to fatigue from higher F_es.

Recovery generally increases the longer one waits after exposure. However, under a broad range of I, F_e, and D conditions, the recovery curve is often diphasic, with a short-term increase in the TTS during the early stages of recovery.

There are also methodological considerations to note in trying to make sense of the mass of fatigue data. First, reliable threshold determination is time-consuming and reflects not only the sensitivity of the receptor system, but such nonsensory factors as practice, motivation, the psychophysical procedure used, and chance fluctuations. If, then, one expects to use the differences between pre and post-exposure thresholds as an accurate index of the change in the auditory system, the effects of these nonauditory factors must be reduced to a minimum. The problems of practice and motivation are reasonably easy to handle and introduce little error — one needs to use well-practiced Ss, and to motivate them adequately (money is useful). The desirability of using well-practiced subjects is sometimes questioned on the grounds that repeated exposures may change their susceptibility — i.e., the ear might conceivably become "toughened up" by such exposures. However, studies concerned with this question have generally (although not invariably) found little evidence of such a change in susceptibility (Hirsh and Ward, 1952; Loeb and Fletcher, 1963; Riach et al., 1964). Where changes have been evident, as in the Loeb and Fletcher study, it appears that decreases in TTS as with repeated exposures reflect the conditioning of the acoustic reflex rather than any increase in the ear's resistance to fatigue.

In selecting a psychophysical testing procedure, the experimenter is faced with the problem of catching the postexposure threshold "on the run." The recovery process is continuous and is quite rapid immediately after cessation of the fatiguing stimulus. For the determination of individual data, this problem has apparently been solved by the use of the method of adjustment with a motor-driven recording attenuator. With such a procedure, momentary fluctuations in the subject's measured threshold because of variations in his attention, etc., are assumed to balance out. It is possible that the rate of recovery very early in the recovery period may be too great to follow correctly, and constant errors may thus result. Lightfoot (1955) determined test-retest reliabilities for the procedure at various recovery times up to nine minutes. He found generally satisfactory reliability coefficients that were as good during the early part of the recovery curve as during later portions. An unpublished study of ours also collected reliability data (on twelve normal subjects) at RIs ranging from 1 to 19 minutes ($F_e = 2000$ Hz; $F_t = 2800$ Hz; $I = 105$ dB SL; pulsed test tones). The coefficients are very high at the 2 through 11 minute RIs: they run from 0.88 to 0.90. The reliability decreased at the 1 minute (r = .78) and 19 minute (r = .70) RIs (the decrease at 19 minutes results from a reduction in intersubject variance as the TTS approaches zero). In contrast to these values, Loeb and Fletcher

(1963) found far lower reliability coefficients for a F_t of 4000 Hz. Since subjects were not highly practiced in either study, this difference is puzzling; however, if Loeb and Fletcher used continuous test tones, the differences might indicate the difficulty subjects have in tracing such a signal.

Although the recording attenuator serves quite satisfactorily for the determination of individual thresholds, group testing usually requires other procedures. Several are quite satisfactory (Hirsh and Ward, 1952; Ward et al., 1958; Harris, 1959, 1961). Although no one has yet systematically investigated the extent to which testing procedures lead to differences in results, it is quite possible that divergences among some of the studies may be due to differences in the testing procedures (cf., Hirsh and Bilger, 1955; Hood, 1950; and Harris, 1953 with respect to the recovery "bounce").

A. Recovery Time

Recovery time is the source of much difficulty in comparing studies of fatigue because, during the RI, TTS changes constantly. Consequently, in describing how variations in I, D, F_e, or F_t affect the TTS, it is necessary to specify the RI at which TTS was obtained. Although some experimenters have averaged TTS over a considerable period of time (Harris, 1959), many specify the amount of TTS at some particular temporal point on the recovery curve. Unfortunately, different experimenters use different points, and this has made comparisons of many of the studies difficult since we have little evidence of the extent to which a given TTS at a given point on the recovery curve uniquely defines the curve—and if it does, how various TTS values along the curve can be computed. Although Ward et al. (1958) have derived reasonably satisfactory mathematical functions describing recovery curves over a fairly wide range of fatigue levels, based on the TTS_2 value (TTS after two minutes of recovery), their data are limited to a few F_ts and cannot be extrapolated to recovery times of less than two minutes because of the complex shape of the early recovery curve.

It is unfortunate that so many different points along the recovery curve have been used in specifying fatigue. It would certainly be desirable to agree upon some common recovery times so that future studies could be more meaningfully compared. TTS_2 or TTS_5 would probably be quite satisfactory, since at such RIs neural adaptation has disappeared and the recovery rate is gradual enough for the determination of reliable thresholds.

If one were to generalize the most representative recovery curve, it would be a negatively accelerating function of time-after-exposure. However, this description is an oversimplification, since under many conditions the curve is not monotonic. Furthermore, the parameters of the function change for different levels of fatigue. Therefore, the exact shape of the recovery curve under various conditions of fatigue has been studied extensively.

Hirsh and Ward (1952) and Hirsh and Bilger (1955) found, as have many others, that recovery from the large, immediate TTS is often followed by a "bounce"—a reversal in the direction of recovery, particularly for higher frequencies. Thus, a valley when $RI = 1$ minute, followed by a bounce at the two-minute RI, is characteristic of many recovery curves (Fig. 1). More than a single recovery function appears to be operating, and Hirsh and Bilger proposed a dual re-

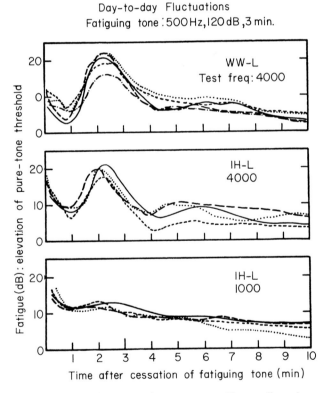

Figure 1 Recovery curves illustrating the two-minute "bounce"; each set of curves represents retests under identical conditions. Note the difference in bounce size at 1000 and 4000 Hz. Exposure: 500 Hz at 120 dB SPL for three minutes. (Hirsh and Ward, 1952. By permission from *Journal of the Acoustical Society of America*.)

covery process: an initial, rapid, but short-lived recovery process (R-1) that is evident for only the first minute or so, followed by a monotonic, negatively accelerated function (R-2). Disappearance of R-1 is evidenced by the bounce. Some authors have suggested cyclical changes at later stages of recovery, but the variations are quite small and may only reflect changes in the listener's attention.

If the initial TTS is not too great, R-1 may *overshoot* the original threshold level, and a temporary sensitization occurs (Hughes, 1954; Hughes and Rosenblith, 1957). When the initial TTS is higher, R-1 is still evident, but is not large enough to produce hypersensitivity. As a rough approximation, the size of the bounce (i.e., the extent to which the R-1 process serves to facilitate hearing) seems to be relatively constant in size (Hirsh and Bilger, 1955). However, just as there is a lower fatiguing intensity for the elicitation of the bounce, so there is an upper limit—one determined by fatigue so severe that the sensitizing R-1 process cannot evidence itself (Jerger, 1956).

The physiological changes that may underlie the R-1 process remain speculative. However, since the oxygen-recovery overshoot (Misrahy *et al.*, 1958c) (with its accompanying supernormal APs and CMs) as well as the increase in the AP that has been found following fatiguing stimulation (Rosenblith *et al.*, 1950; and Hughes and Rosenblith, 1957), occur at time intervals similar to the valley that precedes the bounce, they are clearly candidates for the honor (Fig. 2). Conceivably, the rapidly increasing oxygen supply may result in a temporary increase in the excitability of the hair cells or nerve cells, and since supernormal CMs are not found with the supernormal APs that follow fatiguing stimulation (Hughes and Rosenblith, 1957), the nerve cells appear to be the most likely source of the R-1 process (Hirsh and Bilger, 1955). Also, Hinchcliffe (1957) found that tinnitus appears and disappears at times corresponding generally to the development of the valley and the bounce of the recovery curve. Since this phenomenon suggests an increase in neural activity, it also supports the conclusion that the nerve cells are the basis of the R-1 response.

A second type of sensitization is often evident at relatively long *RI*s. It appears as a slightly improved postexposure threshold for frequencies lying below the depressed area of the fatigue audiogram (Fig. 3). Because of its longer duration, this change probably does not indicate any dynamic recovery process per se; rather, it may represent an improvement in the detection of those signals near the frequencies to which the ear is making subnormal responses (also see Fletcher, 1957).

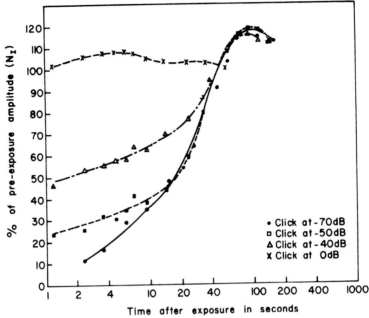

Figure 2 Neural response to clicks following exposure to a 200-Hz tone at 105 dB SPL for 30 sec. Note the supernormal N_1 responses at 100 sec recovery time; the effect of exposure decreases as the clicks increase in intensity. (Rosenblith, 1950. By permission from *Journal of the Acoustical Society of America.*)

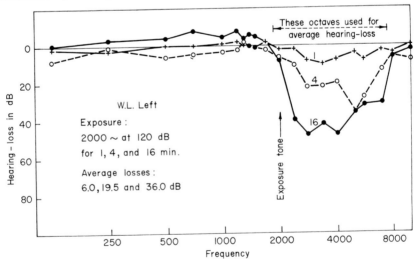

Figure 3 Audiogram of a fatigued ear. Note the improved thresholds below the frequencies at which fatigue is evident. (Davis *et al.*, 1950. By permission from *Acta Oto Laryngologica.*)

After the initial bounce (i.e., from 2 minutes on), the recovery rate is approximately proportional to log RI; it is also proportional to the TTS_2 (Ward *et al.*, 1958) (Fig. 4). However, although the recovery curves tend to converge, the tendency is by no means complete. Ward (1963) developed several equations that fit the data quite well.

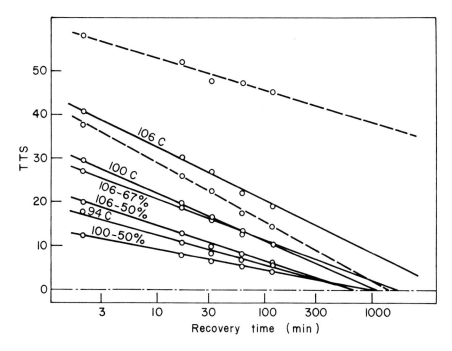

Figure 4 Recovery curves based on TTS measurements ranging from 2 to 112 minutes. Parameters are the SPL of the fatiguing noise and the proportion of time it was on; C indicates a continuous exposure. The logarithmic recovery rate is clearly evident. Note the partial tendency for the curves to converge. (Ward *et al.*, 1958. By permission from *Journal of the Acoustical Society of America*.)

For several of the conditions represented in Fig. 4, recovery times are greater than 16 hours. Such a long period suggests that more than the normal metabolic restorative processes are involved. Perhaps recoveries from tissue alteration are occurring—for example, the return to normal of disarranged or damaged hair cells, or of Reissner's membrane.

That the recovery function is proportional to log RI applies only with certain fatigue limits. The upper limit lies at a TTS_2 of 40 to 50 dB; above this level, recovery is much slower, and Ward (1960b) suggested that in this extreme range, elastic limits have been exceeded. However, we would propose that even with the less severe losses that do not exceed a TTS_2 of 40 dB, recovery times of some 16 or more hours also demonstrate tissue alterations resulting from stimulation that exceeds the tissues' elastic limits. Such changes may increase in severity when TTS_2 reaches 40 to 50 dB, but the change in the recovery slope is not abrupt enough to require the assumption of a completely new set of alterations.

In summary, initial recovery is a complex function, but for RIs greater than 2 minutes, it is within limits, linearly related to log RI. Thus, when dealing with fatigue that is severe enough to require more than a few minutes for recovery, it is wise to determine the TTS at an RI greater than 2 minutes, and, if possible, to determine it at two or more RIs. From these multiple determinations, a reasonably accurate plot of TTS_n for all values of $n > 2$ would be possible, and the comparison of studies that use different RIs to report fatigue severity would become a more reasonable task.

B. Intensity of the Fatiguing Stimulus

Obviously, increasing the intensity (I) of the fatiguing stimulus should produce an increase in the TTS. Although it generally does, there are some exceptions. They suggest the existence of a variety of changes that underly TTS and that develop at different Is. Three ranges of I are of particular interest. The first is the low I range in which $F_t = F_e$ increases little if at all as a function of I (Fig. 5), and decreases in a symmetrical fashion above and below F_e. At such levels, adaptation rather than fatigue may be the source of the observed TTSs (Caussé and Chavasse, 1947; Selters, 1964). Under such conditions, the TTS may be only a special case of loudness decrement, which has been found to be relatively invariant with adapting I (Hood, 1950).

The second I range is that in which one finds the maximum TTS shifting above F_e; eventually, as I continues to increase, the maximum TTS is found one-half octave and more above F_e (Fig. 5). At these levels, and with $F_t > F_e$, TTS is quite clearly a positive function of I. The positive function makes it probable that fatigue as well as adapting changes are taking place. The upward frequency shift, on the other hand, may have more than a single explanation. It probably results from the constantly changing mechanical characteristics of the basilar membrane. Because stiffness increases toward the basal end, the elastic limits become more and more restricted, and tissue altera-

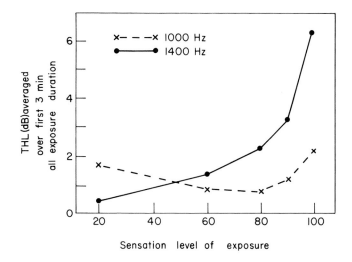

Figure 5   Increase in TTS (THL) as a function of intensity increase ($F_e = 1000$ Hz).
Note the lack of any increase in TTS below 80 dB when $F_t = F_e$. When F_t is one-half
octave above F_e, growth is continuous and becomes greater than that found at the exposure frequency. Note too the function's acceleration. (Hirsh and Bilger, 1955. By
permission from *Journal of the Acoustical Society of America*.)

tions from approaching or exceeding these limits become more likely.
Consequently, the decrease in the response of the basilar membrane
on the high-frequency side of the point of maximum response may be
more than offset by the decrease in its elastic limits. Whether the upward shift of the maximum TTS results exclusively from the mechanical characteristics of the basilar membrane is unknown; however,
since the stiffer portions are more subject to permanent damage from
intense stimulation, it is probable that they are also more susceptible
to reversible tissue alterations.

The third I range is that in which the accelerating increase in TTS
becomes most marked. Although the overall function tends to accelerate positively for $F_t > F_e$ one generally finds some I range through
which the acceleration is particularly large. This maximum may indicate the onset of damaging fatigue (Rüedi and Furrer, 1946; Hood,
1950; Hirsh and Bilger, 1955; Epstein and Schubert, 1957; and
Lawrence and Yantis, 1957). If so, then the recovery time should also
accelerate as should the rate at which fatigue effects accumulate with
increased duration of exposure — even minor and reversible tissue
damage will probably not recover as rapidly as the metabolic changes
that underlie auditory fatigue. In addition, if this "critical" intensity

does result in pathological processes, recruiting phenomena should emerge, together with other types of hearing changes that reflect tissue damage in the cochlea. Epstein and Schubert (1957) investigated these matters using an exposure frequency of 4000 Hz. Although recruitment and marked acceleration of TTS were evident for intensities of 80 dB and greater, they did not find any acceleration in times of recovery. However, since their recovery-rate index was obtained during the first minute after cessation of the fatiguing exposure, it may have been obtained too early to permit accurate prediction of total recovery time. Finally, in this I range, the effect of increasing the fatiguing D should differ from that for a nondamaging I; indeed, these stimuli, if continued long enough, might result in permanent threshold shifts (PTS). Ward *et al.* (1958), studying the effect of various durations and intensities of broad-band noise, found that TTS grows in proportion to the logarithm of exposure time, at a rate that is also proportional to the extent that I exceeds some base value. The study was not designed to test whether, at intensities below this base value, TTS ceases to grow continuously with D but the results suggest this possibility.

Thus, it appears that, as I is increased, additional functional alterations appear. At low intensities, the TTS is reasonably well restricted to the frequency of the fatiguing stimulus, is relatively small, and is not much affected by the intensity or duration of the fatiguing stimulus. It may well be that the TTSs observed over this I range reflect neural changes and, possibly, changes in the metabolic conditions of the cochlea, all of which recover quite rapidly. These changes could probably be considered "normal" (nonpathological) in every sense of the word. However, as the intensity of the fatiguing tone increases, the TTS effect broadens toward frequencies above the fatiguing frequency, becomes more closely related to I and D, and recovery time becomes proportional to TTS_2. At some intensity level (or levels), the changes in auditory function begin to reflect slow-recovering tissue and/or chemical changes that are pathological or prepathological in nature. In all probability (both on a rational basis and on the basis of experimental findings), the various changes do not show up at the same intensity levels, and the search for *the* critical level of intensity that clearly separates damaging from nondamaging stimulation is a futile one.

Two interesting exceptions in the expected positive relation between I and TTS should be noted. The first is the fact that when

$F_t = F_e$, an I of 20 dB SL results in larger TTSs than do Is of 80 dB and greater (Lierle and Reger, 1954; Hirsh and Bilger, 1955) (Fig. 6). The reversal is short-lived, and the recovery curves often cross. Although small, this reversal does illustrate the danger of using TTSs observed very shortly after cessation of the exposure tone as indices of long-term fatigue effects. In general, such a reversal means that the TTS resulting from the higher I recovers faster than the TTS following the 20 dB I, and Fig. 6 may illustrate the recovery curves of two essentially different processes—i.e., *adaptation* for the 20 dB I, and moderate *fatigue* (with its attendant sensitizing R-1 process) for the higher Is.

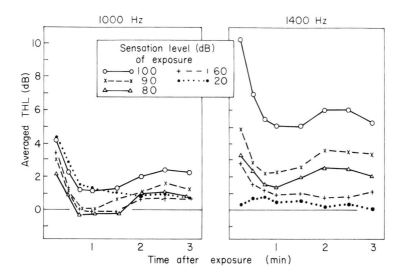

Figure 6   Recovery curves for exposures at different intensities ($F_e = 1000$ Hz); the two sets of curves are for F_ts of 1000 and 1400 Hz. When $F_t = 1000$ Hz, the initial TTS for the 20 dB exposure is large; since recovery from this level of exposure is a monotonically decreasing function, it *crosses* the recovery curves for exposures to intensities of 80 dB and higher, which bounce. Note the greater TTS obtained at 1400 Hz. (Hirsh and Bilger, 1955. By permission from *Journal of the Acoustical Society of America*.)

The second reversal of the expected positive function occurs at Is above 110 dB SPL (Davis *et al.*, 1950; Miller, 1958b) and at RIs greater than one minute. Such reversals are not general (Trittipoe, 1958), but have been observed for frequencies above 2000 Hz when D has been brief. Since the reversal is found at intensities well above those that trigger the aural reflex, and since it is found at high frequencies, there is some question as to whether this reversal is due to the reflex. It is difficult to explain: because of the short exposures involved, the phenomenon is limited to relatively small TTSs.

C. Duration

Except when it results from high intensity impulse stimuli, fatigue develops gradually. Consequently, its development has been explored in a number of studies, with I, F_e, and F_t as parameters. Unfortunately, there is no study or group of studies that describe TTS growth over more than a limited range of D, I, and F conditions.

Hood (1950), using 100-dB SL tones, and the same frequency for fatiguing and test tones, investigated TTS growth at frequencies from 500 to 4000 Hz for durations ranging from 100 to 320 sec. He found that TTS (measured 10 sec after cessation of the fatiguing tone) increases as a linear function of log D (i.e., it is negatively accelerated). Davis *et al.* (1950) measured TTSs at several F_ts above F_e and for longer RIs; they also reported that growth is negatively accelerated. Harris (1953) however (using a 750-Hz fatiguing tone and a 1000-Hz test tone) investigated TTS_2 growth over exposure durations of 30 sec to 15 minutes, and found that TTS growth is generally a linear function of D. Ward *et al.* (1958) determined TTS_2 growth to noise for periods ranging from 12 to 108 minutes at overall levels of 88 through 106 dB SPL. In this study, growth of TTS was found to be generally proportional to log D with (from extrapolation to shorter durations) an apparent "indifference" time below which TTS_2 is zero; further, the slope of their growth function increases for higher intensities and is, in fact, proportional to the number of decibels by which the fatiguing noise exceeds a "critical intensity" (Fig. 7).

These and other studies show that TTS growth is linearly proportional to log D except for frequencies below 2000 Hz, particularly when the fatiguing stimulus is noise or a rapidly interrupted tone (Ward, 1963). Under these latter conditions, the aural reflex serves to protect the ear and growth rate is reduced until the reflex has relaxed (this relaxation time is a function of the I and character of the stimulus).

Ward's study raises two obvious questions: what is the growth function like at intervals less than 12 minutes, and what is it like at intervals greater than 108 minutes? If one assumes, as Ward did in extrapolating the growth curves to exposure intervals of less than 12

$$TTS_2 = A \left(\log_{10} T \right) + B$$

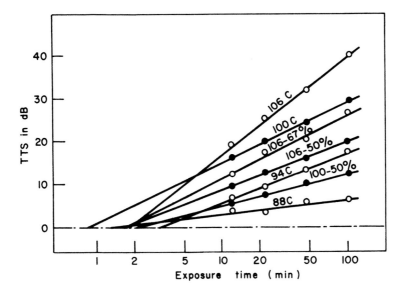

Figure 7 Growth of TTS_2 for F_t of 4000 Hz; parameters are the SPL of the fatiguing noise and the proportion of time it was on; C indicates a continuous exposure. Since TTS was not measured at durations of less than twelve minutes, the extrapolations to shorter durations cannot be accepted completely; in all probability the curves level off as they approach zero TTS. (Ward *et al.*, 1958. By permission from *Journal of the Acoustical Society of America*.)

minutes, that the log D relation holds over all durations, then the curves reach a negative value at zero exposure time. This paradoxical situation may mean that the first elements to be fatigued are the most sensitive ones that respond to physiological noise anyway and, consequently, contribute little to the detection of external signals. If, however, the growth curves had been empirically extended to the shorter durations, they probably would have become asymptotic to the zero TTS level. Consequently, the curves as extrapolated downward in Fig. 7 underestimate the size of the TTS_2 for short exposures. As a matter of fact, Ward *et al.* (1958) suggested that the log functions probably do not extend below a D of five minutes. In any event, growth curves plotted in log-D units probably accelerate during the first few minutes of fatiguing exposure.

The second unanswered question concerns the nature of the curves beyond 108 minutes. It is clear that TTS_2 cannot increase indefinitely since it cannot possibly exceed complete and utter deafness. Besides this limitation, it is possible that, for moderate intensity levels, growth may level off before PTS occurs. Such upper duration limits have not been explored extensively — in part because PTS often becomes a significant consideration, and in part because the practical difficulties of long testing sessions discourage such studies. In one study, Harris (1961) investigated TTS growth to intermittent stimulation for 30 hours. An asymptote of about 10 dB TTS was reached after 13 hours of exposure, so it is clear that studies seeking to determine the D at which a TTS of any significant size would level off would have to extend over several days.

A number of other studies have been concerned with the cumulative aspects of fatigue. As to be expected (and as indicated in Fig. 7), TTS growth rate increases with fatiguing intensity, although the nature of the intensity-duration relation is not a simple multiplicative one, which should not be too surprising in view of the fact that TTS is an accelerating function of intensity. Possibly the best way to illustrate the $I \times D$ relation is with equal TTS contours as illustrated in Fig. 8 (see Harris, 1959, for similar functions; also Spieth and Trittipoe, 1958, for a limited set of $I \times D$ conditions). Note that greater increases in exposure intensity are needed to produce given TTS at shorter durations than at longer durations. Put in more familiar hearing-damage language, as the duration of the fatiguing noise is increased, the effect of intensity increases.

Several studies have been concerned with the growth of TTS in a partially recovered ear. If one assumes that, during exposure, recovery processes are set up to oppose the fatiguing processes, the question of re-exposing a partially recovered ear is seen to be merely a special case of the situation in which the fatiguing exposure is continuous. Ward et al. (1959b) investigated TTS growth as a function of the TTS still existing after the ear was allowed to recover partially. They found that if such existing TTS were considered simply as the additional exposure time needed to produce it, growth could be predicted from the functions shown in Fig. 7. Further, when the recovery times and re-exposure times are relatively short, growth is proportional to the duty cycle, which suggests that the recovery and growth characteristics of fatigue interact in an additive manner, although their rates may be inversely proportional. A second question is whether recovery rate is proportional to the degree of existing fatigue, whether fatiguing stimulation is occurring or not. Put in another manner, the question amounts to whether the recovery rate is exclusively

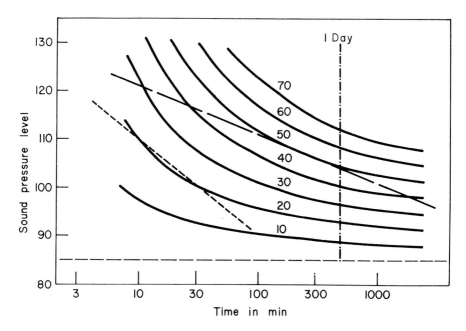

Figure 8 Intensity-duration combinations producing equal TTS$_2$s. The parameter is the TTS size in dB. Note that for the shorter durations, the effect of increasing intensity is smaller than it is for the longer durations. (Ward *et al.*, 1958. By permission from *Journal of the Acoustical Society of America*.)

a function of the severity of the existing fatigue. In view of the negatively accelerating recovery curve and growth curve, this notion does not appear to be unreasonable.

A study supporting this hypothesis involved the determination of TTS growth when the exposure level was suddenly decreased (Ward *et al.*, 1960). The results appear in Fig. 9. The ear was exposed for 30 minutes to a 105 dB SPL tone after which the intensity was decreased to 95 dB. TTS growth under these changing conditions is shown in the upper curve. The dip in the curve shows that when the weaker exposure tone was presented, the recovery process rate was greater than the fatiguing process rate for the weaker stimulus. Eventually, the recovery rate decreased until the fatigue rate balanced, and then exceeded it. Such a function suggests that the recovery rate is proportional to the TTS whether the ear is being stimulated or not. Further, rate of fatigue growth is related to exposure intensity, so if TTS growth curves (to stimuli not intense enough to produce PTS) were allowed to continue to their asymptotic levels, these levels should be proportional to the intensity of the fatiguing stimulus.

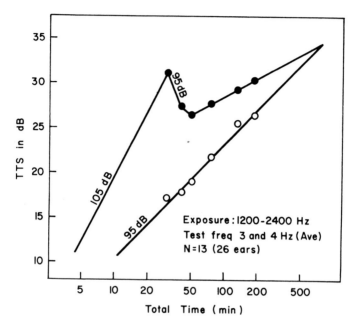

Figure 9 Growth of TTS₂s when the fatiguing intensity is suddenly decreased (upper curve). Note that, during the initial portion of the exposure at the reduced intensity, recovery processes are greater than fatiguing processes. (Ward *et al.*, 1960. By permission from *Journal of the Acoustical Society of America.*)

Another interesting situation concerns the effect of exposing the ear to fatiguing stimulation either as soon as the ear has returned to normal, or immediately following an exposure too weak to produce a TTS. If Ward *et al.* (1958) are correct in suggesting their initial fatigue effects are unmeasurable because they involve units so sensitive that their responses are masked by physiological noise, then it is probable that increased TTS would result in either of the two conditions indicated above. Harris (1955) investigated the first situation by re-exposing the ear as soon as it recovered to TTS = 0; he found that the TTS then increased in size. Trittipoe (1958, 1959) and Ward (1960a) investigated the second situation. Although Trittipoe did find some TTS increments following exposure to "nonfatiguing" tones, Ward found the effects to be virtually nonexistent. But his data indicate a very slight TTS increase if the higher intensity fatiguing exposure is continued for only three minutes before TTS is measured. These results are of little practical importance in predicting TTS growth over an extended D, but they still lend tentative support to the conclusion that initial fatigue effects may affect the most sensitive physiologically masked units, and there may be an extremely limited "latent" fatigue effect.

D. Frequency

The ear is more subject to fatigue at the higher frequencies, at least up to around 4000 to 6000 Hz. Thus, when the fatiguing stimulus is a broad band noise, maximum TTSs are found at these high frequencies (Hirsh and Ward, 1952; Miller, 1958a; Ward et al., 1958), and when it is a pure-tone, TTS is found to increase as F_e increases (Davis et al., 1950; Ward et al., 1959a). Further, maximum TTSs appear at frequencies above F_e. The ear's greater susceptibility to high-frequency fatiguing stimulation should not be too surprising in view of its greater tendency to permanent high frequency damage; both probably result from the greater stiffness of the high frequency portions of the basilar membrane and, possibly, the more limited response areas of these portions.

It has usually been assumed that generalizations concerning the effects of various factors on TTS apply accurately to PTS as well. This assumption is reasonable in view of the facts that both TTS and PTS are due to tissue changes along the basilar membrane, and that both tend to be greatest in the $4000-6000$-Hz region. However, most PTSs result from exposure to noise or to impulsive stimuli, both of which contain frequency components of considerable range whose intensities at the cochlear level are a function of the ear's conductive characteristics. Further, most PTSs develop as a result of chronic exposure to such complex stimuli rather than from a single, short but intense exposure.

However, when the ear is exposed to stimuli intense enough to cause a PTS after a relatively short exposure, the frequency characteristics of the PTS may differ from that produced by similar stimuli of lower I. Thus Miller et al. (1963), using bands of noise to produce PTS, found that the PTS and TTS audiograms do not agree — maximum

PTS occurs at lower frequencies than maximum TTS. Elliott and Mc-Gee (1965) also found that PTSs resulting from intense pure-tone stimulation range far below F_e, with damage often extending to the apical end of the basilar membrane. It appears then, that agreement between TTS and PTS audiograms may be good if the PTS has developed from long term exposure. But if the ear is exposed to an intensity capable of producing a PTS after only a short exposure, a quite different hearing loss pattern may occur, particularly with respect to its spread to frequencies below F_e. Interestingly, Davis predicted in 1957 that permanent hearing losses from chronic exposure to noise might well differ from those resulting from a single exposure.

E. Other Changes in Hearing

In addition to its threshold shift, the fatigued ear exhibits several other changes. Several investigators have reported shifts in the pitch of tones. Davis et al. (1960), using F_ts up to 4000 Hz reported that for a limited range of frequencies above F_e, there is an upward shift. Rüedi and Furrer (1946) also noted pitch shifts, but reported that for F_es above 4000 Hz, the direction of the shift is downward; Elliott et al. (1964), however, did not find the downward pitch change. The upward shift when $F_t > F_e$ is not too surprising in view of the skewed shape of the response curve along the basilar membrane; the F_t tone probably activates the relatively unaffected higher frequency receptor units. Figure 10 illustrates the manner in which the effect probably occurs.

In addition to pitch shifts, Davis et al. (1950) reported other qualitative changes. Their subjects said that tones within one-half octave above F_e sounded "noisy," "rough," or "buzzing." Other experimenters have reported the development of tinnitus after cessation of the fatiguing stimulus (Hinchcliffe, 1957).

With complex signals, the relatively greater susceptibility to fatigue of the higher frequency receptor units becomes evident. Hirsh and Ward (1952), for example, reported that clicks sound "thud-like" — an indication that the lower frequency components of the click reappear before the higher frequency components.

Other changes include the development of recruitment (Davis et al., 1950; Békésy, 1960; Riach et al., 1964) and changes in the temporal integration of short tone bursts (Jerger, 1955). Both of these changes suggest hair cell dysfunction.

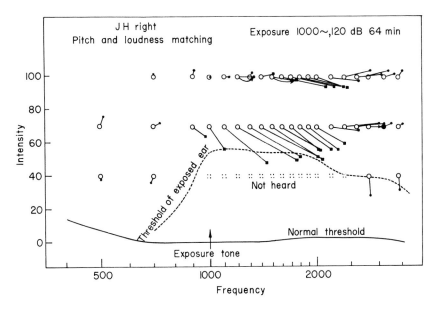

Figure 10 Pitch and loudness matching with a fatigued ear. The open circles represent the frequency and intensity of tones to the fatigued ear. These tones were matched by tones (solid figures) to the unfatigued ear. Note the upward pitch shift; note also that differences in matching intensities decrease at higher intensities, a reflection of the fatigued ear's recruitment. (Davis *et al.*, 1950. By permission from *Acta, Oto Laryngologica.*)

III. ADAPTATION

A. Methodological Considerations

Interest in the effects of moderate or of high I stimuli has not been confined to measurements obtained after the sound has been terminated. Indeed, a large number of studies have concerned themselves with sensitivity changes that occur *during* such stimulation. Measures of loudness decrement have generally been employed, and have usually been labeled "perstimulatory fatigue" or "adaptation." The latter is the term we shall use in this discussion.

Many techniques (see Small, 1963) have been devised for measuring adaptation in its development, asymptotic state, and recovery. Depending on the adaptation state with which one is concerned, different techniques may be appropriate. Thus, the simultaneous dichotic loudness balance (SDLB) technique, since it entails no interruption of the adapting stimulus, is the best yet devised for measuring the developmental course of adaptation. However, when interest is centered on the point of maximum adaptation, then the methods called asymptotic localization and the moving phantom (Wright, 1960), which entail adapting the ear to its asymptotic state before testing begins, hold certain advantages. Finally, the methods of intensive and phase localization are more appropriate for measuring recovery from adaptation, for in each method, the stimulus is first terminated before measurement of adaptation is begun.

The SDLB technique is the one that has been most frequently used for measuring all of the aspects of adaptation. Both pre and post-adaptation balances are made in the usual manner. During the adaptation period, however, the test ear, i.e., the one being adapted, is continuously stimulated while the control ear is only periodically stimulated for balancing purposes. Most studies have used a 15-sec balancing period followed by a 45-sec rest period for the control ear. At the end of a test run, the average of the preadaptation intensities in the control ear is compared to the perstimulatory and poststimulatory values. Any observed difference in the intensity necessary to obtain a balance is taken as a measure of the degree of adaptation in the test ear.

Within the general framework of the SDLB technique, several variations have been developed. Hood (1950) explored adaptation with a tracking procedure in which the subject during each balancing period continuously adjusts the intensity presented to the control ear by means of a recording attenuator so as to maintain a loudness match between the ears. Palva (1955) and Small and Minifie (1961) also used this tracking method. In 1955, Egan introduced the method of fixed intensity (Fig. 11), in which the subject, during each balancing period, adjusts the intensity of the comparison tone in discrete steps so as to obtain a single loudness match. He also devised a modification, the method of varied intensity (Fig. 11), because subjects reported that the tone to the continuously stimulated ear becomes duller and more noise-like with the passage of time, thereby increasing the difficulty of making loudness matches. As a result of these qualitative changes, the subjects began to rely on an internal standard partially independent of the loudness of the adapting stimulus. In the method of varied intensity, the level in the test ear is varied each time a loudness match is to be made, thus minimizing the subject's tendency to form an internal standard. In comparing these methods, Egan found a greater amount of adaptation (10 dB) for the method of varied intensity.

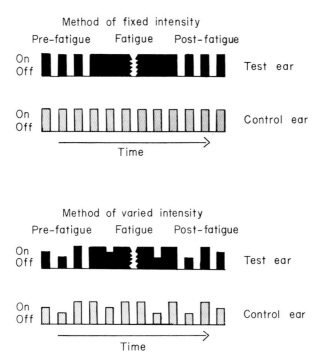

Figure 11 Schematic presentation of methods of fixed and varied intensity. The bars indicate when the stimulus is on. The height of the bars indicates the relative intensity of the stimulus. In the method of fixed intensity, the stimulus presented to the test ear always has the same intensity. In the method of varied intensity, the stimulus presented to the test ear for a given balance may have one of several intensities. In both methods, the intensity of the stimulus presented to the control ear is adjusted by the subject during each balancing period.

That method in turn has been modified so that only practice sessions and the preadaptation balances are made at varying intensities. No comparison of this modified method with either the fixed or varied intensity methods has been made, so it is not known whether the modified method is any more sensitive than the fixed intensity method.

Regardless of the specific method of presentation, the SDLB technique has serious drawbacks. First, Békésy and Rosenblith (1951) reported that crossover (the effect of stimulating one ear with an earphone on the contralateral ear) occurs at 40 to 50 dB SL in the frequency range from 100 to 10,000 Hz. Since adaptation occurs at intensity levels of 15 to 20 dB SL, any study that employs a fatiguing stimulus at 70 dB SL or greater may cause adaptation in the control ear as well as in the test ear (though to a lesser degree). Procedurally, little can be done to handle such crossover phenomena, and indeed, if the relation between adaptation and the intensity of the adapting stimulus is linear, as has been suggested (Hood, 1950; Carterette, 1956; Jerger, 1957), then the only problem crossover presents is that of underestimating the extent of adaptation at the higher intensity levels. However, if the relation is in any way nonlinear, the true datum is completely obscured.

Second, maintaining a continuous tone in the control ear during a loudness match can be detrimental. Considering this aspect, Hood (1950) had his subjects make continuous loudness balance tracings for five minutes. He concluded that whatever change takes place during continuous stimulation does so slowly; this conclusion seems hardly justified by his data.

More recently, Small and Minifee (1961) investigated the effect of the duration of the comparison tone. The on- and off-times of the comparison stimulus were varied in 10-sec intervals from 10 to 50 sec in all combinations that do not exceed 60 sec. They found that for off-intervals less than 30 sec, the duration of the comparison tone is inversely related to the degree of adaptation. However, when 30 sec or more elapse between comparison tones, the on-time of the comparison tone becomes insignificant (Figs. 12 and 13). Note however, that durations of less than 10 sec were not investigated, so conclusions based on this study are severely limited—particularly since considerable adaptation occurs during the initial 10 sec of exposure. Such rapid adaptation has been demonstrated by two procedures. The first, asymptotic localization, involves median plane localizations obtained with 1 sec pulses to the control ear; subjects are asked to report whether the image is located to the right, to the left, or in the median plane under both normal and maximally adapted states. Using these 1 sec pulses, Wright (1960) observed 50 dB of adaptation where studies involving adjustment procedures with tones of 10 sec and longer (Egan, 1955; Jerger, 1957) reported only 20 dB. The second method involved a "moving phantom." Here, the ear is again adapted to its asymptotic state before measurement begins. The procedure consists of determining the time necessary for a sustained tone, led to the control ear and judged initially to be toward that side of the median plane, to move to a central position. Since time intervals are the units of measurement, a comparison with the methods that use intensity is all but impossible. Nevertheless, the moving phantom method demonstrates quite clearly that significant adaptation can occur in less than 10 sec (Fig. 14).

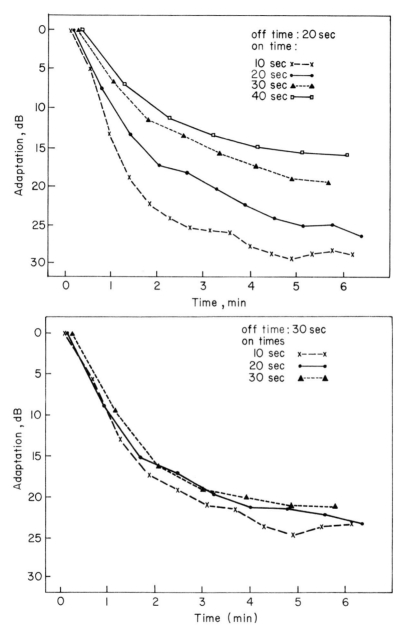

Figure 12   Figures 12 and 13 show the temporal course of adaptation obtained by a
Figure 13   tracking procedure with comparison tones of various on-off times. Each
data point is the average of two judgments from each of eleven subjects. The stimulus
was a 4000-Hz tone presented at 75 dB SL. (Small and Minifie, 1961. By permission
from *Journal of the Acoustical Society of America*.)

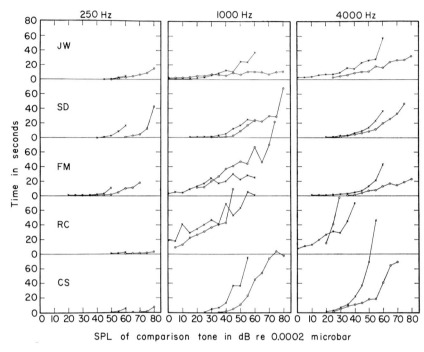

Figure 14 The time required for a moving phantom to reach the median plane for each of five subjects tested at 250, 1000, and 4000 Hz. The parameters are 80-dB (open circles) and 60-dB (crosses) adapting stimuli. (Wright, 1960. By permission from *Journal of the Acoustical Society of America.*)

Third, with the SDLB technique, one must ask whether the matches are based solely on loudness comparisons since tones of the same frequency and loudness, when led to the two ears, fuse into a single sound image that lies in the median plane. In the SDLB technique, however, intensity is varied by the subject, and as it varies, so does location. Therefore, the subject, though instructed to make loudness balances, may use localization cues. The question then follows as to what contribution each aspect of simultaneous stimulation makes to measured adaptation. Egan (1955) studied loudness balances made with tones of the same frequency — 800 Hz — and tones of differing frequencies — 800 and 1000 Hz. In the latter cases, the balance is determined only by loudness cues since each tone is localized at its respective ear. Figure 15 shows Egan's finding that measured adaptation is independent of the influence of localization. But when Egan and Thwing (1955) compared three methods, the results indicated otherwise. The methods were (a) SDLB, (b) delayed balance (Wood, 1930), in which the comparison tone is presented to the control ear immediately after the adapting stimulus is terminated, and (c) intensive

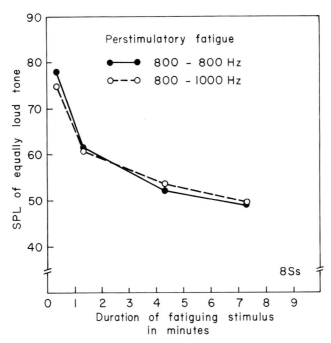

Figure 15 Adaptation of an 800-Hz tone at an intensity of 80 dB SPL obtained with the method of varied intensity. The intensity of an equally loud comparison tone of either 800 or 1000 Hz is shown as a function of the duration of the adapting stimulus. (Egan, 1955. By permission from *Journal of the Acoustical Society of America*.)

localization, in which the intensity of the comparison stimulus necessary for a median plane judgment is ascertained. These three methods respectively are dependent on (a) loudness and localization cues, (b) loudness cues alone, and (c) localization cues alone. Figure 16 presents the adaptation observed with each method, but the results cannot be interpreted unequivocably because the methods vary in more aspects than just the cues they furnish. For instance, although the delayed balance method provides pure loudness judgments, it may be subject to time errors. And the intensive localization method involves terminating the stimulus (although it is turned back on for the judgment). The exact contribution made by each of these two

kinds of cues has not yet been satisfactorily assessed. Thus one cannot safely conclude that the method that involves both loudness and
localization cues actually measures the most adaptation.

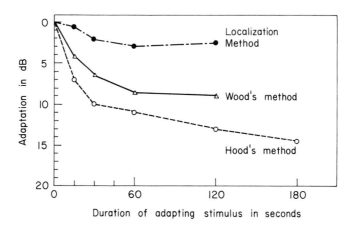

Figure 16   Adaptation as measured by three methods; Hood's method is the SDLB
technique. (Egan and Thwing, 1955. By permission from *Journal of the Acoustical
Society of America.*)

B. Findings

Growth. Putting aside the inherent methodological problems, we
can proceed to the data that have been gathered on the phenomenon
of adaptation. In general, its course of development is one of negative
acceleration, with the greatest rate of adaptation occurring during the
first one or two minutes (Fig. 15), and the asymptotic level being
reached anywhere from three to seven minutes after the onset of the
adapting stimulus. Most of the recovery from adaptation occurs within one minute, and recovery is complete within two minutes. Additionally, adaptation has a roughly linear relation to the intensity and
little or no relation to the frequency of the adapting stimulus.

Although the developmental course of adaptation is well established, the values found at any particular point on that curve vary
widely between investigators. The extent of the discrepancies can
be seen in Fig. 17. By far the most divergent results are those of Hood
(1950) and Palva (1955). Both used a tracking procedure in obtaining
the loudness matches, but their attentuation rates differed. Palva
used a motor-driven attenuator with a rate of 2.3 dB per sec for the
presentation of the stimulus to the control ear, and Hood used a

manually operated attenuator with a rate governed by the subject. That the attenuation rate may in some manner account for this divergence is supported by the fact that Small and Minifie (1961) using a rate of 5 dB per sec (greater than Palva's, but less than Hood's) obtained adaptation of an intermediate value. In light of the various studies, even a general statement about the values for any point along the development curve of adaptation would be misleading. Further, methodological studies are sorely needed so that the absolute degree of adaptation may be determined more accurately.

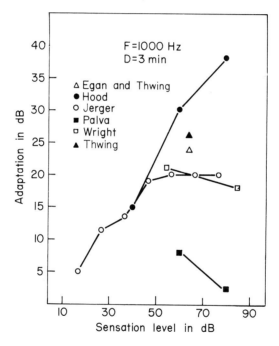

Figure 17 Comparison of the amount of adaptation obtained by six different investigators. All points represent adaptation for a 1000-Hz tone after three minutes of continuous stimulation. (Jerger, 1957. By permission from *Journal of the Acoustical Society of America*.)

Intensity. Just as the values used in describing adaptation are in conflict, so is the relation of adaptation to the intensity of the adapting stimulus. For a continuous pure tone, Hood (1950) found a roughly linear relation over the range of intensity values he investigated (Fig. 17). Jerger (1957), too, demonstrated a linear relation, at least from

10 dB to 60 dB SL, but above this level, the function flattens out (Fig. 17). Additionally, in those studies that investigated only two intensities (Palva, 1955; Wright, 1960), there is no increase in adaptation as a function of the adapting intensity.

To summarize, for those studies that have data points in common (Hood, 1950; Palva, 1955; Jerger, 1957; and Wright, 1960), only Hood showed a substantial increase in the degree of observed adaptation beyond the 60-dB level. Two speculations as to why this leveling off occurred present themselves. First, if crossover does operate so as to cause adaptation in the control ear and there is a linear relation between adaptation and intensity, then a leveling off of observed adaptation would occur at approximately the 70-dB point. This sort of speculation is, of course, restricted by the fact that two studies (Hood, 1950; Carterette, 1956) did show a linear relation continuing above 60 dB.

Another likely explanation of the observed leveling off of adaptation at 60 dB lies in the fact that the data are plotted in intensity units rather than in subjective loudness units. Carterette (1956) found a linear relation only when he made just such a transformation. Although a general statement might be that adaptation and the intensity of the adapting stimulus are linearly related, the upper limit of this function remains in doubt. More evidence is needed before such a statement can be made with confidence.

Adaptation can be measured at intensity levels other than that of the adapting stimulus. This aspect has been investigated only by adapting the test ear at one intensity and measuring adaptation at a lower intensity. The opposite procedure has received no attention. The effect of adapting at one intensity and measuring adaptation at a lower intensity was first investigated by Hood (1950), who exposed the ear to a 100-dB SL tone and then measured adaptation at sensation levels extending from 20 dB through 100 dB. The adaptation he found was similar to that seen with lower adapting intensities; in fact, the values were the same as if the adapting and test intensities were identical. It appears that adaptation when measured at any given intensity, is determined by that test intensity — at least when it is lower than the adapting intensity. Egan (1955) provided further experimental support when he adapted at 80-dB SPL and tested at 60-, 70-, and 80-dB SPL; he found decreasing amounts of adaptation as the test intensity was lowered. Hood (1950) offered a theoretical interpretation: he postulated that for any test intensity, there is a receptor group whose size is proportional to that intensity; the amount of adaptation, then, reflects the size of the receptor group so long as the adapting *I* is equal to or greater than the test intensity.

Still another aspect of intensity—the effect of concentration of energy—can be studied by using narrow- or broad-band noise for the adapting stimulus. Carterette (1956) compared several bands of noise and a 1500-Hz tone using the methods of fixed and variable intensity, with 50-, 70-, and 90-dB SPL adapting stimuli. The results indicate that adaptation tends to increase as bandwidth increases, at least for the 90-dB SPL intensities (Fig. 18). Apparently, as the available energy is spread over a broader frequency range, it adapts a larger receptor group. An exception to this tendency is evident in Fig. 18, where it will be noted that pure tone stimulation produces the greatest adaptation, which suggests the development of fatigue.

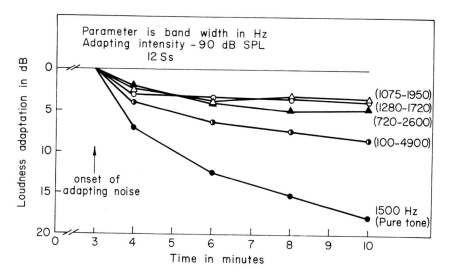

Figure 18 Temporal course of adaptation as a function of the duration of the adapting stimulus. Each point is based on two measures for each of twelve subjects. (Carterette, 1956. By permission from *Journal of the Acoustical Society of America*.)

Interruption Rate. Carterette (1955) measured adaptation to a noise that was interrupted at rates varying from 1 to 12.4 per sec, with a 50 percent duty cycle. First, he observed that, with total energy equal to that in a continuous adapting noise, the continuous noise produces more adaptation. Second, as interruption rate increases, the degree of adaptation also increases. Carterette suggested that, as interruption rate is increased, the time for recovery is shortened and, thus, cumulative effects may be produced. However, the period of adaptation is likewise reduced. Apparently recovery processes suffer relatively more from the increase in interruption rate than do the adapting processes; thus there must be either a latency in the onset of the recovery processes or an initial recovery rate lower than the initial adapting rate. Certainly, these findings again emphasize that too little is known of the initial stages of adaptation and recovery.

Frequency. Two aspects of the frequency parameter merit discussion. First, does adaptation vary as a function of the frequency of the adapting stimulus, and second, does adaptation at one frequency spread to neighboring frequencies. Considering the first aspect, Jerger (1957) found a slight tendency for adaptation to increase as frequency increases from 125 Hz to 1000 Hz, but to remain approximately constant for frequencies from 1000 through 8000 Hz. Confirming evidence is lacking, since most studies have confined themselves to one frequency. Of those studies that used two or more frequencies (Hood, 1950; Palva, 1955), differences in adaptation as a function of the adapting frequency were not reported.

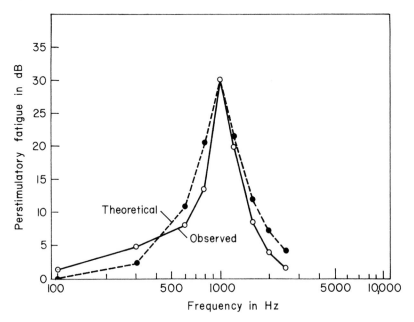

Figure 19 Observed and theoretical frequency gradients of adaptation. The observed gradient is based on maximal adaptation to a 1000-Hz tone, presented at 80 dB SPL. (Thwing, 1955. By permission from *Journal of the Acoustical Society of America.*)

As for the spread of adaptation to neighboring frequencies, there has been only one comprehensive study (Thwing, 1955). Apparently adaptation, at least for 1000 Hz at 80-dB SPL, has its maximum effect at the adapting frequency, with continuously lower degrees of adaptation observed on both sides until at 100 Hz and 2500 Hz, it has completely disappeared (Fig. 19). Thwing suggested that adaptation is proportional to the extent to which excitation patterns of the adapting and comparison stimuli overlap. A theoretical curve based on this hypothesis is shown in Fig. 19; it is symmetrical just as the data points are. Whether adaptation is always greatest at the adapting frequency, irrespective of frequency and intensity, is not known. The collection of such data would be of value in its own right, but additionally, would provide an evaluation of Thwing's hypothesis.

C. Asymptotic Level

Intensity and, to a much lesser extent, frequency both act to determine the temporal course of adaptation and in particular the point at which its asymptotic state is reached. Originally, Hood (1950) reported that adaptation is complete within 3 to 3.5 minutes regardless of the intensity or frequency of the adapting stimulus. However, later studies confirmed this finding only for intensities up to 60 dB SL, or frequencies up to 1000 Hz (Jerger, 1957). Above these values, the frequency effect is negligible, and the degree of adaptation observed becomes primarily a function of the intensity of the adapting stimulus. Also, at these higher levels, as the intensity increases, the point at which the asymptote is reached is further delayed. In general, for the higher intensities, the point of maximum adaptation is reached between five and seven minutes (e.g., see Figs. 12, 13, 15, 16, and 18), although increases in adaptation are reported beyond this point at a considerably slower rate. For example, Carterette (1956) reported that adaptation was still increasing at seven minutes when the intensity of the adapting stimulus was 90 dB SPL. That the asymptote is not reached in three minutes in most studies, except at lower intensities and lower frequencies, is most likely attributable to the addition of fatigue processes.

Recovery. The chief difficulty in measuring recovery from adaptation is that the commonest technique (SDLB) involves restimulation of the test ear during the recovery process. Also, the first postadaptation balance has been taken at approximately one minute after the adapting stimulus has been terminated. Thus the recovery process, curtailed by measurement difficulties, is poorly known. Among those investigators who have used the SDLB technique (Egan, 1955; Thwing, 1955; Wright, 1959), it is generally agreed that recovery is rapid, with far more recovery taking place in the first minute than in any comparable period thereafter. For example, Egan reported first-minute recovery of about 70 percent, Thwing reported 80 percent, and Wright reported 75 percent. The most interesting aspect of these data is that, regardless of the extent of adaptation at asymptote, a similar proportion of recovery takes place in the first minute. Not one of these investigators reported more than 6 or 7 dB adaptation after 60 sec, even though adaptation at asymptote was as high as 30 dB. Further recovery occurs during the second minute and, with the exception of one report (Wright, 1960, who observed between 3 and 8 dB of adaptation at the three-minute point), the evidence suggests that the functional characteristics of the ear are restored by the third minute.

The SDLB technique gives no information about the course of recovery during the first minute, and since this time period includes most of the recovery, other techniques are more appropriate. The method of intensive localization is preferred because restimulation is minimized. In this method, the intensity necessary for a median-plane localization is determined by having the subject report if the fused image is to the left, to the right, or in the center while brief stimuli are presented. The intensity necessary for a "center" judgment *before* adaptation is compared with the intensity necessary *after* adaptation. Since restimulation is brief, certainly the effect of restimulation is minimized, and the course of recovery during the first minute can be ascertained.

Békésy (1960, pp. 357–358) using this method with stimuli of 0.2 sec duration, found that 80 percent of the recovery occurs during the first 5 sec; almost complete recovery occurs within 10 sec. Since the initial level of adaptation was low (15 dB), it is not possible to generalize these findings. Once again, we must close the discussion with the comment that more work needs to be done before definitive statements can be made.

REFERENCES

von Békésy, G. (1951). DC potentials and energy balance of the cochlear partition. *J. Acoust. Soc. Am.*, **23**, 576–582.
von Békésy, G. (1960). *Experiments in hearing.* McGraw-Hill, New York.

von Békésy, G. and Rosenblith, W. A. (1951). The mechanical properties of the ear. In S. S. Stevens (Ed.). *Handbook of experimental psychology.* pp. 1075-1115. Wiley, New York.

Butler, R. A., Honrubia, V., Johnstone, B. M., and Fernández, C. (1962). Cochlear function under metabolic impairment. *Ann. Otol. Rhinol. Lar.,* **71,** 648-656.

Carterette, E. C. (1955). Perstimulatory auditory fatigue for continuous and interrupted noise. *J. Acoust. Soc. Am.,* **27,** 103-111.

Carterette, E. C. (1956). Loudness adaptation for bands of noise. *J. Acoust. Soc. Am.,* **28,** 865-871.

Caussé, R. and Chavasse, P. (1947). Études sur la fatigue auditive. In H. Piéron (Ed.) *L'Année psychologique.* Vols. 43-44 for 1942-1943, pp. 265-298. Presses Universitaires de France, Paris.

Davis, H. (1957). Biophysics and physiology of the inner ear. *Physiol. Rev.,* **37,** 1-49.

Davis, H., Morgan, C. T., Hawkins, J. E., Jr., Galambos, R., and Smith, F. W. (1950). Temporary deafness following exposure to loud tones and noise. *Acta Oto-Lar., Suppl.* **88.**

Davis, H. and Associates (Benson, R. W., Covell, W. P., Fernández, C., Goldstein, R., Katsuki, Y., Legouix, J.-P., McAuliffe, D. R., and Tasaki, I.) (1953). Acoustic trauma in the guinea pig. *J. Acoust. Soc. Am.,* **25,** 1180-1189.

Derbyshire, A. J. and Davis, H. (1935). The action potentials of the auditory nerve. *Am. J. Physiol.,* **113,** 476-504.

Egan, J. P. (1955). Perstimulatory fatigue as measured by heterophonic loudness balances. *J. Acoust. Soc. Am.,* **27,** 111-120.

Egan, J. P. and Thwing, E. J. (1955). Further studies on perstimulatory fatigue. *J. Acoust. Soc. Am.,* **27,** 1225-1226 (L).

Elliott, D. N. and McGee, T. M. (1965). Effect of cochlear lesions upon audiograms and intensity discrimination in cats. *Ann. Otol. Rhinol. Lar.* **74,** 386-408.

Elliott, D. N., Sheposh, J., and Frazier, L. (1964). Effect of monaural fatigue upon pitch matching and discrimination. *J. Acoust. Soc. Am.,* **36,** 752-756.

Epstein, A. and Schubert, E. D. (1957). Reversible auditory fatigue resulting from exposure to a pure tone. *Archs. Otolar.,* **65,** 174-182.

Fletcher, J. L. (1957). Pure-tone thresholds following stimulation by narrow-band filtered noise. *Psychol. Monogr.,* **71** (4).

Gisselsson, L. and Sørensen, H. (1959). Auditory adaptation and fatigue in cochlear potentials. *Acta Oto-Lar.,* **50,** 391-405.

Harris, J. D. (1953). Recovery curves and equinoxious exposures in reversible auditory fatigue following stimulation up to 140 dB plus. *Laryngoscope,* **63,** 660-673.

Harris, J. D. (1955). On latent damage to the ear. *J. Acoust. Soc. Am.,* **27,** 177-179 (L).

Harris, J. D. (1959). Auditory fatigue following high frequency pulse trains. *U.S. Nav. Med. Res. Lab. Rep. 306.*

Harris, J. D. (1961). Temporary threshold shift following 60 hours of 3.5 kc pulses at 90-100 SPL. *U.S. Nav. Med. Res. Lab. Memo. Rep. 61-9.*

Hinchcliffe, R. (1957). Threshold changes at 4 kc/s produced by bands of noise. *Acta Oto-Lar.,* **47,** 496-509.

Hirsh, I. J. and Bilger, R. C. (1955). Auditory-threshold recovery after exposures to pure tones. *J. Acoust. Soc. Am.,* **27,** 1186-1194.

Hirsh, I. J. and Ward, W. D. (1952). Recovery of the auditory threshold after strong acoustic stimulation. *J. Acoust. Soc. Am.,* **24,** 131-141.

Hood, J. D. (1950). Studies in auditory fatigue and adaptation. *Acta Oto-Lar., Suppl.* **92.**

Hughes, J. R. (1954). Auditory sensitization. *J. Acoust. Soc. Am.*, **26**, 1064–1070.

Hughes, J. R. and Rosenblith, W. A. (1957). Electrophysiological evidence for auditory sensitization. *J. Acoust. Soc. Am.*, **29**, 275–280.

Huizing, H. C. (1948). The relation between auditory fatigue and recruitment. *Acta Oto-Lar., Suppl.* **78**

Jerger, J. F. (1955). Influence of stimulus duration on the pure-tone threshold during recovery from auditory fatigue. *J. Acoust. Soc. Am.*, **27**, 121–124.

Jerger, J. F. (1956). Recovery pattern from auditory fatigue. *J. Speech Hear. Disorders*, **21**, 39–46.

Jerger, J. F. (1957). Auditory adaptation. *J. Acoust. Soc. Am.*, **29**, 357–363.

Lawrence, M. and Yantis, P. A. (1957). Overstimulation, fatigue, and onset of overload in the normal human ear. *J. Acoust. Soc. Am.*, **29**, 265–274.

Lierle, D. M. and Reger, S. N. (1954). Further studies of threshold shifts as measured with the Békésy-type audiometer. *Trans. Am. Otol. Soc.*, **42**, 211–227.

Lightfoot, C. (1955). Evaluation of threshold tracing audiometry as a method for studying effects of strong acoustic stimulation. *U.S.A.F. Sch. Aviat. Med., Proj. 21-1203-0001, Rep. 8.*

Loeb, M. and Fletcher, J. L. (1963). Temporary threshold shift in successive sessions for subjects exposed to continuous and periodic intermittent noise. *J. Aud. Res.*, **3**, 213–220.

Miller, J. D. (1958a). Temporary hearing loss at 4000 C.P.S. as a function of a three-minute exposure to a noise of uniform spectrum level. *Laryngoscope*, **68**, 660–671.

Miller, J. D. (1958b). Temporary threshold shift and masking for noise of uniform spectrum level. *J. Acoust. Soc. Am.*, **30**, 517–522.

Miller, J. D., Watson, C. S., and Covell, W. P. (1963). Deafening effects of noise on the cat. *Acta Oto-Lar., Suppl.* **176**

Misrahy, G. A., Arnold, J. E., Mundie, J. R., Shinabarger, E. W., and Garwood, V. P. (1958a). Genesis of endolymphatic hypoxia following acoustic trauma. *J. Acoust. Soc. Am.*, **30**, 1082–1088.

Misrahy, G. A., De Jonge, B. R., Shinabarger, E. W., and Arnold, J. E. (1958b). Effects of localized hypoxia on the electrophysiological activity of cochlea of the guinea pig. *J. Acoust. Soc. Am.*, **30**, 705–709.

Misrahy, G. A., Shinabarger, E. W., and Arnold, J. E. (1958c). Changes in cochlear endolymphatic oxygen availability, action potential, and microphonics during and following asphyxia, hypoxia, and exposure to loud sounds. *J. Acoust. Soc. Am.*, **30**, 701–704.

Palva, T. (1955). Studies on per-stimulatory adaptation in various groups of deafness. *Laryngoscope*, **65**, 829–847.

Riach, W. D., Elliott, D. N., and Frazier, L. (1964). Effect of repeated exposure to high-intensity sound. *J. Acoust. Soc. Am.*, **36**, 1195–1198.

Rosenblith, W. A. (1950). Auditory masking and fatigue. *J. Acoust. Soc. Am.*, **22**, 792–800.

Rosenblith, W. A., Galambos, R., and Hirsh, I. J. (1950). The effect of exposure to loud tones upon animal and human responses to acoustic clicks. *Science*, **111**, 569–571.

Rüedi, L. and Furrer, W. (1946). Physics and physiology of acoustic trauma. *J. Acoust. Soc. Am.*, **18**, 409–412.

Selters, W. (1964). Adaptation and fatigue. *J. Acoust. Soc. Am.*, **36**, 2202–2209.

Shimizu, H., Konishi, T., and Nakamura, F. (1957). An experimental study of adaptation and fatigue of cochlear microphonics. *Acta Oto-Lar.*, **47**, 358–363.

Small, A. M. (1963). Auditory adaptation. In James Jerger (Ed.) *Modern developments in audiology.* Academic Press, New York.

Small, A. M. and Minifie, F. D. (1961). Effect of matching time on perstimulatory adaptation. *J. Acoust. Soc. Am.,* **33**, 1028–1033.

Spieth, W. and Trittipoe, W. J. (1958). Intensity and duration of noise exposure and temporary threshold shifts. *J. Acoust. Soc. Am.,* **30**, 710–713.

Thwing, E. J. (1955). Spread of perstimulatory fatigue of a pure tone to neighboring frequencies. *J. Acoust. Soc. Am.,* **27**, 741–748.

Tonndorf, J. and Brogan, F. A. (1952). Two forms of change in cochlear microphonics: parallel shifts in stimulus intensity and truncation of gradient curves. *U.S.A.F. Sch. Aviat. Med., Proj. 21-27-001, Rep. 6.*

Trittipoe, W. J. (1958). Residual effects of low noise levels on the temporary threshold shift. *J. Acoust. Soc. Am.,* **30**, 1017–1019.

Trittipoe, W. J. (1959). Residual effects at longer pre-exposure durations. *J. Acoust. Soc. Am.,* **31**, 244 (L).

Ward, W. D. (1960a). Latent and residual effects in temporary threshold shift. *J. Acoust. Soc. Am.,* **32**, 135–137.

Ward, W. D. (1960b). Recovery from high values of temporary threshold shift. *J. Acoust. Soc. Am.,* **32**, 497–500.

Ward, W. D. (1963). Auditory fatigue and masking. In J. F. Jerger (Ed.) *Modern developments in audiology.* Academic Press, New York.

Ward, W. D., Glorig, A., and Sklar, D. L. (1958). Dependence of temporary threshold shift at four kc on intensity and time. *J. Acoust. Soc. Am.,* **30**, 944–954.

Ward, W. D., Glorig, A., and Sklar, D. L. (1959a). Temporary threshold shift from octave-band noise: Applications to damage-risk criteria. *J. Acoust. Soc. Am.,* **31**, 522–528.

Ward, W. D., Glorig, A., and Sklar, D. L. (1959b). Temporary threshold shift produced by intermittent exposure to noise. *J. Acoust. Soc. Am.,* **31**, 791–794.

Ward, W. D., Glorig, A., and Selters, W. (1960). Temporary threshold shift in a changing noise level. *J. Acoust. Soc. Am.,* **32**, 235–237.

Wever, E. G. and Lawrence, M. (1955). Patterns of injury produced by overstimulation of the ear. *J. Acoust. Soc. Am.,* **27**, 853–858.

Wever, E. G. and Smith, K. R. (1944). The problem of stimulation deafness. *J. Exp. Psychol.,* **34**, 239–245.

Wood, A. G. (1930). Quantitative account of the course of auditory fatigue. Unpublished master's thesis, Univ. of Virginia.

Wright, H. N. (1959). Auditory adaptation in noise. *J. Acoust. Soc. Am.,* **31**, 1004–1012.

Wright, H. N. (1960). Measurement of perstimulatory auditory adaptation. *J. Acoust. Soc. Am.,* **32**, 1558–1567.

Chapter Five

Critical Bands

FOREWORD

Nowhere in auditory theory or in acoustic psychophysiological practice is there anything more ubiquitous than the critical band. It turns up in the measurement of pitch, in the study of loudness, in the examination of acoustic annoyance, in the investigation of the intelligibility of speech, in the analysis of masking and fatiguing signals, in the perception of phase, and even in the determination of the pleasantness of music. And likely, in one way or another, it will be part of our final understanding of how and why we perceive anything that reaches our ears. Students of vision have no such omnipresent entity to worry and console them. The other senses lack the mysteriousness of this unseen—perhaps nonexistent—but pervasive auditory filter. Bertram Scharf has worked closely with the critical-band and critical-ratio concepts throughout his professional life. In this chapter, he has covered many of the processes into which the critical band enters, and all of the theoretical bases necessary for an understanding of the band's ubiquity.

157

Critical Bands

Bertram Scharf[*]

I. INTRODUCTION

The concept of the critical band relates to so much of what concerns the psychoacoustician — thresholds, loudness, pitch, binaural masking, musical consonance, speech, etc. — that a single report cannot cover everything. Therefore, I have written this chapter primarily to cover the *empirical* critical band — its experimental bases, its dependence on duration, its relation to other auditory functions, and its application to various models — and to describe the mechanisms that may underlie it.

As a purely empirical phenomenon, the critical band is that bandwidth at which subjective responses rather abruptly change (Feldtkeller, 1955; Feldtkeller and Zwicker, 1956; Zwicker *et al.*, 1957; Zwicker, 1960; Scharf, 1961b). Thus the loudness of a band of noise at a constant sound pressure remains constant as the bandwidth increases up to the critical band; then loudness begins to increase. In another type of experiment, the threshold of a narrow band of noise lying between two masking tones remains constant as the frequency separation between the tones increases until the critical band is reached; then the threshold of the noise drops precipitously. In these and other experiments, the measurement of the critical band requires manipulation of bandwidth. Measured in this manner, the critical band turns out to be remarkably alike in many kinds of experiment.

Often, the critical-band concept is used, not to summarize, but to

°Department of Psychology, Northeastern University, Boston, Massachusetts.

analyze the results of an experiment or to supplement an auditory model (Marill, 1956; Green, 1958a,b; Swets *et al.*, 1962; Durlach, 1964). So used, the critical band refers to a filtering process assumed to take place within the auditory system. Calculations of the bandwidth of the internal filter depend on somewhat arbitrary assumptions about the mode of operation of the filter (Green, 1958a,b) and its shape (Swets *et al.*, 1962; Mathews and Pfafflin, 1965). These calculated bandwidths have seldom been the same as the empirically measured ones.

Fletcher (1940) originally used the term "critical band" to refer to both calculated and directly measured values. The measurements were sketchy and inconclusive. The calculations were based on the hypothesis that when a white noise just masks a tone, only a relatively narrow band of frequencies surrounding the tone—and equal to it in power—does the masking; sound energy outside the band contributes little or nothing. Since the size of this hypothetical masking band is estimated from the experimentally measured signal-to-noise ratio at the pure-tone threshold, the obtained estimates are now called "critical ratios." Critical ratios and critical bands are related in a simple fashion.

I will try to maintain a clear distinction between directly measured critical bands and indirectly derived bandwidths such as the critical ratio. The term critical band is reserved for the direct measurements.

II. THE CRITICAL BAND AS AN EMPIRICAL PHENOMENON

The initial measurement of the critical band and much of the subsequent work have been carried out by Zwicker and Feldtkeller and their colleagues in Stuttgart. Additional measurements come from laboratories in East Germany, the Netherlands, and the United States. Figure 1 summarizes most of these results and shows how the critical bandwidth changes as a function of its center frequency; the solid curve represents the data obtained by Zwicker (from Feldtkeller and Zwicker, 1956), the triangles those obtained by Greenwood (1961b), and the squares those from my own laboratory. Table I provides the best approximations of critical bandwidths from the majority of data now available. It is a valuable guide in the planning of experiments and in the analysis of data. However, these values are probably reliable only within about ± 15 percent, owing to the variability within and among subjects.

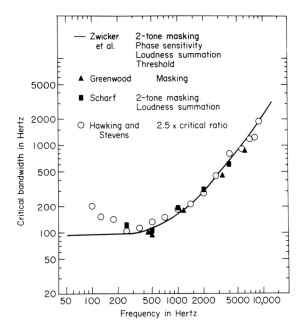

Figure 1 Critical bandwidth as a function of the frequency at the center of the band. The solid line is a smoothed average of measurements by Zwicker and his colleagues. Triangles (Greenwood, 1961a) are based upon masking by narrow bands of noise. Squares are averages obtained by the author. Circles are the published signal-to-noise ratios of Hawkins and Stevens (1950) converted to hertz and multiplied by 2.5. (By permission from *Journal of the Acoustical Society of America.*)

A. Loudness of Complex Sounds

Many experiments have dealt with the loudness of noise bands or of multitone complexes as a function of Δf (bandwidth or overall frequency separation) under a variety of conditions (Zwicker and Feldtkeller, 1955; Bauch, 1956; Zwicker *et al.*, 1957; Scharf, 1959a,b, 1961a, 1962; Niese, 1960, 1961; Port, 1963). All showed that the loudness of a subcritical complex sound of invariant intensity is largely independent of Δf – it is about as loud as an equally intense pure tone lying at the band's center frequency. Only when Δf exceeds the critical band does the loudness of the complex begin to increase. Since most of these experiments were concerned more with loudness summation than with the critical band per se, only a couple (Zwicker and Feldtkeller, 1955; and Zwicker *et al.*, 1957) provide precise estimates of the critical band. Figure 2 shows the results for bands of noise

TABLE I
EXAMPLES OF CRITICAL BANDWIDTH

Number	Center frequency (Hz)	Critical band (Hz)	Lower cutoff frequency (Hz)	Upper cutoff frequency (Hz)
1	50	–	–	100
2	150	100	100	200
3	250	100	200	300
4	350	100	300	400
5	450	110	400	510
6	570	120	510	630
7	700	140	630	770
8	840	150	770	920
9	1,000	160	920	1,080
10	1,170	190	1,080	1,270
11	1,370	210	1,270	1,480
12	1,600	240	1,480	1,720
13	1,850	280	1,720	2,000
14	2,150	320	2,000	2,320
15	2,500	380	2,320	2,700
16	2,900	450	2,700	3,150
17	3,400	550	3,150	3,700
18	4,000	700	3,700	4,400
19	4,800	900	4,400	5,300
20	5,800	1,100	5,300	6,400
21	7,000	1,300	6,400	7,700
22	8,500	1,800	7,700	9,500
23	10,500	2,500	9,500	12,000
24	13,500	3,500	12,000	15,500

centered geometrically at 1000 Hz and set at the sound pressure levels shown on the curves. At all the levels tested except the lowest, loudness is constant up to a bandwidth of about 160 Hz.*

---

*At sensation levels between about 10 and 15 dB, the loudness of a single critical band changes almost in direct proportion to intensity, so that increasing the spread of energy from one to two critical bands, for example, produces two component bands each half as loud as the original single band. The total loudness equals that of the original band, and so loudness does not increase with bandwidth even beyond the critical band. Below about 10 dB, loudness decreases with bandwidth beyond the critical band (Scharf, 1959a). Also, near the masked threshold, loudness is independent of bandwidth (Scharf, 1961a).

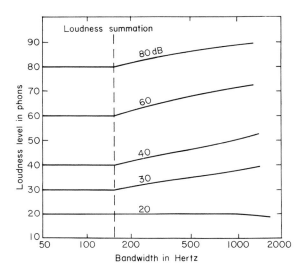

Figure 2   The loudness level of a band of noise centered at 1000 Hz measured as a function of the width of the band. The parameter is the effective sound pressure level of the noise. The dashed line shows that the critical bandwidth at which loudness begins to increase is the same at all the levels tested. (Adapted from Feldtkeller and Zwicker, 1956, p. 82. By permission from S. Hirzel Verlag.)

Figure 3 shows that the critical band can be estimated from the data of individual subjects as well as from averages. Six subjects matched the loudness of two-tone complexes with variable Δfs to a reference two-tone complex with a Δf of 220 Hz. Each component of the standard complex was set to 50 dB SPL. The ordinate of Fig. 3 is the difference between the overall sound pressure levels of the comparison complex and the experimental complex. Each symbol represents a single judgment by a subject using a sone potentiometer to adjust the level of either the comparison (C) or the experimental complex ([). For four of the six subjects, loudness began to increase with Δf at the critical bandwidth (300 Hz at a center frequency of 2000 Hz). For the other two subjects, loudness first began to increase at Δfs of 400 and 500 Hz. Similar measures at center frequencies of 250, 500, 1000, and 4000 Hz were combined with measures of two-tone masking for the same six subjects and plotted as the squares in Fig. 1. (Although the size of the critical band varies among listeners, no broad systematic study of the intersubject, intrasubject, or interexperiment variability is yet available.)

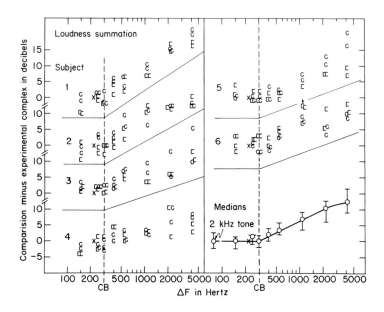

Figure 3 Loudness summation as a function of the frequency separation, Δf, in a two-tone complex centered at 2000 Hz. Individual judgments by each of six subjects are in separate blocks. Crosses are drawn at the Δf (220 Hz) of the comparison complex. Medians and interquartile ranges of the combined data show that loudness begins to increase when the Δf of the experimental complex exceeds the critical band.

The role of the critical band in loudness summation was also demonstrated in experiments that varied the number of components in multitone complexes (Scharf, 1959b), the intensity relations of the components (Scharf, 1962), or the level of a background masking noise (Scharf, 1961a). The critical band was studied in earphone listening, both monaural and binaural, and under free-field conditions (Niese, 1960, 1961). Port (1963) and Zwicker (1965b) investigated it in terms of the summation of loudness at short durations. Of all the measures of the critical band, those concerning the summation of loudness are the most reliable, involving as they do a dozen reports from four laboratories.

B. Narrow-Band Masking

Until the general nature of the critical band was clarified, the concept was most often applied to experiments on masking. Fletcher (1940) defined the critical band as that band of frequencies within a masking noise that alone contributes to the masking of a pure tone at the center of the band. Fletcher's definition led to two types of experiment. One measures the masking of pure tones in wide-band noise and yields the critical ratio; the other samples the masked threshold of tones in the presence of bands of noise of different widths. If a masking band exists, the tone should become more difficult to detect as the noise bandwidth is increased up to the critical band. Further increases in bandwidth should not raise the threshold. Fletcher (1940) published preliminary results of the second type of experiment, but they were too variable, and too few bandwidths were sampled to provide a reliable measure. Since 1940, measurements of the masking of pure tones as a function of the bandwidth of the masking noise have been made by Schafer *et al.* (1950), Feldtkeller and Zwicker (1956), Hamilton (1957), and Bos and de Boer (1966), but Greenwood (1961a) provided the most comprehensive data.

In his experiments, Greenwood used the Békésy tracking method to measure the masked threshold of pulsed tones as a function of frequency. The masking noise was varied in width, spectrum level, and frequency location. At sensation levels below about 50 to 60 dB, the threshold of a pure tone increases as its frequency approaches the center frequency of the noise band. When the width of the noise band is subcritical or critical, the threshold reaches a maximum near the center and then begins to decrease, describing a triangular plot as shown in three quadrants of Fig. 4. When the noise is supercritical, the threshold curve has a flat top and is trapezoidal as shown in the upper right-hand quadrant of Fig. 4. At sensation levels above 50 dB, the subcritical and critical bands also produce flat-topped curves, but they are narrower than the curves produced by supercritical bands. As Greenwood pointed out, this change in shape *does not mean* that the critical bandwidth changes as a function of level, for a change occurs only when the bandwidth is subcritical. Supercritical bands do not produce curves that change shape. Moreover, the threshold of the maximally masked tone (near the center frequency) increases at all levels in direct proportion to the increase in the bandwidth of the masking noise up to, but not beyond the critical band. Greenwood (1961b) published estimates of the critical band at the five frequencies at which he located his noise bands. Four of these values were precise enough to reproduce as the triangles in Fig. 1. The agreement of his data with the other data is very good.

Greenwood's data do present some problems, however. The invariance of the signal-to-noise ratio within the critical band does not agree with other data. Moreover, these ratios were often 4 to 7 dB

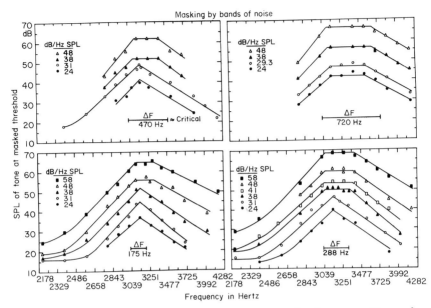

Figure 4 Masked threshold of a pure tone as a function of its frequency. The masker is a band of noise whose width is different in each quadrant, and whose spectrum level is the parameter of the curves. Results are for one subject. Equal distances along the abscissa represent approximately equal fractions of a critical band. (Adapted from Greenwood, 1961a. By permission from *Journal of the Acoustical Society of America*.)

smaller than those reported by Zwicker (1958, 1963a) from extensive measurements with narrow-band maskers. They are also smaller than expected from the relation between the critical band and critical ratio. These discrepancies may have been caused partly by a 40-Hz gap in Greenwood's masking noises. This narrow gap could also have caused overestimation of the critical bandwidth near 1000 Hz, although not at higher frequencies (Green, 1965), but the possibility seems unlikely—such a frequency-dependent distortion would grossly alter the shape of Greenwood's function (see Fig. 1) relating critical bandwidth to frequency. Moreover, in a similar series of measurements, Feldtkeller and Zwicker (1956) reported similar results, but at only one center frequency.

The experiments by Greenwood (1961a) and by Feldtkeller and Zwicker (1956) are unique for having measured complete masked audiograms for bands of noise of varying width. All the other experiments reviewed in this section measured threshold only at or near the center frequency of the masking bands.

Hamilton (1957), using a forced-choice procedure, measured the masked threshold of an 800-Hz tone as a function of the bandwidth of the masking noise. He found that the threshold increases as bandwidth increases from 19 Hz to about 145 Hz (the critical band at 800 Hz), and thereafter remains constant as bandwidth increases up to 1100 Hz. The coincidence of Hamilton's critical-band measurement with Zwicker's is the more striking because Hamilton was apparently unaware of Zwicker's publications. Hamilton's experiments have been replicated and confirmed by van den Brink (1964a).

Schafer *et al.* (1950) used bands of synthetic noise composed of tones 1 Hz apart to mask tones at three different frequencies. This masked threshold first rises and then remains approximately constant as the bandwidth increases. The transition from a rising to a constant threshold is too gradual, however, to permit more than a rough estimate of the critical band. The authors' estimates were about half as large as Greenwood's and Hamilton's, but the data could fit the larger values almost as well. This experiment illustrates the difficulty of trying to measure a subjective discontinuity and the disadvantage of limiting the relevant measurements to the center frequency.

The same difficulty and limitation are apparent in the data of Bos and de Boer (1966), who measured their own thresholds at five center frequencies as a function of masker bandwidth. Nevertheless, their combined data, although rather irregular, indicate that the masked threshold becomes independent of the bandwidth of the masker for values near Zwicker's critical bandwidths. Bos and de Boer ascribed much of the difficulty in this type of measurement to the amplitude fluctuations in narrow-band noise. At narrow widths, the masking noise is so similar to the signal that a difference limen for intensity is measured. To prove their point, they measured intensity discrimination for their masking noises, and showed that the DL and the masked threshold vary as a function of bandwidth in about the same way, especially within the critical band. De Boer (1962) also pointed out that, in the results of Hamilton (1957), Swets *et al.* (1962) and, to a lesser extent, Schafer *et al.* (1950), the masked threshold of a pure tone increases with bandwidth at about the same rate as does the difference limen for narrow-band noise. The rate of increase is about 1.5 dB per doubling of bandwidth, which also means that the signal-to-noise ratio at threshold decreases with bandwidth up to the critical band and thereafter continues to decrease at a more rapid rate.

Despite the apparent confusion of intensity discrimination and masking, masking by narrow-band noise can provide adequate estimates of critical bandwidth, as evidenced by the overall agreement of Greenwood's, Hamilton's, and van den Brink's measures with all the other measures of the critical band.

C. Two-Tone Masking

Zwicker (1954) used a different approach to the precise measurement of the critical band in masking. He took the threshold of a narrow-band noise in the presence of two tones, one on either side of the noise. Increasing the difference in frequency, Δf, between the two tones leaves the masked threshold of the noise unchanged until a critical Δf is reached, whereupon the threshold falls sharply and continues to fall as Δf increases. One of Zwicker's figures (for masking tones at 50 dB SPL) is reproduced as Fig. 5. Thresholds with only a single masking tone are also shown. Measurements were carried out in this manner at eight frequencies ranging from about 90 to 9000 Hz and are included in the solid curve of Fig. 1.

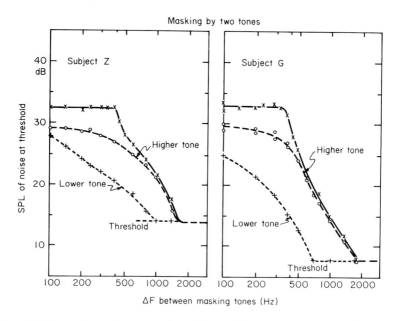

Figure 5 The masking of a narrow band of noise by two pure tones as a function of their frequency separation, Δf. Xs are the threshold values measured in the presence of both tones, circles in the presence of the high tone alone, and crosses in the presence of the low tone alone. Absolute threshold in the quiet is also shown. (Adapted from Zwicker, 1954. By permission from *Acustica*.)

Greenwood (1961a) also used a two-tone complex to mask a narrow band of noise. He took masked audiograms for the noise as a function of the Δfs between the masking tones. Subcritical Δfs give unimodal audiograms; supercritical Δfs give bimodal audiograms with a dip near the middle frequency. These results fully corroborate Zwicker's (1954) results, as do those of Scholl (1962b), who used two narrow bands of noise to mask a sinusoidal signal. Green (1965), however, measured much wider critical bands when he used two tones to mask a third tone lying between them. Only part of the difference from previous results was due to the combination of sinusoidal maskers and a sinusoidal signal, for Green also measured a wider critical band, although not so much wider, when he used the same stimulus configuration as Zwicker (1954) with a narrow-band noise as the signal. Probably the critical factor, as Green suggested in his conclusion, was the 77 dB SPL. Zwicker (1954) had used masking levels of 40, 50, 60, and 80 dB SPL, and his results were least regular at 80 dB. Greenwood (1961a) and Scholl (1962b) used masker levels of 52.5 dB and 60 dB SPL.

I also noted the importance of the masker level in some unpublished experiments. I used one pair of tones to mask a second pair lying within 30 to 100 Hz of each other or to mask a narrow-band noise. As the subject tracked the signal, the masking tones moved gradually apart in frequency. The six subjects usually showed fairly distinct breaks in their threshold curves at Δfs that, on the average, closely approximated the critical band in each of the five frequency regions tested. But this neat relation did not hold for 87 dB SPL masking tones. There, the masked threshold decreased gradually with increasing Δf both inside and outside the critical band, just as did Green's (1965) thresholds over a comparable range of Δfs. Consequently, only data collected at 57 dB SPL have been combined with loudness-summation data to give the squares of Fig. 1. The breakdown in the critical-band measurements at high levels may well be caused by harmonic distortion in the ear and by the emergence of combination and difference tones.

D. Threshold of Complex Sounds

Just as the energy outside of a critical band may not contribute to the masking of a signal within that band, it also may not contribute to the audibility of a complex sound. Gässler (1954) did the basic experiments, measuring the threshold of a multitone complex composed of from 1 to 40 sinusoids evenly spaced 10 or 20 Hz apart. As each tone was added to the complex, the overall sound pressure level at threshold remained constant up to the critical bandwidth; i.e., with the addition of each new tone the levels of the original tones were decreased. When tones were added beyond the frequency limits of the critical band, the overall sound pressure level of the complex increased. Similar results were obtained when a background noise was introduced (Fig. 6), and when bands of white noise were substituted for

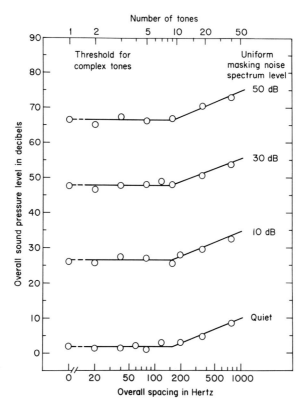

Figure 6 Threshold of complex tones as a function of their overall spacing. Parameter is the spectrum level of a uniform masking noise. The number of tones in the complex is given at the top. (Data are from Gässler, 1954. By permission from *Acustica*.)

the multitone complexes. The results indicate that the total energy necessary for a sound to be heard remains constant so long as the energy is confined to a single critical band.

E. Phase Sensitivity

Although the ear is not markedly adept at distinguishing phase relations, such an ability does appear to account for differences in the detectability of amplitude modulation (AM) and frequency modulation (FM) when the principal modulation products fall within a single critical band. Zwicker (1952) showed that the ear can detect the AM of a pure tone more readily than the FM. The difference holds, however, only at low modulation frequencies; it disappears as the frequency increases. The sensitivity to FM and AM becomes the same when the frequency separation between the sidebands of the three-tone spectrum (produced by modulation) is equal to the critical band. Since the complexes produced under AM and those produced under FM are essentially the same except with respect to phase relations (provided the frequency change is restricted to a narrow range), we may assume that the ear detects AM more easily than FM because it is more sensitive to the phase relations under AM, but only when the Δf of the complex is less than a critical band. When Δf is greater than a critical band, there is no difference in sensitivity to AM and FM, implying that, beyond the critical band, the phase relations within the complex no longer serve as significant cues. As in other types of experiments, the critical band does not vary with the sound pressure level.

Earlier, Mathes and Miller (1947) found that clearly audible AM and FM first begin to sound alike when modulation frequencies reach values equal to about 40 percent of the carrier frequency. These frequencies are considerably higher than those at which Zwicker (1952) found AM and FM to be equally detectable. Apparently the "usual" critical band is measurable only in the *detection* of modulation, not in the suprathreshold sensations.

F. Musical Consonance

The critical band also has its esthetic side. Plomp and Levelt (1962, 1965) asked musically naive subjects to judge the pleasantness of two-tone complexes on a seven-point scale. Amazingly, the mean judgments of pleasantness or consonance were fairly constant when the two tones (each at 60 dB SPL) were separated by more than a critical band but starting at the critical bandwidth, the mean rating rapidly declined as the two tones moved closer together. Consonance reached its lowest value at a frequency separation of about

0.2 critical bands. At still narrower separations, consonance increased somewhat, probably owing to audible beats. Figure 7 shows the results at five center frequencies; arrows indicate the critical bandwidth as measured by Zwicker. Agreement is excellent at all center frequencies except 250 Hz: two tones separated by more than a critical band are judged more pleasant or consonant than two tones within the same critical band.

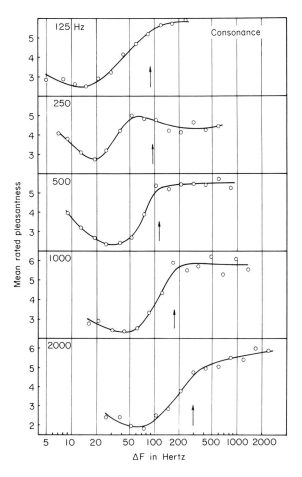

Figure 7 The rated pleasantness or consonance of a two-tone complex as a function of the frequency separation, Δf, between the tones. Parameter is the geometric mean of the two tones. Arrows indicate the critical bandwidth. (Adapted from Plomp and Levelt, 1962, by permission from the authors.)

Using their subjects' ratings and the critical-band measures, Plomp and Levelt (1965) calculated the consonance of two chords, each comprising six partials, as a function of the frequency separation. They found consonance peaks at the simple frequency ratios — octave, fifth, fourth, etc. — the usually accepted consonants in music. Analyzing actual musical compositions, they found that a composition by Bach has a greater mean distance between adjacent simultaneously sounded frequencies than does a modern composition by Dvořák. But in both compositions, the mean distance between adjacent frequencies is the same function of center frequency as is the critical band, although the distance is somewhat smaller in absolute value.

In a much earlier study, Mayer (1894) had twelve musicians judge musical consonance. The frequency separations at which two tones were first judged to be steady (consonant?) are generally smaller than those of Plomp and Levelt. In a second procedure, Mayer manually interrupted the output of a tuning fork and resonator in order to determine the lowest interruption rate at which the tone sounded steady. This "threshold" rate increases as a function of frequency; in terms of the modulation products, the separation between the carrier frequency and the nearest side-band also increases with the tone's frequency. The relation is similar to that observed by Mayer between his two-tone complexes and their center frequency (Greenwood, 1961b).

G. Discrimination of Partials in a Complex Tone

Plomp (1964) offered still another demonstration of the coalescence between two tones lying within the same critical band. He determined the ear's capacity to analyze a twelve-tone complex into its sinusoidal components. Each component or partial was at a loudness level of 60 phons. In one series of measurements, the partials were harmonically related and in another series they were not. The listener judged which of two pure tones was a component of the complex. One of the tones was always at the same frequency as one of the partials; the other lay half way between that frequency and the frequency of the next higher partial. Plomp calculated the critical bandwidth on the assumption that the highest distinguishable partial is separated from its neighbor by at least one critical band. So, for example, with a fundamental frequency of 250 Hz, 6.5 partials can be distinguished 75 percent of the time in the harmonic complex. This means that, up to 1625 Hz (6.5 × 250 Hz), a separation of 250 Hz between two partials is sufficient for them to be distinguished, but at higher frequencies, 250 Hz is not sufficient. In the same manner, Plomp obtained estimates of the critical band using twelve fundamental frequencies. Above 1000 Hz, Plomp's estimates coincide with the other critical-band measures, but below 1000 Hz, his estimates are about two-thirds as large.

III. CRITICAL RATIOS

A. In Man

Prior to the direct measures of the past decade, indirect estimates of the critical band were based mostly upon the masking of pure tones by wide-band noise. This approach originated with Fletcher (1940) and with Fletcher and Munson (1937), who suggested that a pure tone masked by a white noise is in effect masked by only a narrow, "critical" band of frequencies surrounding the tone, and that the power in this band is equal to the power in the tone. Given the masked threshold and these two assumptions, the "critical band" is easily calculated. Its width in hertz is the ratio of the intensity of the tone to the intensity per cycle of the noise. This ratio is now called the *critical ratio* to distinguish it from the directly measured critical band. The formula for a critical ratio is:

$$CR \text{ in dB} = T - L_{ps} \qquad (5\text{--}1)$$

where T is the threshold in decibels of the pure tone, and L_{ps} is the spectrum level of the wide-band noise. It follows that

$$CR \text{ in Hz} = \text{antilog} \quad (10^{-1} \times CR \text{ in dB}) \qquad (5\text{--}2)$$

Calculated in this manner, critical ratios in man turn out to be about 2.5 times smaller than the critical band (except below 200 Hz), and are a parallel function of frequency. The difference in absolute size disappears if we replace the hypothesis that the signal-to-noise ratio at the critical bandwidth is 0 dB, by the justifiable hypothesis that it is −4 dB (i.e., a ratio of 2.5). Fletcher (1940) based the original equal-power hypothesis on data that have proved misleading. He found that bands of noise only 30 Hz wide, centered at seven different frequencies, just masked a tone lying at the center frequency and having the same intensity. He assumed that the same signal-to-noise ratio of 0 dB holds at all subcritical bandwidths. Later results (Bauman *et al.*, 1953; Hamilton, 1957; Swets *et al.*, 1962, and van den Brink, 1964a) show that the signal-to-noise ratio at very narrow bandwidths is not the same as at the critical band. Hamilton (1957), for example, found that the signal-to-noise ratio decreased from about 0 dB for a band 30 Hz wide to almost −4 dB at the critical bandwidth of 145 Hz (the center frequency was 800 Hz). Greenwood (1961a) and Zwicker (1958) measured critical-band signal-to-noise ratios that vary from −3 to −8 dB.

The variability in this signal-to-noise ratio means that no very stable estimate of the *absolute* size of the critical band can be made from the critical ratio. Nevertheless, the critical ratio does provide a way to compare critical bands as a function of frequency. For example, multiplying the Hawkins and Stevens (1950) critical ratios by 2.5 gives the unfilled circles in Fig. 1. Their deviation at low frequencies may reflect an increase in the signal-to-noise ratio there, as suggested by Greenwood's (1961a) data. More relevant is the fact that these critical ratios are independent of the overall level of the masking noise between 20 and 90 dB SPL. Other measurements of the masking of pure tones by wide-band noise yield similar values for the critical ratio (Bilger and Hirsh, 1956; and Green *et al.*, 1959).

B. In Animals

Animals that have auditory systems similar to man's should have a critical-band mechanism, although the size of the critical band may depend upon the length of the basilar membrane and the encompassed frequency range. No direct measurements of critical bandwidth have been published, but there are several indirect measures (via critical ratios) for cats, rats, and chinchillas.

Figure 8 gives the results of measurements on four cats (Watson, 1963), six chinchillas (Miller, 1964), five to seven rats (Gourevitch, 1965), and four men (Hawkins and Stevens, 1950). In all four species, the critical ratio is invariant over a wide range of masking noise levels. The functions for the first three are similar in shape to man's and therefore resemble his critical-band function (see Fig. 1). This resemblance suggests that the mechanism underlying the critical band (and the critical ratio) is the same in these animals as in man.

To use these measured critical ratios to calculate critical band-

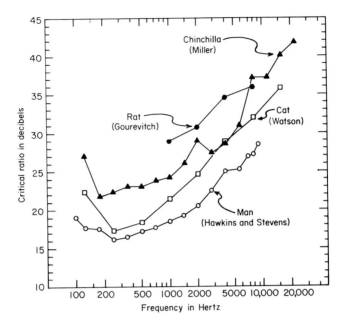

Figure 8   The critical ratio measured in four species as a function of the frequency of the masked tone. The critical ratio is the difference between the spectrum level of the wide-band masking noise and the level of the just masked tone.

widths, we need only assume that critical bands in animals are approximately 2.5 times wider than their critical ratios, as in man. Then the critical band at center frequencies above 500 Hz is two to three times wider in the cat than in man, four to nine times wider in the chinchilla, and about ten times wider in the rat. Adding 4 dB to the critical ratios at 1000 Hz, for example, gives critical-band estimates of 175 Hz in man, 360 Hz in the cat, 670 Hz in the chinchilla, and 1950 Hz in the rat. Such large differences are not unexpected since the frequency ranges handled by these species vary from under 20,000 Hz in man to about 100,000 Hz in the rat while the length of the basilar membrane varies from about 35 mm in man to about 10 mm in the rat. The differences among the estimated bandwidths are greatly reduced when the critical bands are converted to lengths on the basilar membrane. These conversions are made with functions that relate position of maximum stimulation along the basilar membrane to frequency (Békésy, 1960a, pp. 442 and 507) or with data obtained from lesions induced on the basilar membrane (Schuknecht,

1953). In the human, the cat, and the rat,* the estimated critical band at 1000 Hz covers from 1 to 2 mm of basilar membrane.

These results suggest that the cochleas of these animals may be approximate scale models of each other (Békésy and Rosenblith, 1951; Greenwood, 1961b). Now direct measurements of the critical band, such as in two-tone masking, are needed to check the critical-ratio estimates and also to check the irregularities in Fig. 8.

IV. THE CRITICAL BAND AS AN INTERNAL FILTER

Detection theorists use a hypothetical critical band to account for data on the detectability of signals in noise. This band represents an assumed internal process; it is anchored only indirectly to stimulus measures. It indicates the size and sometimes the shape of the internal filter that would be required in an ideal observer to yield results similar to those obtained with humans. Fletcher's (1940) critical-ratio concept also involved an internal mechanism operating to "filter out" that part of the masking noise not adjacent to the signal frequency.

Swets *et al.* (1962) made ingenious use of the detection model. They reasoned that, since the detectability of a fixed signal depends on how much noise reaches the detector, the width of the internal filter lying between the noise source and the detector can be estimated by comparing changes in detectability (a) when the noise is varied in bandwidth, and (b) when its bandwidth is kept broad, but its power is varied. When bandwidth is varied, they assumed, the internal filter and the real external filter work in series to reduce the noise power reaching the detector. Then "the change in the noise power at the detector . . . . can be determined indirectly if it is assumed that the changes produced by varying an external filter on the noise are comparable to changes produced by simply varying the power of a broad-band noise." Thus "the changes in the detectability index which are produced by external filtering can be translated into changes in noise power at the detector" (pp. 110–111). Given the size of the external filter, the size of the internal filter necessary to achieve these changes at the detector could then be calculated. In this manner, the results from three listeners yielded values for the internal filter that averaged 41, 79, and 95 Hz depending upon the

---

*Most probably also in the chinchilla, as inferred from measurements of D. H. Eldredge (personal communication).

shape — single tuned, Gaussian, or rectangular — assumed for the filter. Since the critical band is 160 Hz at 1000 Hz, no simple correspondence between the empirical critical band and the internal filter seemed forthcoming. However, the assumption that varying an external filter has the same effect on detectability as varying the power of a wideband noise was not supported by the data. According to this assumption, halving the bandwidth of the narrow-band noise should result in the same increase in detectability as reducing the power in the wide-band noise 3 dB, but examination of the data reveals that halving the bandwidth is comparable to reducing the broad-band noise by 1.5 dB. Hamilton (1957) also measured a 1.5-dB threshold decrease per halving of bandwidth. This slow change in threshold at narrow bandwidths is probably caused by factors unrelated to the critical-band mechanism — factors such as the fluctuations in narrowband noise that make the masker sound like the signal (Hamilton, 1957; Bos and de Boer, 1966). Thus, if only the critical-band mechanism were operating, detectability would increase twice as fast with decreasing bandwidth. The same detectability measured with a 10-Hz wide noise band, for example, should occur with a 20-Hz wide band. So the values for the internal filter calculated by Swets et al. could be doubled. In that case the internal filter, taken as equivalent to a Gaussian filter, is the same width (158 Hz at 1000 Hz, measured at the half-power points) as the critical band.

In another type of experiment, the evaluation of the internal filter is based upon measurements of the detectability of two or more tones as a function of their frequency separation. Such experiments measure the critical bandwidth directly, under the assumption that two tones separated by more than a critical band are more difficult to detect than two tones within the same band (cf. Gässler, 1954). This assumption has at times been borne out (Marill, 1956; van den Brink, 1964b), but more often no critical frequency separation has appeared (Schafer and Gales, 1949; Veniar, 1958; Green, 1958b). Disparate results are not surprising since the difference between the thresholds of a subcritical two-tone complex and a supercritical complex could not amount to more than 3 dB.[*] The interpretation of the divergent

---

[*]Greenberg and Larkin (1966) may have surmounted this difficulty. They instructed subjects to listen for a tone of known pitch. Then they presented tones at other frequencies as well, without informing the subjects. Detection was about as good when the unfamiliar tones were within the same critical band as the familiar one, and was worse when they were outside it. This result suggests that a listener can be primed to attend to tones within a single critical band to the partial exclusion of other tones.

results, however, has been in terms of several alternative models of the internal filter: a single filter of fixed width that can scan the incoming signals, a filter of variable size, and multiple filters operating simultaneously. Swets (1963), in summarizing these and many other results, concluded that "evidence for involvement of cognitive factors makes it seem clear that the number, the frequency locations, and the widths of the critical bands which are operative in a given auditory task reflect to a substantial extent the strategy of listening that is adopted by the observer for that particular task" (p. 429). In this context, "critical bands" should read internal filters. Central or cognitive factors doubtless contribute heavily to the variance in critical-band measurements, but the seven experiments described in Section II succeeded, despite large variability, in obtaining a remarkably consistent set of measurements of the critical band. So, despite the manipulations one performs with the hypothetical internal filters in order to accommodate a theory, the fact remains that the empirical critical band summarizes a great variety of data.

V. CRITICAL BANDS AT SHORT DURATIONS

The experiments described in Section II used stimuli whose duration exceeded 150 or 200 msec, and for them, the size of the critical band (and the critical ratio) is well established. A major question concerns the constancy of the critical bandwidth as duration is shortened. If the critical band is the same size at very short and at long durations, the ear's frequency selectivity might be based on rapid mechanical events. If, on the other hand, the critical band is wider (or nonexistent) at very short durations, the frequency selectivity might be a neural process that requires a certain build-up time. Not only would such information be relevant to a physiological model of the critical-band mechanism, but it is also needed to clarify threshold measurements and loudness judgments for brief tones, since all such measurements involve a redistribution of energy — effective signal bandwidth increases with decreasing duration.

Several threshold experiments (Hamilton, 1957; Scholl, 1962a,b; Zwicker, 1965a,b) indicated wider critical bands at durations under 100 msec than are usually measured at longer durations. These results suggest an altered critical-band mechanism that could also account for many of the data on wide-band and narrow-band masking at short durations (Elliott, 1965; Zwicker, 1965a,b). However, an altered mechanism is not implied by loudness measurements; they show that the critical band is independent of duration (Port, 1963; Zwicker, 1965a,b).

A. Threshold at Short Durations

Most studies of the relation between threshold and duration deal with either tones or white noise. Inferences about the critical band are possible from these studies because the spectrum of a tonal signal widens with decreasing duration, but the confounding of duration with changes in spectrum requires caution in the interpretation of the data. Moreover, the spectrum can seldom be precisely specified. Several studies varied duration and bandwidth independently, thus giving a firmer basis for critical-band measurement. In some experiments, the effective duration of the masking sound was varied; in others, the duration of the signal was varied.

Masker Duration Varied. To determine the effect of masker duration on the critical band, Scholl (1962b), Zwicker (1965b), and Elliott (1965) measured the masked threshold of a signal whose onset was delayed for a variable time period relative to the masker's onset. In such experiments, the signal's duration must be short. Otherwise, the total "effective" masker duration (signal delay plus signal duration) cannot be made short enough. Both Scholl and Zwicker also varied the masker's bandwidth.

Scholl's (1962b) masker was two third-octave bands of noise lasting 500 msec and lying on either side of a 2000-Hz tonal signal. Figure 9 shows the threshold of the 3-msec tone pulse as a function of the frequency separation, Δf, between the noises; the delay time, t, is the parameter. If the critical band is the value of Δf at which the threshold began to go down, then as t decreases from 300 to 3 msec, the critical Δf grows from almost 300 Hz, the steady-state value, to 750 Hz. Results are similar for tones at 500 and 6000 Hz.

Zwicker's (1965b) masker was a single band of white noise of variable width. The signal, at the center frequency of the band, was a 4800-Hz tone lasting 2 msec or a 1000-Hz tone lasting 5 msec. As expected, at long delays, the threshold remains constant as bandwidth increases beyond the steady-state critical band. At short delays, however, the threshold rises as the masker widens well beyond this value. So with a supercritical masking noise, threshold increases with decreasing delay time, but with a critical (or, presumably, subcritical) masker, threshold is independent of delay time. Elliott (1965) obtained similar results.

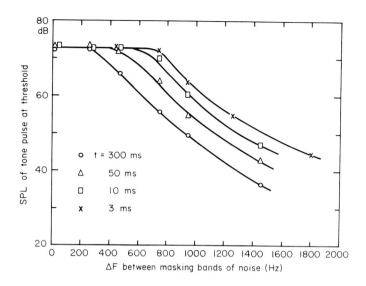

Figure 9 Masked threshold of a 3-msec, 2000-Hz tone as a function of the frequency separation between two narrows bands of masking noise. The parameter is the delay, t, of the onset of the tone relative to the onset of the noise. (Adapted from Scholl, 1962b. By permission from *Acustica*.)

These findings suggest that a larger part of a supercritical masking noise contributes to masking at short durations than at long durations. Scholl's (1962b) straightforward interpretation of these findings was that the critical-band mechanism requires a build-up time — his data suggest a time constant of about 10 msec. Accordingly, one would expect a tone outside the frequency limits of a narrow-band masker to have a higher threshold at short delays, owing to increased interaction between signal and noise. Elliott (1965) measured the threshold of a tone pulse masked by narrow-band noise as a function of frequency and delay time, and, except at low frequencies, confirmed this expectation. The resulting masked audiograms, however, show no flattening at the top as Greenwood's (1961a) did when his narrow-band masker was wider than the critical band. So if the critical-band mechanism does operate with a wider filter at short durations, the change is not equivalent to an increase in stimulus bandwidth; we cannot trade effective masker duration for masker bandwidth. Shortening signal delay is more like decreasing the slopes — spreading the skirts — of a narrow-band masker. In this connection, it is interesting to note that, at short delays, Zwicker (1965b) found no threshold ele-

vation or "overshoot" in the masking of a 2-msec, 5000-Hz signal by
a narrow-band noise, one critical band wide and centered at 2900 Hz
—nor did Zwicker and Wright (1963) in the masking of 10-msec tone
pulses by a narrow-band noise centered at 1000 Hz. Their narrow-
band filters were much sharper than the one used by Elliott, and at
1000 Hz, the pulse's rise/fall times were longer. A measurable overshoot seems to require, among other things, a filter with an attenuation slope gradual enough so that flattening in the auditory system
raises the internal noise level enough to affect the threshold of an
off-center tone.

The assumption of reduced frequency selectivity at short delays is
consistent with some of Zwicker's (1965a) other data. He showed that
the threshold of a white-noise signal masked by white noise is independent of signal delay. As the bandwidth of the signal narrows, an
overshoot appears and grows until it equals the overshoot measured
with a tonal signal, a reasonable result since reduced frequency selectivity should mean that a larger portion of a wide-band masker contributes to masking narrow-band signals at short delays. A wide-band
signal would already be masked at long delays by much of the wide-
band masker, so that reducing frequency selectivity by shortening signal delay should not produce a threshold elevation. However,
Zwicker (1965b) did measure an overshoot for a wide-band signal
when he introduced a frequency gap of about 1000 Hz in the white-
noise masker. That part of the white-noise signal lying in the gap
seems to determine detectability, and as the delay time is reduced,
the threshold rises because more of the white-noise masker interacts
with signal energy in the gap. A similar overshoot was measured for
a tonal signal lying in the gap.*

*The overshoot for the tone masked by white noise with a gap is only a few decibels
more than for the tone masked by white noise without a gap. According to Zwicker
(1965b), this similarity is contrary to the notion of reduced frequency selectivity at
short durations. He reasoned that opening a gap around a tone should reduce the
threshold more at long delays (where selectivity is supposed to be fully developed)
than at short delays. Such a differential effect would enhance the usual overshoot
found with a wide-band masker. This reasoning may be valid for narrow gaps but
seems inappropriate to wide gaps. If the gap is so wide that the noise is totally removed, then the insertion of the "gap" must reduce the threshold *more* at short delays than at long, because the threshold of a tone in the quiet is necessarily independent of "delay time" relative to a nonexistent noise, whereas the threshold of a
tone in white noise decreases with increasing delay. The amount of overshoot for a
tone masked by a white noise with a gap should depend on the width of the gap, with
the greatest overshoot occurring in a gap around one critical band wide and the least

In summary, the experiments on the role of effective masker duration suggest that critical bandwidth is larger at short durations. The inference that the widening of the critical band is caused by reduced frequency selectivity at short durations is supported by most of the results both with narrow-band and with wide-band masking.

Signal Duration Varied. What happens to the critical band when the effective masker duration is relatively long and the *signal* duration is shortened? In his experiment on the masking of an 800-Hz tone as a function of masker bandwidth, Hamilton (1957) also varied signal duration. At durations of 25 and 50 msec, threshold energy continued to increase with masker bandwidth up to a larger bandwidth than at longer signal durations. This result means that the critical band at short signal durations is wider even when the masker precedes the signal by a presumably long time. (Hamilton did not specify the signal delay time, but it was probably at least 500 msec in his 2-sec noise bursts.)

Scholl (1962a) varied signal duration and *signal* bandwidth. He measured the masked threshold of bands of noise of different durations as a function of their bandwidth. The masker was a uniform noise. At 3 msec, threshold remains approximately constant as bandwidth increases, which is quite different from what happens at 500 msec. There, the threshold rises with bandwidth beyond the critical band (Gässler, 1954); it also rises at 10 and 50 msec, but not as much. This experiment showed that the critical band widens with decreasing signal duration until at 3 msec it disappears. (Creelman, 1961, also found that the masked threshold of short trains of damped sinusoids is independent of bandwidth.)

These data, like those obtained with short masker durations, fit the hypothesis that the ear's frequency selectivity is poorer at short durations. When the signal duration is very short, all the signal energy, within and without the steady-state critical band, contributes to detectability, and threshold becomes independent of bandwidth. Consequently, at brief masker durations, threshold should remain independent of bandwidth since the ear ought to analyze neither the masker nor the signal — only the overall signal-to-noise ratio should matter. Zwicker (1965a) made these measurements with a 2-msec signal delayed 2 msec relative to the onset of a wide-band masker.

---

in very wide gaps. Until these predictions are tested, it is not clear whether Zwicker's results for a single gap of intermediate size support the hypothesis of reduced selectivity at short delays.

The threshold was not constant, but *decreased* with increasing band-width.

Another difficulty concerns the implication in Scholl's (1962a) experiments that the ear analyzes the noise and signal independently. Despite a long signal delay during which the ear has time to develop full frequency selectivity for the masking noise, the ear apparently has to start building its selectivity from scratch in order to handle a short-duration signal when it comes on. The resolution of these difficulties calls for more data and better theory. For now, let us see what relevant data can be culled from the literature on temporal summation.

Most experiments on temporal summation vary signal duration, but neither signal nor masker bandwidth. Nevertheless these experiments may be relevant to the critical band. Assuming that the ear is a perfect temporal integrator with a time constant of about 200 msec (Zwis-locki, 1960), we can distinguish two possibilities: (a) if the critical bandwidth increases with decreasing duration, then threshold energy should remain constant below 200 msec even at durations so short that much of the signal energy falls outside the steady-state critical band (this simple prediction assumes that the critical bandwidth increases more rapidly than the effective bandwidth of the signal); and (b) if the critical bandwidth does not change with duration, then threshold energy should begin to increase at durations where significant energy falls outside the steady-state critical band (this prediction is based on Gässler's [1954] finding that energy outside the maximally intense critical band does not contribute to detection).

Many studies (Garner, 1947; Garner and Miller, 1947; Gales and Wilcott, 1954; Feldtkeller and Oetinger, 1956; Green *et al.*, 1957; Hamilton, 1957; Plomp and Bouman, 1959; Miskolczy-Fodor, 1959, 1960; Békésy, 1960a; Goldstein and Kramer, 1960; Plomp, 1961; Scholl, 1962a; Zwicker and Wright, 1963; van den Brink, 1964a; Dallos and Olsen, 1964; Sheeley and Bilger, 1964; Zwicker, 1965a) have reported on the relation between duration and the threshold of pure tones both in the quiet and in noise. Most of these studies showed that the constant-energy law holds, even for the shortest durations used. However, not every investigator used durations short enough to spread energy outside the steady-state critical band, thereby permitting a clear distinction between a constant and an increasing critical bandwidth. Garner (1947), Green *et al.* (1957), Hamilton (1957), Plomp and Bouman (1959), Miskolczy-Fodor (1960), Plomp (1961), and Sheeley and Bilger (1964) all found an increase in threshold energy, but at different durations. Among these studies, only Garner's (1947) measured an increase in threshold energy at a duration corresponding to a normal-sized critical band. The others found that energy began to increase at such long durations (e.g., 10 to 50 msec in Plomp and Bouman's study) that the effective bandwidth of the signal was quite narrow. So in these experiments, the short-duration critical band, measured indirectly, appears to be narrower than normal — certainly not wider.

However, the prediction of a wider critical band was fulfilled in at least four studies covering frequencies from 250 to 4000 Hz (Feldtkeller and Oetinger, 1956; Scholl, 1962a; Zwicker and Wright, 1963; van den Brink, 1964a). In all four, the energy threshold of tone masked by wide-band noise remains constant down to durations briefer than 10 msec. Thus, at short durations, the ear appears able to integrate energy over more than a single, normal-sized critical band. Zwicker (1965a) also found no change in the energy threshold for a 5000-Hz tone down to 2 msec, but he did find a small increase for a 1000-Hz tone.

No ready explanation for the discordant findings is at hand. But differences among subjects and procedures probably play a more important role at short than at long durations.

Measurements of wide-band noise threshold as a function of duration are more consistent. These studies (Garner, 1947; Miller, 1948; Feldtkeller and Oetinger, 1956; Miskolczy-Fodor, 1959; Green, 1960; Scholl, 1962a; Small *et al.*, 1962) showed that the threshold energy in a wide-band noise *decreases* below about 200 msec. One simple interpretation is that an enlarged critical band at short duration permits a larger portion of the noise spectrum to contribute to detectability than can contribute at longer durations.

It is interesting to note that Plomp's (1961) analysis of his own data on the threshold of periodic tone pulses also implies a decrease in critical bandwidth with increasing duration. Jeffress (1964) too computed (from the data of Green *et al.*, 1957) values for the "effective" bandwidth of an assumed internal filter, which decreases in size with increasing duration.

B. Loudness at Short Durations

Recall that the loudness of long-duration stimuli increases with bandwidth beyond the critical band (except near threshold); within the critical band, loudness is approximately independent of spectral distribution, provided overall level is constant. So if the critical band is larger at 5 than at 200 msec (as most threshold measurements seem to indicate), the loudness of a 5-msec band of noise should increase less with bandwidth than that of a band of noise 200 msec or longer. But Port (1963) found that the loudness of a 5-msec noise increases with bandwidth just as the loudness of a 1200-msec noise does (Fig. 10). At the widest bandwidth, the difference between the noise and an equally loud 2000-Hz tone was 18 dB at both durations. Port obtained this result with a loudspeaker and three noise bursts per second. Zwicker (1965b) obtained similar results using an earphone and a burst frequency of one per second. In more recent experiments, I found that the loudness of a simultaneous pair of equally loud tones is the same function of frequency separation whether the tones last 5 msec or 300 msec.

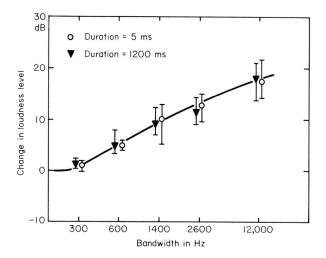

Figure 10   The change in the loudness level of noise bands at two durations as a function of bandwidth. The bands were centered at 2000 Hz. The briefer noise was at 50 dB SPL, and the longer noise at 40 dB. (Adapted from Port, 1963. By permission from *Acustica*.)

Since the relation between loudness and bandwidth is independent of stimulus duration, it follows that the critical band is independent of duration. It also follows that the loudness of subcritical stimuli, such as pure tones, and of supercritical stimuli should vary in the same way as a function of duration. Port (1963) showed that the loudness of each remains constant when duration is reduced below 70 msec, provided sound energy is held constant. Of course, if duration were reduced so much that the energy in subcritical stimuli were spread beyond the critical band, less energy should then be required for constant loudness. Neither Port's nor most other studies used durations brief enough to bear on this question.

Zwicker (1966) measured the same relation between loudness and duration as did Port, and for both a pure tone and wide-band noise, but earlier studies often did not. Some (Munson, 1947, and Small *et al.*, 1962) reported that as duration decreases, sound energy must be increased to maintain constant loudness; others (Miller, 1948; Garner, 1949; Békésy, 1960a) reported that energy must be decreased. Niese (1957, 1959) confirmed Port's constant-energy rule for both tones and white noise, but he measured a shorter time constant. These studies with their divergent outcomes do not suggest, however, that the loudness of subcritical and supercritical stimuli depends in different ways on duration. Rather, they show how difficult it is to measure loudness as a function of duration. Reichardt (1965) described the difficulties that beset such attempts; individual subjects differ widely not only in their judgmental criteria but also seem to have different time constants. It is easier to measure loudness summation at a single duration as a function of bandwidth, as Port, Zwicker, and I have done, and come up with consistent results about the critical band.

The direct measurements, although limited, give no evidence for an increased critical bandwidth at short durations, which is certainly surprising, since *threshold* measurements have shown that the critical band increases with decreasing duration. However, some of the same threshold measurements have also shown that the masked audiogram for narrow-band stimuli changes little or not at all as a function of duration (Zwicker and Wright, 1963; Elliott, 1965; Zwicker, 1965b). If the masked audiogram changes little, so does the excitation pattern derived from it. Since we assume that loudness depends closely on the excitation pattern (Fletcher and Munson, 1937; Zwicker and Scharf, 1965), the invariance of the excitation pattern as a function of duration is congruent with the finding that loudness changes with bandwidth in about the same way at short and long durations. The problem becomes one of understanding how the patterns manage to remain the same at short durations, while the critical band widens. Before I speculate further about the critical-band mechanism and the ear's frequency selectivity, let me make this simple empirical summary: in threshold measurements, the critical band appears to widen with decreasing duration below about 100 msec; in loudness measurements, it appears to remain constant.

VI. CORRELATES OF THE CRITICAL BAND

The critical-band function bears a close resemblance in form to several other functions of frequency: the place of maximal displacement on the basilar membrane, the difference limen for frequency, and the mel scale of pitch (Békésy and Rosenblith, 1951). Probably the pivotal relation is to the location on the basilar membrane. This relation makes it appear that critical bands as well as difference limens and equal mel intervals correspond to constant distances on the basilar membrane. The critical band corresponds to about 1.3 mm along the basilar membrane if we assume 24 critical bands (up to 16,000 Hz) laid end to end on a basilar membrane 32 mm long. The correspondence, however, tends to break down at low frequencies. Zwislocki (1965) suggested that a better correspondence obtains between these various psychophysical measures—critical bands, mels, and difference limens—and neural density in the cochlea. Each critical band, for example, corresponds to about 1300 neurons.

Although useful and provocative, the assumptions that critical bands correspond to equal distances or to a constant number of neurons must be considered tentative because of the uncertainties in the measurement of frequency localization on the basilar membrane. (Indeed, Fletcher, 1953, suggested that the critical band may be more closely related to the *width* of the basilar membrane at a given point than to its length.) Despite this reservation, critical bands vary little in terms of their corresponding distances on the basilar membrane, quite in contrast to their large changes in size when measured in hertz. Measured in mels, the size of the critical band also varies little, from 100 mels at low center frequencies to 180 mels at high (Stevens and Volkmann, 1940). The mel scale is not accurate enough, however, to distinguish 100 from 180 mels at opposite ends of the scale, so that the pitch range of the critical band may in fact be fairly constant, perhaps approximating 150 mels. Measured in numbers of frequency-difference limens, the critical band is once again fairly constant, comprising approximately 60 difference limens at all center frequencies. Watson (1963) noted that, in the cat, the critical ratio is equal to about 20 difference limens as measured by Elliott *et al.* (1960); hence the cat's critical *band,* as derived in Section III B, would be about 50 difference limens. These correlations imply a common mechanism underlying critical-band analysis, pitch perception, and frequency discrimination. It would therefore be of fundamental interest to compare directly, for example, the effects of shortened durations or of various types of hearing impairment on these phenomena. The data available show that both pitch perception and frequency discrimination deteriorate at durations shorter than 100 to 200 msec (Stevens and Davis, 1938). It remains to be tested whether this deterioration is consistent with the increased critical bandwidth suggested by threshold measurements at short durations.

VII. APPLICATIONS OF THE CRITICAL BAND

A. A Model of Loudness Summation

Zwicker (1958, 1963a) developed a system based on the critical band for the objective calculation of loudness. This system also serves as a model of loudness summation that brings order to a large and complex set of data (Zwicker and Scharf, 1965). Essentially, the model permits the conversion of the physical spectrum of a given sound into a psychological "spectrum" in which frequency is replaced by "tonalness" and amplitude by specific loudness. Tonalness is related to frequency by the critical-band function. A unit of tonalness corresponds in width to a critical band, but it is called a Bark (after the German acoustician Barkhausen) and replaces the critical band in order to distinguish it, a measure of assumed sensory events, from the critical band. Such a distinction is necessary since there is seldom a one-to-one correspondence between the number of critical bands in the acoustical stimulus and the number of Barks in its psychological representation. For example, an ideal pure tone represented by a single line on the physical spectrum is represented on the psychological spectrum by a curve spreading over several units of tonalness (this spread is inferred from the masking audiogram produced by a pure tone). The loudness per Bark or specific loudness is related to amplitude by a formula based on Stevens' power law (Stevens, 1957). Integration of specific loudness yields a value for the total loudness in sones.

The critical band not only contributes a rational unit of measurement to the model, but it also permits the precise determination of the loudness patterns produced by pure tones. Normally these patterns are derived from the masking pattern of the sound whose loudness is to be calculated. When the sound is a pure tone, however, beating between it and the pure-tone probe precludes measurements of masking near the tone and its harmonics. Substituting a critical or subcritical band of noise for the pure tone in the masking measurements avoids this problem. If the noise is centered on the tone's frequency and is equally intense, a masking pattern results that, except for the absence of the irregularities caused by beating, is essentially the same as that produced by the tone (Zwicker, 1956; Ehmer, 1959).

B. Threshold Model

Zwicker (1956) developed a model for the calculation of the threshold of pure tones and of noise, both masked and unmasked. The model rests on his (1956, 1962) finding that a change of 1 dB in the intensity of a critical or subcritical band of noise is just detectable (except at low frequencies where a larger change is required). The modulation of the lower cutoff frequency of a wide-band noise also becomes detectable when the lowest critical band within the noise undergoes a change of 1 dB. In terms of the tonalness scale, a change in either amplitude or frequency becomes noticeable as soon as the excitation changes at least 1 dB over at least 1 Bark. Excitation, like specific loudness, is derived from masking patterns and can be thought to represent neural activity.

The concepts of excitation and tonalness are elaborated elsewhere (Zwicker, 1958; Feldtkeller, 1963; Zwicker and Scharf, 1965), but an example of a straightforward application of the model can be useful. Scholl (1963) predicted within 1 dB the threshold of a truck horn masked by an internal-combustion engine. He first measured the sound pressure level of each component critical band of the wide-band engine noise; then he analyzed the signal, also a wide-band noise, into its component critical bands. The masked threshold predicted for the horn is equal to the signal level that brings at least one of the signal's component critical bands to within 6 dB of the masker level in the same band. (When the level difference is 6 dB, the excitation over 1 Bark changes by the required 1 dB.) In these particular calculations, conversion to the tonalness scale and the Bark was not necessary because the spectra of both the signal and masker covered the whole audible frequency range.

This example is simpler than most, because it can be solved without taking account of the increased size of the difference limen at low frequencies and of the bandwidth of the signal. The detectability of a signal also appears to increase with the number of component critical bands or Bark units lying almost within 6 dB of the masker. In the model, the reduced sensitivity at low frequencies is handled by adding an appropriate amount to the measured levels of the affected critical bands within the masker. The role of the number of near-threshold critical bands is handled by subtracting an appropriate value from the calculated overall masked threshold. Both of these correction factors are published in Scholl's (1963) paper; it also describes the whole model and shows how it can be extended to short-duration and pulsed signals.

C. Speech

The role, if any, of the critical band in the perception of speech remains obscure even though the initial measurements of the critical ratio were closely related to a search for a meaningful analysis of the speech spectrum (Fletcher, 1953, p. 293). French and Steinberg (1947), measuring the intelligibility of speech passed through low and high-cutoff filters, found that 20 adjacent frequency bands contribute about equally to intelligibility when each approximates a critical band. The width of the 20 bands does not grow as rapidly with frequency above 1500 Hz as does the critical bandwidth. However, as French and Steinberg pointed out, such results apply *in detail* only to the particular recording system, loudspeakers, listeners, and speech materials used.

Since these first encouraging results, no other investigation of the possible role of the critical band in speech was published until a report by Morton and Carpenter (1963). They thought that the formants of speech can be identified in the absence of a prominent peak, provided that the two most intense harmonic components are at least one critical band apart. Measurements with complex tones derived from pulse trains supported the notion and led to the study of stimuli comprising two sinusoids. Morton and Carpenter tested the hypothesis that a change in the energy distribution of two tones lying within the same critical band is more difficult to perceive than a corresponding change in two tones separated by more than one critical band. They reasoned that the ear tends to integrate the energy lying within a critical band, thus obscuring variations in energy distribution. Their preliminary results, collected at a single center frequency with only three frequency separations, support the hypothesis. Measurements collected by Chaves and Scharf (1966) with six to nine frequency separations at each of four center frequencies, give a different picture. They showed that it is usually more difficult to detect an intensity difference between two tones close or far apart in frequency than between two tones separated by some intermediate distance, roughly equal to the critical bandwidth. The effect of Δf is clearest when the lower-frequency component is more intense than the higher-frequency component. The difference between the two studies probably stems from Chaves and Scharf's use of more experienced subjects. The implication for speech recognition may be that formants are easiest to identify when harmonics are separated by about one critical band.

One may also attack the problem of speech intelligibility by filtering the signals to determine which components are required for correct identification. Most published studies used filter widths too large to be relevant to critical bands (see Kryter, 1960). But Castle (1964a) found that isolated vowels passed through third-octave filters "were often correctly recognized when only a single formant frequency was presented to the listeners" (p. 149). Does this fact mean that the listener's ability to identify simple speech sounds is unimpaired by the suppression of components outside the critical bandwidth? Obviously many more data are needed, including measurements of the effect of small variations in the location and width of the filters (which was not part of Castle's work with vowels). In a related study, however, Castle (1964b) measured the intelligibility of words passed through filters varied in width and sharpness. Even with the spectrum reduced to the width of a single critical band (240 Hz at a center frequency of 1560 Hz), the intelligibility score was 25 percent with sharp filtering. A higher score under such severe filtering could not be expected for word stimuli whose spectra change rapidly over time. It must be that the critical-band mechanism can follow the frequency transformations that are necessary for recognition of the complete word. Perhaps careful adjustment of the filtering to the spectrum of a stable signal such as an isolated vowel (e.g., centering the passband on the appropriate formant frequency) would yield much higher intelligibility scores.

Still another approach to the investigation of the critical band in speech is Zwicker's (1963b). He built an electronic analog of the ear; the device includes an analysis of the spectrum into critical bands. These critical bands, unlike the ear's, are at fixed frequencies. Nevertheless, preliminary investigation (with numbers as the speech input) indicate that the relevant information is retained when the signal is filtered and otherwise transformed. The presence of the original speech information in the output of the analog model is tested by converting the output into a pulse sequence that stimulates the "listener's" forearm via 24 vibrators. Subjects can learn to distinguish the digits 0 through 9. What effect a change in the width and location of the analog's filtering system would have on the information content of the output cannot be measured with this apparatus. Although Zwicker's analog does not demonstrate that the ear actually makes use of its critical-band mechanism in the perception of speech, the fact that a spectral analysis into critical bands does not remove the original information lends some support to such a notion.

D. Critical Bands in Impaired Ears

The measurement of critical bandwidth in impaired ears may provide evidence for the locus of the critical-band mechanism and also may clarify some of the perceptual difficulties associated with hearing loss. On an a priori basis, it seems reasonable that, if the critical-band mechanism were primarily cochlear, any gross disturbance of the cochlea might very well vitiate the operation of the mechanism.

De Boer (1961) was the first to report direct measures of the critical band in a pathological ear — one apparently suffering a cochlear lesion. He measured the threshold of pure tones masked by bands of noise of varying width, and also the threshold of bands of noise in the quiet. The patient showed strong evidence of an enlarged critical band. Later, De Boer (personal communication, 1964) used a different technique on a number of patients: he measured the masked threshold of a pure tone located in a gap of white noise as a function of the width of the gap (Webster *et al.*, 1952). These measures also led him to conclude that patients with a cochlear impairment generally show increased critical bands.

Support for de Boer's conclusion comes from Langenbeck (1951), who reported that, of 263 clinically examined ears, those with inner-ear lesions and a loss exceeding 40 dB at their best frequency had a lower threshold for a uniform masking noise (similar to white noise) than for any pure tone. In contrast, the normal ear has a threshold about 10 dB higher for a uniform masking noise than for a middle-frequency tone (Gässler, 1954; Scholl, 1962a), and this difference is explained by the ear's inability to use more than one or two critical bands for the detection of the noise. If the critical band were enlarged, then the threshold of the noise relative to that of the tone would be reduced. (Such a finding in normal ears for short-duration tones and noises is also attributed to an increased critical band.)

However, indirect measurements based on critical ratios (calculated from wide-band masking) do not indicate a widened critical band in impaired hearing. Palva *et al.* (1953), reviewing the literature on noise audiometry, noted that some reports show increased masking (increased critical ratio) in perceptual deafness and other reports do not; the only firm conclusion was that the critical ratio is normal in conductive deafness. Their own study of 81 ears, normal and pathological, shows no significant differences among several types of pathology in the masking effect of a 100-dB white noise on any frequency ranging from 250 to 8000 Hz. This finding, supported by Jerger *et al.* (1960), suggests that the critical band of masking is usually not enlarged in any common auditory pathology. More recently, Simon (1963) measured increased critical ratios in nine ears with cochlear impairment, particularly at 4000 Hz, where loudness recruitment was present. Nevertheless, the weight of evidence indicates that the critical ratio is not increased in cochlear impairment.

A study of loudness summation in impaired ears (Scharf and Hellman, 1966) yielded a less equivocal picture than the threshold measurements. In ears with cochlear impairment and an average hearing loss of 65 dB, the critical band was much wider than normal, for loudness did not change with Δf increasing even up to six or seven normal-sized critical bands. (In ears with conductive impairment, the critical band in loudness summation was normal.) Measures of narrow-band masking, however, revealed no significant increase in the spread of masking and excitation at the low sensation levels tested—such an increase would be expected if the ear's frequency selectivity were grossly altered. This normal spread of excitation on which loudness is thought to be directly dependent led to the conjecture that in cochlear pathology the critical-band mechanism might be disturbed at a level beyond the formation of the excitation patterns.

VIII. THE CRITICAL-BAND MECHANISM

The critical-band mechanism appears to discriminate between sound energy within a single critical band and energy outside the band, thus permitting the auditory system to treat subcritical stimuli alike with respect to threshold, masking, loudness, and harmonic discrimination. The mechanism is analogous to a set of band-pass filters with variable center frequencies. This analogy has been commonly used in the interpretation of critical-band data, especially in signal-detection theory. Two immediate questions are where and how the filtering takes place.

The locus of the critical-band mechanism is probably peripheral, perhaps right in the cochlea as suggested by the similarity between the critical-band function and the function relating frequency to locus on the basilar membrane. Some empirical support comes from Niese's (1960) demonstration that the increase of loudness with bandwidth cannot occur interaurally: for example, loudness does not increase when the frequency separation between two narrow bands of noise exceeds critical bandwidth unless both noises are led to the same ear. In contrast, of course, are the experiments on the binaural masking of pure tones. These studies show the dependency of the masked threshold, and therefore of the critical ratio, on phase relation between the two ears. This effect may reflect a change either in critical bandwidth or in the signal-to-noise ratio within the critical band.

More compelling support for a peripheral locus for the critical-band mechanism comes from Békésy's (1960b, 1962) investigations of inhibition in the eye and on the skin where small stimulus gradients are transformed into sharply circumscribed areas of sensation surrounded by areas of inhibition. Békésy called the combined area of sensation and inhibition the neural inhibitory unit. Zwislocki (1965) calculated that this neural unit in the ear corresponds to the critical band. Both he and Békésy related the neural unit to lateral inhibition in the receptor organ itself; in the ear this interpretation implicates the neural network in the cochlear partition. Békésy (1962) suggested that many of the similarities, including the presence of a neural unit in the eye, ear, and skin, are related to the fact that the retina, the basilar membrane, and the skin are sense organs with large surface areas. "In addition, there are similarities in the nerve supplies of their end organs, which show highly developed lateral interconnections with neighboring end organs. These lateral interconnections seem to be responsible for lateral inhibition. . . ." (Békésy, 1962, p. 1003). In this context, van den Brink's (1964b) report of a fundamental similarity between the ear's and the eye's detection of spatially separated narrow stimuli is noteworthy. Van den Brink measured the threshold of two 10-Hz bands of noise as a function of frequency separation, and of two points of light as a function of spatial separation. At large separations, the probability of hearing or seeing the stimuli is predictable on the assumption that the two components have independent effects. As the separation decreases, the probability of detection increases slowly until it reaches a plateau. Close together, the components apparently interact and behave more like a single stimulus at a higher energy level. The form of the function relating the probability of detection to stimulus separation is remarkably alike in the eye and ear. Moreover, interaction between the two noises begins at a frequency separation of one critical band.

If the critical-band mechanism seems likely to be a form of lateral inhibition in the cochlea, then this neural process must be very rapid. Otherwise, the steady-state critical band would probably not be measurable in loudness summation at durations as brief as 1 msec. Békésy (1965, p. 460) said that lateral "inhibition must be effective within a few milliseconds" to account for the ability of the ear and other sense organs to localize a stimulus within 1 msec. But then lateral inhibition may not be the only basis for the critical-band mechanism, (certainly mechanical filtering on the basilar membrane plays a role). Threshold measurements at short durations, which have shown a widening of the critical band, may force us to postulate additional neural filtering at higher stages in the auditory system — filtering that affects loudness and detectability differently. Models to account for such differential handling of loudness and detectability may not be difficult to build, but the data at short durations are still too few to warrant the effort.

Meanwhile, the critical-band mechanism seems to be one stage of a multistage filtering process — or it may comprise the whole chain. The role of central or cognitive factors in the chain is not clear. We do not know whether central processes alter the critical-band mechanism as suggested by Swets (1963) or whether central factors affect only the handling of the information already coded by a wholly stimulus-dependent critical-band mechanism.

IX. SUMMARY

At the critical bandwidth, listeners' responses to complex sounds change. In seven different kinds of experiments — on loudness summation, narrow-band masking, two-tone masking, threshold, phase sensitivity, musical consonance, and harmonic discrimination — listeners react one way when the stimuli are wider than the critical band and another way when the stimuli are narrower. In all seven, the width of the critical band is the same function of its center frequency and is mostly independent of sound pressure.

Closely related to the critical band is the critical ratio, a measure of the signal-to-noise ratio for a pure tone just masked by a wide-band noise. The critical band and the critical ratio vary similarly as a function of frequency, but the critical band is about 2.5 times larger. This difference disappears if we discard the incorrect assumption that the critical band of noise contained within the wide-band masker and the just masked tone are equally intense. Data show that the critical band must be more intense than the tone by about 4 dB, which is equivalent to a ratio of 2.5 and means that the same critical band applies to wide-band masking as to other types of masking.

Critical ratios have been measured in animals as well as in man. In the cat, rat, and chinchilla, they are approximately the same function of frequency as in man, although considerably larger. Moreover, in all four species, the calculated critical bandwidth seems to correspond to the same distance, 1 to 2 mm, on the basilar membrane.

At durations under 100 msec, threshold measurements indicate a wider critical band, but measurements of loudness summation indicate a normal-sized critical band. Insufficient data are available to resolve this seeming contradiction and other difficulties concerning the critical band at brief durations.

The critical band has proved useful in models of loudness and threshold. Possible specification of its role in speech may be at hand. Also, investigations that suggest an enlarged critical band in cochlear deafness may provide new insight into auditory pathology.

Although little is known about the critical-band mechanism as a physiological process, many data have been analyzed in terms of a critical band that acts like a filter somewhere within the auditory system. The similarity of the critical-band function to the mel scale of pitch, to the just noticeable difference scale of frequency, and especially to the function relating position on the basilar membrane to frequency, suggests that the critical-band mechanism may be part of a multistage process that includes both mechanical filtering on the basilar membrane and neural filtering (such as by lateral inhibition in the neural network of the cochlea). A complex process is also suggested by the measurements of the critical band at short durations.

ACKNOWLEDGMENT

The author appreciates the careful reading of the manuscript by D. D. Greenwood, A. W. Mills, E. Zwicker, and J. J. Zwislocki who suggested a number of improvements. Preparation of this chapter was supported by a grant from the Department of U.S. Public Health Service.

REFERENCES

Bauch, H. (1956). Die Bedeutung der Frequenzgruppe für die Lautheit von Klängen. *Acustica*, **6**, 40–45.

Bauman, R. C., Dieter, C. L., Lieberman, G., and Finney, W. J. (1953). The effects of very narrow band filtering on the aural recognition of pulsed signals in noise backgrounds. *J. Acoust. Soc. Am.*, **25**, 190 (A).

von Békésy, G. (1960a). *Experiments in hearing*. McGraw-Hill, New York.

von Békésy, G. (1960b). Neural inhibitory units of the eye and skin. Quantitative description of contrast phenomena. *J. Opt. Soc. Am.*, **50**, 1060–1070.

von Békésy, G. (1962). Lateral inhibition of heat sensations on the skin. *J. Appl. Physiol.*, **17**, 1003–1008.

von Békésy, G. (1965). Inhibition and the time and spatial patterns of neural activity in sensory perception. *Ann. Otol. Rhinol. Lar.*, **74**, 445–462.

von Békésy, G. and Rosenblith, W. A. (1951). The mechanical properties of the ear. In S. S. Stevens (Ed.) *Handbook of experimental psychology*. Wiley, New York.

Bilger, R. C. and Hirsh, I. J. (1956). Masking of tones by bands of noise. *J. Acoust. Soc. Am.*, **28**, 623–630.

de Boer, E. (1961). Measurement of the critical band-width in cases of perception deafness. *Proc. III Int. Congr. Acoust.* **1**, 100–102. Elsevier, Amsterdam.

de Boer, E. (1962). Note on the critical bandwidth. *J. Acoust. Soc. Am.*, **34**, 985–986 (L).

Bos, C. E. and de Boer, E. (1966). Masking and discrimination. *J. Acoust. Soc. Am.*, **39**, 708–715.

van den Brink, G. (1964a). Detection of tone pulse of various durations in noise of various bandwidths. *J. Acoust. Soc. Am.*, **36**, 1206–1211.

van den Brink, G. (1964b). Experiment on cochlear summation. *J. Acoust. Soc. Am.*, **36**, 1213–1214 (L).

Castle, W. E. (1964a). *The effect of selective narrow-band filtering on the perception of certain English vowels*. Mouton, The Hague.

Castle, W. E. (1964b). Effects of selective narrow-band filtering on the perception by normal listeners of Harvard PB–50 word lists. *J. Acoust. Soc. Am.*, **36**, 1047 (A).

Chaves, J. F. and Scharf, B. (1966). Critical bands and the discrimination of intensity relations in two-tone complexes. *J. Acoust. Soc. Am.*, **39**, 1262 (A).

Creelman, C. D. (1961). Detection of complex signals as a function of signal bandwidth and duration. *J. Acoust. Soc. Am.*, **33**, 89–94.

Dallos, P. J. and Olsen, W. O. (1964). Integration of energy at threshold with gradual rise-fall tone pips. *J. Acoust. Soc. Am.*, **36**, 743–751.

Durlach, N. I. (1964). Note on binaural masking-level differences at high frequencies. *J. Acoust. Soc. Am.*, **36**, 576–581.

Ehmer, R. H. (1959). Masking by tones vs. noise bands. *J. Acoust. Soc. Am.*, **31**, 1253–1256.

Elliott, D. N., Stein, L., and Harrison, M. J. (1960). Determination of absolute-intensity thresholds and frequency-difference thresholds in cats. *J. Acoust. Soc. Am.*, **32**, 380–384.

Elliott, L. L. (1965). Changes in the simultaneous masked threshold of brief tones. *J. Acoust. Soc. Am.*, **38**, 738–746.

Feldtkeller, R. (1955). Über die Zerlegung des Schallspektrums in Frequenzgruppen durch das Gehör. *Elektron. Rdsch.*, **9**, 387–389.

Feldtkeller, R. (1963). Lautheit und Tonheit. *Frequenz,* **17,** 207-212.

Feldtkeller, R. and Oetinger, R. (1956). Die Hörbarkeitsgrenzen von Impulsen verschiedener Dauer. *Acustica,* **6,** 489-493.

Feldtkeller, R. and Zwicker, E. (1956). *Das Ohr als Nachrichtenempfänger.* S. Hirzel, Stuttgart.

Fletcher, H. (1940). Auditory patterns. *Rev. Mod. Phys.,* **12,** 47-65.

Fletcher, H. (1953). *Speech and hearing in communication* (2nd ed.). Van Nostrand, Princeton, New Jersey.

Fletcher, H. and Munson, W. A. (1937). Relation between loudness and masking. *J. Acoust. Soc. Am.,* **9,** 1-10.

French, N. R. and Steinberg, J. C. (1947). Factors governing the intelligibility of speech sounds. *J. Acoust. Soc. Am.,* **19,** 90-119.

Gales, R. S. and Wilcott, R. C. (1954). The effect of envelope shape on the masked threshold of short bursts of tone. *J. Acoust. Soc. Am.,* **26,** 944 (A).

Garner, W. R. (1947). The effect of frequency spectrum on temporal integration of energy in the ear. *J. Acoust. Soc. Am.,* **19,** 808-815.

Garner, W. R. (1949). The loudness and loudness matching of short tones. *J. Acoust. Soc. Am.,* **21,** 398-403.

Garner, W. R. and Miller, G. A. (1947). The masked threshold of pure tones as a function of duration. *J. Exp. Psychol.,* **37,** 293-303.

Gässler, G. (1954). Über die Hörschwelle für Schallereignisse mit verschieden breitem Frequenzspektrum. *Acustica,* **4,** 408-414.

Goldstein, R. and Kramer, J. C. (1960). Factors affecting thresholds for short tones. *J. Speech Hear. Res.,* **3,** 249-256.

Gourevitch, G. (1965). Auditory masking in the rat. *J. Acoust. Soc. Am.,* **37,** 439-443.

Green, D. M. (1958a). Detection of signals in noise and the critical band concept. Tech. Report No. 82, *Electron. Def. Group, University of Michigan.*

Green, D. M. (1958b). Detection of multiple component signals in noise. *J. Acoust. Soc. Am.,* **30,** 904-911.

Green, D. M. (1960). Auditory detection of a noise signal. *J. Acoust. Soc. Am.,* **32,** 121-131.

Green, D. M. (1965). Masking with two tones. *J. Acoust. Soc. Am.,* **37,** 802-813.

Green, D. M., Birdsall, T. G., and Tanner, W. P., Jr. (1957). Signal detection as a function of signal intensity and duration. *J. Acoust. Soc. Am.,* **29,** 523-531.

Green, D. M., McKey, M. J., and Licklider, J. C. R. (1959). Detection of a pulsed sinusoid in noise as a function of frequency. *J. Acoust. Soc. Am.,* **31,** 1446-1452.

Greenberg, G. Z. and Larkin, W. D. (1966). Frequency-selective detection of signals in noise. *J. Acoust. Soc. Am.,* **39,** 1247 (A).

Greenwood, D. D. (1961a). Auditory masking and the critical band. *J. Acoust. Soc. Am.,* **33,** 484-502.

Greenwood, D. D. (1961b). Critical bandwidth and the frequency coordinates of the basilar membrane. *J. Acoust. Soc. Am.,* **33,** 1344-1356.

Hamilton, P. M. (1957). Noise masked thresholds as a function of tonal duration and masking noise band width. *J. Acoust. Soc. Am.,* **29,** 506-511.

Hawkins, J. E., Jr. and Stevens, S. S. (1950). The masking of pure tones and of speech by white noise. *J. Acoust. Soc. Am.,* **22,** 6-13.

Jeffress, L. A. (1964). Stimulus-oriented approach to detection. *J. Acoust. Soc. Am.,* **36,** 766-774.

Jerger, J. F., Tillman, T. W., and Peterson, J. L. (1960). Masking by octave bands of noise in normal and impaired ears. *J. Acoust. Soc. Am.*, **32**, 385–390.

Kryter, K. D. (1960). Speech bandwidth compression through spectrum selection. *J. Acoust. Soc. Am.*, **32**, 547–556.

Langenbeck, B. (1951). Neues zur Praxis und Theorie der Geräuschaudiometrie. *Z. Lar. Rhinol. Otol.*, **30**, 423–441.

Marill, T. (1956). Detection theory and psychophysics. *M.I.T. Res. Lab. Electron. Tech. Rep. 319*.

Mathes, R. C. and Miller, R. L. (1947). Phase effects in monaural perception. *J. Acoust. Soc. Am.*, **19**, 780–797.

Mathews, M. V. and Pfafflin, S. M. (1965). Effect of filter type on energy-detection models for auditory signal detection. *J. Acoust. Soc. Am.*, **38**, 1055–1056 (L).

Mayer, A. M. (1894). Researches in acoustics. *Lond. Edinb. Dubl. Phil. Mag.*, **37**, *ser. 5*, 259–288.

Miller, G. A. (1948). The perception of short bursts of noise. *J. Acoust. Soc. Am.*, **20**, 160–170.

Miller, J. D. (1964). Auditory sensitivity of the chinchilla in quiet and in noise. *J. Acoust. Soc. Am.*, **36**, 2010 (A).

Miskolczy-Fodor, F. (1959). Relation between loudness and duration of tonal pulses. I. Response of normal ears to pure tones longer than click-pitch threshold. *J. Acoust. Soc. Am.*, **31**, 1128–1134.

Miskolczy-Fodor, F. (1960). Relation between loudness and duration of tonal pulses. II. Response of normal ears to sounds with noise sensation. *J. Acoust. Soc. Am.*, **32**, 482–486.

Morton, J. and Carpenter, A. (1963). Experiments relating to the perception of formants. *J. Acoust. Soc. Am.*, **35**, 475–480.

Munson, W. A. (1947). The growth of auditory sensation. *J. Acoust. Soc. Am.*, **19**, 584–591.

Niese, H. (1957). Vorschlag für die Definition und Messung der Deutlichkeit nach subjektiven Grundlagen. *HochfrequenzTech. Elektroakust.*, **65**, 4–15.

Niese, H. (1959). Die Trägheit der Lautstärkebildung in Abhängigkeit vom Schallpegel. *HochfrequenzTech. Elektroakust.*, **68**, 143–152.

Niese, H. (1960). Subjektive Messung der Lautstärke von Bandpassrauschen. *Hochfreq-Tech. Elektroakust.*, **68**, 202–217.

Niese, H. (1961). Die Lautstärkebildung bei binauralem Hören komplexer Geräusche. *HochfreqTech. Elektroakust.*, **70**, 132–141.

Palva, T., Goodman, A., and Hirsh, I. J. (1953). Critical evaluation of noise audiometry. *Laryngoscope*, **63**, 842–860.

Plomp, R. (1961). Hearing threshold for periodic tone pulses. *J. Acoust. Soc. Am.*, **33**, 1561–1569.

Plomp, R. (1964). The ear as a frequency analyzer. *J. Acoust. Soc. Am.*, **36**, 1628–1636.

Plomp, R. and Bouman, M. A. (1959). Relation between hearing threshold and duration for tone pulses. *J. Acoust. Soc. Am.*, **31**, 749–758.

Plomp, R. and Levelt, W. J. M. (1962). Musical consonance and critical bandwidth. *Proc. IV Int. Congr. Acoust.*, paper P55. Harlang and Toksvig, Copenhagen.

Plomp, R. and Levelt, W. J. M. (1965). Tonal consonance and critical bandwidth. *J. Acoust. Soc. Am.*, **38**, 548–560.

Port, E. (1963). Über die Lautstärke einzelner kurzer Schallimpulse. *Acustica*, **13**, 212–223.

von Reichardt, W. (1965). Zur Trägheit der Lautstärkebildung. *Acustica*, **15**, 345–354.

Schafer, T. H. and Gales, R. S. (1949). Auditory masking of multiple tones by random noise. *J. Acoust. Soc. Am.*, **21**, 392–398.

Schafer, T. H., Gales, R. S., Shewmaker, C. A., and Thompson, P. O. (1950). The frequency selectivity of the ear as determined by masking experiments. *J. Acoust. Soc. Am.*, **22**, 490–497.

Scharf, B. (1959a). Critical bands and the loudness of complex sounds near threshold. *J. Acoust. Soc. Am.*, **31**, 365–370.

Scharf, B. (1959b). Loudness of complex sounds as a function of the number of components. *J. Acoust. Soc. Am.*, **31**, 783–785.

Scharf, B. (1961a). Loudness summation under masking. *J. Acoust. Soc. Am.*, **33**, 503–511.

Scharf, B. (1961b). Complex sounds and critical bands. *Psychol. Bull.*, **58**, 205–217.

Scharf, B. (1962). Loudness summation and spectrum shape. *J. Acoust. Soc. Am.*, **34**, 228–233.

Scharf, B. and Hellman, R. P. (1966). A model of loudness summation applied to impaired ears. *J. Acoust. Soc. Am.*, **40**, 71–78.

Scholl, H. (1962a). Über die Bildung der Hörschwellen und Mithörschwellen von Impulsen. *Acustica*, **12**, 91–101.

Scholl, H. (1962b). Das dynamische Verhalten des Gohörs bei der Unterteilung des Schallspektrums in Frequenzgruppen. *Acustica*, **12**, 101–107.

Scholl, H. (1963). Über ein Objektives Verfahren zur Ermittlung von Hörschwellen und Mithörschwellen. *Frequenz*, **17**, 125–133.

Sheeley, E. C. and Bilger, R. C. (1964). Temporal integration as a function of frequency. *J. Acoust. Soc. Am.*, **36**, 1850–1857.

Simon, G. R. (1963). The critical bandwidth level in recruiting ears and its relation to temporal summation. *J. Aud. Res.*, **3**, 109–119.

Small, A. M., Brandt, J. F., and Cox, P. G. (1962). Loudness as a function of signal duration. *J. Acoust. Soc. Am.*, **34**, 513–514 (L).

Stevens, S. S. (1957). On the psychophysical law. *Psychol. Rev.*, **64**, 153–181.

Stevens, S. S. and Davis, H. (1938). *Hearing*. Wiley, New York.

Stevens, S. S. and Volkmann, J. (1940). The relation of pitch to frequency: A revised scale. *Am. J. Psychol.*, **53**, 329–353.

Swets, J. A. (1963). Central factors in auditory frequency selectivity. *Psychol. Bull.*, **60**, 429–440.

Swets, J. A., Green, D. M., and Tanner, W. P., Jr. (1962). On the width of critical bands. *J. Acoust. Soc. Am.*, **34**, 108–113.

Veniar, F. A. (1958). Signal detection as a function of frequency ensemble. *J. Acoust. Soc. Am.*, **30**, 1020–1024.

Watson, C. S. (1963). Masking of tones by noise for the cat. *J. Acoust. Soc. Am.*, **35**, 167–172.

Webster, J. C., Miller, P. H., Thompson, P. O., and Davenport, E. W. (1952). The masking and pitch shifts of pure tones near abrupt changes in a thermal noise spectrum. *J. Acoust. Soc. Am.*, **24**, 147–152.

Zwicker, E. (1952). Die Grenzen der Hörbarkeit der Amplitudenmodulation und der Frequenzmodulation eines Tones. *Acustica*, **2**, 125–133.

Zwicker, E. (1954). Die Verdeckung von Schmalbandgeräuschen durch Sinustöne. *Acustica*, **4**, 415–420.

Zwicker, E. (1956). Die elementaren Grundlagen zur Bestimmung der Informations-
kapazität des Gehörs. *Acustica*, **6**, 365–381.

Zwicker, E. (1958). Ueber psychologische und methodische Grundlagen der Lautheit.
Acustica, **8**, 237–258.

Zwicker, E. (1960). Über die Rolle der Frequenzgruppe beim Hören. *Ergebn. Biol.*,
23, 187–203.

Zwicker, E. (1963a). Ueber die Lautheit von ungedrosselten und gedrosselten Schal-
len. *Acustica*, **13**, 194–211.

Zwicker, E. (1963b). Möglichkeiten zur Spracherkennung über den Tastsinn mit
Hilfe eines Funktionsmodells des Gehörs. *Elektron. Rechenanl., Beih.* **7**, 239–244.

Zwicker, E. (1965a). Temporal effects in simultaneous masking by white-noise bursts.
J. Acoust. Soc. Am., **37**, 653–663.

Zwicker, E. (1965b). Temporal effects in simultaneous masking and loudness. *J.
Acoust. Soc. Am.*, **38**, 132–141.

Zwicker, E. (1966). Ein Beitrag zur Lautstärkemessung impulshaltiger Schalle. *Acustica*, **17**, 11–22.

Zwicker, E. and Feldtkeller, R. (1955). Ueber die Lautstärke von gleichförmigen Ger-
äuschen. *Acustica*, **5**, 303–316.

Zwicker, E. and Scharf, B. (1965). A model of loudness summation. *Psychol. Rev.*, **72**,
3–26.

Zwicker, E. and Wright, H. N. (1963). Temporal summation for tones in narrow-band
noise. *J. Acoust. Soc. Am.*, **35**, 691–699.

Zwicker, E., Flottorp, G., and Stevens, S. S. (1957). Critical bandwidth in loudness
summation. *J. Acoust. Soc. Am.*, **29**, 548–557.

Zwislocki, J. (1960). Theory of temporal auditory summation. *J. Acoust. Soc. Am.*, **32**,
1046–1060.

Zwislocki, J. (1965). Analysis of some auditory characteristics. In R. D. Luce, R. R.
Bush, and E. Galanter (Eds.) *Handbook of mathematical psychology*. Vol. 3, pp. 1–
97. Wiley, New York.

Chapter Six

Cochlear Mechanics and Hydro-dynamics

FOREWORD

Basic to an understanding of the process underlying hearing is an understanding of the ways in which an acoustic signal is transformed and transduced into a series of neural impulses. This chapter by Juergen Tonndorf is designed to expose the transformation process up to the point where it ceases to be mechanical. Tonndorf's work in this country has been almost totally concerned with the mechanical events that take place in ears (and in ear models) prior to the final transduction into neuro-electric waves and impulses. He is especially interested in the periodicity-pitch problems and has taken a strong stand regarding their solution through mechanical demodulation in the cochlea. At the same time, he has touched on the continuing concern of many theorists regarding what kinds of filtering and sharpening mechanisms exist in the auditory system. Since we are able to distinguish pitches and pitch changes easily even when the traveling-wave patterns for the stimulating tones seem identical, some sort of differentiating process must be at work. Tonndorf has made the case for his own favorite mode of differentiation.

Cochlear Mechanics
and Hydro-dynamics

Juergen Tonndorf[*]

I. INTRODUCTION

The cochlea converts acoustic signals into neural signals that are then further processed within the auditory nervous system. However, before this neural transduction takes place, the signals undergo a number of transformations. This chapter is concerned with the mechano-acoustic events occurring within the cochlea following the displacement of the stapes footplate after an acoustic signal. Some of these events are more than mere "transformations" and, strictly speaking, constitute the beginning of auditory processing.

Applying the principles that Fourier[†] set forth in his famous paper

---

[*]Otolaryngology Department, College of Physicians and Surgeons, Columbia University, New York.

[†] H. S. Carslaw (1950) gives the following historical account: Fourier presented his paper *"La theorie analytique de la chaleur"* to the French Academy originally in 1811. Although he was awarded the prize, the paper was not considered worthy to be included in the *Memoires*. The judges included LaPlace, Lagrange, and Legendre, his actual predecessors. Fourier then wrote, and published in 1822, a larger treatise under the same title. In 1824, after he himself had become secretary to the *Academie,* he had the original paper of 1811 published officially in its *Memoires.* This story shows that the significance of an important new contribution is often not recognized by contemporaries, even the experts. New ideas take time to sink in. Furthermore, it should be noted that Fourier's original paper did not deal with the analysis of complex vibrations, but with problems of heat flow.

of 1824, G. S. Ohm postulated in 1843 that the ear performs a Fourier analysis upon the incoming signal—a logical assumption since a listener is able to discern the various partials of a complex tone. Helmholtz in 1863, endorsed Ohm's "acoustic law" and at the same time suggested a *mode* by which the cochlea might execute the required analysis. According to his "place theory," high frequencies are received at the base of the cochlea, near the windows. As the frequency becomes lower, this place moves systematically farther toward the apex. Thus, place, in Helmholtz's opinion, represents frequency.

He also indicated a *mechanism* by which the cochlea might perform this frequency analysis. He knew that the basilar membrane is narrower at its basal end and wider at the apical one and further, that it is made up of transverse fibers. He assumed these fibers to be under tension. Such a system, when stimulated by a given frequency, would form a local displacement maximum at the place of resonance.

There was, of course, some criticism of these hypotheses. Seebeck (1841), a contemporary of Ohm's, studied the perception of complex tones produced by a siren. He felt that some of his results were incompatible with the assumption of a Fourier analysis, but rather indicated a *waveform* or *time analysis.* It is a curious fact that Ohm (1843), who apparently did not conduct acoustic experiments of his own, cited Seebeck's findings in support of his own thesis. Seebeck (1843) in turn wrote a rebuttal, but it found little attention in his own time. Apparently, the Fourier principle with its clear-cut mathematical formulation was too powerful to be put aside. In recent times, Schouten (1938, 1940a, 1940b), Small (1955), de Boer (1956), Schouten *et al.* (1962), and others have taken up Seebeck's experiments again, confirmed his results, and expanded upon his concepts.

Occasional other criticisms appeared. M. Wien (1905) argued that Helmholtz's assumption of sharp local resonances in the human ear (required by the sharp frequency differentiation) is incompatible with the demonstrated high damping. Rutherford (1886) suggested that the only task of the cochlea is to act as a mechano-neural transducer, and therefore he relegated the analytical function entirely to the brain in an early "telephone theory." Since 1896, M. Meyer (1928) has used a "hydraulic model" of the cochlea with a nonelastic basilar membrane. This membrane is displaced solely by the shifting fluid columns of the perilymphatic scalae. Ewald (1899, 1903) also employed a simple mechanical model of the cochlea. When properly stimulated, this model produces a wave pattern along its elastic basilar membrane. This pattern is characteristic for each frequency, but there is no systematic relation between frequency and place in this "sound-pattern theory."

Cochlear theory received new impetus in 1928, the year of Békésy's first publication on the subject.* Békésy, like Meyer, Ewald, and others before him, approached the problem by constructing cochlear models; but in contrast to his predecessors, his models were based (*a*) upon dimensional analysis and (*b*) upon measurements of some crucial structural properties of the inner ear.

II. MODELS

A. Dimensional Analysis

Dimensional analysis (Bridgman, 1922) allows the comparison of different-sized similar structures as they respond to a given form of stimulation. For example, the forces acting upon a large ship and upon its smaller model can only be compared meaningfully when the comparison is based upon certain dimensionless constants.

For a given situation, the ratio between the inertial forces acting upon a system and the viscous counter-forces generated by this system may be kept constant by application of the rule expressed in the Reynolds number, R,

$$R = vd\rho / \eta \qquad (6\text{-}1)$$

(v = velocity, d = linear dimension, ρ = density, and η = viscosity). In dimensional terms, this equation becomes

$$R = \frac{LT^{-1} \times L \times ML^{-3}}{ML^{-1}\,t^{-1}} \qquad (6\text{-}2)$$

---

*To be sure, between 1900 and 1928 there were a number of other studies of cochlear function — some of them direct precursors of Békésy's work. The interested reader is referred to Wever (1962) for a review of them.

Although I have made reference in this chapter to Békésy's papers by their actual dates of publication, the reader should be informed that practically *all* of his papers have been collected in his book: *Experiments in Hearing* (1960). (Dr. E. G. Wever translated those that had originally appeared in German.) Other briefer (though less comprehensive) summarizing accounts may be found in Békésy and Rosenblith (1951) and in Békésy's Nobel Lecture (1961).

(L = length, T = time, and M = mass), which is seen to be dimension-less (i.e., independent of the size of the system under consideration). Models thus often bear little resemblance to the original structures they are supposed to represent—a point that is apparent in the usage of two different terms: (*a*) "airplane model," (a scale model that usually cannot fly), and (*b*) "model airplane" (one that can fly but often looks quite different from a large airplane). The Reynolds num-ber is not the only constant used in dimensional analysis, and since some of these constants are mutually exclusive, sometimes several models are built in order to satisfy the various conditions one wants to examine.

In the case of the cochlear models, frequency (f) is of the dimension T^{-1}. Thus, Békésy (1928) modified Equation (6-1) to

$$\rho\, fd^2/\eta = c \tag{6-3}$$

(c = constant). In 1960, I simplified it further to

$$f\, d^2 \propto c, \tag{6-4}$$

provided the density and viscosity of a given model are kept uniform. This relation was borne out by actual measurement. It indicates that as the physical size of a cochlear model — specifically its area factor, d^2, increases, the range of frequencies to which it will respond decreases. This fact greatly facilitates experimentation. Similarly, displacement amplitudes increase with model size so that the extremely small amplitudes in the cochlea can, in a properly chosen model, be "trans-formed" into larger, more easily observed amplitudes (Tonndorf, 1960b).

B. Structural Properties

Békésy's measurements of the ear (since 1928) primarily concerned properties of the basilar membrane. He found that it is indeed an elastic membrane, as most earlier investigators had supposed, but that it is not under the transverse tension that Helmholtz required. In fact, it appears to have no tension in any direction[*] (Békésy, 1941);

---

[*]This point deserves some comment. If the tension of a given membrane is really zero, initially its displacement does not grow in linear relation to the applied signal. Hooke's law does not hold in this case, i.e., the restoring, elastic force varies with the third power of the displacement. (Per illustration, consider the extreme case of a

instead, its stiffness varies exponentially with distance. If d (in cm^3/ dynes) expresses the volume displacement of the basilar membrane resulting from a uniformly applied force and x (in cm) its length, Békésy's measurements can be expressed as

$$d = e^{1.32\ x}.$$

In my own models, I have usually been able to produce gradients for which the exponential multiplier had approximately one-half of the above value, provided the difference in length of the basilar membrane was taken into account (Tonndorf, 1958a).

Békésy simplified his models (Fig. 1) in two respects. First, in preliminary experiments, he found that the volume displacement of the basilar membrane and that of Reissner's membrane are always equal

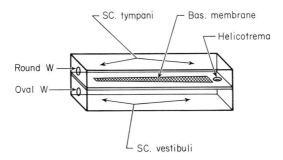

Figure 1 Cochlear model of the Békésy type. This schematic drawing represents the model that I have used in my own experiments. It is very similar to Békésy's original one. It has a transparent lucite shell enclosing two "perilymphatic" scalae. The perilymphatic fluid is a glycerin-water mixture controlled for viscosity. In a model five times larger than a human cochlea, a glycerin-water mixture of 30 centipoises provides approximately the same damping as obtained in a model the size of an actual cochlea with a fluid viscosity of 2 centipoises, which is that of human perilymph. Sandwiched between the two scalae is the cochlear partition, a thin metal frame giving support to the basilar membrane, which is made of latex, and, in typical cases, has an exponential stiffness gradient. Note also the helicotrema and the two cochlear windows. (Tonndorf, 1958a. By permission from *Journal of the Acoustical Society of America*.)

flaccid membrane which is much larger in diameter than would be required by the size of its supporting rim.) It would be more in line with observed facts (e.g., the input/ output function of cochlear microphonics) if the basilar membrane could be shown to have a small, but definite degree of tension, a determination that, experimentally, may not be easy to make. This point was recently brought to my attention by G. G. Harris (Bell Telephone Laboratories).

and that they stay in phase. Furthermore, since the basilar membrane possesses a stiffness gradient but Reissner's membrane is of uniform low stiffness, he concluded that it is the basilar membrane that is of primary functional importance. Therefore, he omitted Reissner's membrane so that the cochlear partition of his models consists only of a "basilar membrane" — an elastic membrane with a stiffness gradient from base to apex. Second, he noted that some lower verebrate animals (e.g., monotremata, birds, and reptiles) already possess a receptor organ that is not unlike the cochlea, but is uncoiled. Such organs function in essentially the same manner as those of higher mammals. The models are therefore simplified by being straight rather than coiled.

C.   Traveling-Wave Concept

Békésy (1928) first established the traveling-wave concept; that is to say, sinusoidal stimulation of his models produced a basilar-membrane displacement that had all the temporal and spatial characteristics of waves traveling continuously from base to apex. These Békésy waves have some distinct properties. As indicated in Fig. 2, the displacement amplitude first increases slowly, and, after going through a maximum, diminishes rapidly with distance. When frequency is altered, the place of the maximal displacement shifts in the

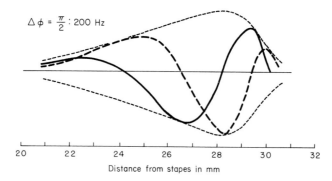

Figure 2   Instantaneous displacement of the partition (solid line) in a cochlear model. Synchronously with the signal, the pattern moves in a wave-like fashion from base to apex (toward the right in this figure). The dotted line represents the long-time average of the amplitude peaks — the so-called envelope. Note the gradual buildup of average amplitude with distance and its rapid decrement beyond the point of maximal displacement. The wavelength decreases monotonically with distance so that at the distal end there are smaller and smaller wavelets. (Tonndorf, 1962b. By permission from *Journal of the Acoustical Society of America*.)

same manner as predicted by Helmholtz's place theory (Fig. 3); i.e., with increasing frequency it moves toward the base of the cochlea. However, the underlying mechanism is not the same.

Figure 3 shows a property of the Békésy model that most clearly shows wave propagation. For the sine-wave signals used, a cumulative negative phase shift occurs with distance along the partition. This shift ultimately reaches a rather high value (I once measured shifts up to -12π during onset events in response to sine-wave signals). Such large values can only occur in traveling-wave events. Within a resonant system (e.g., a Helmholtz model) the maximum is $-\pi$. The phase data of Fig. 3 can also be converted into propagation time to show that the velocity along the partition decreases exponentially with distance.

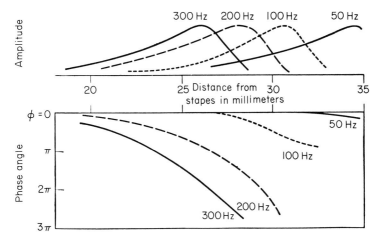

Figure 3 *Top:* Distribution of envelopes and their maxima along the partition for some low-frequency signals (amplitudes normalized). *Bottom:* Cumulative phase lag of the traveling wave relative to the stapedial displacement for the same frequencies. Data from human cadaver specimen. (Békésy, 1947. By permission from *Journal of the Acoustical Society of America*.)

D. Further Model Studies

Most other model studies have taken Békésy's measurements into account. Mechanical models were made by Diestel (1954) and by Tonndorf (1957a); electrical network models were constructed by Peterson and Bogert (1950), by Hauser (1961), and by Völz (1961);

Flanagan (1962) and Khanna *et al.* (1968) used computer models. Mathematical theories, which in essence are abstract models, were proposed by Fletcher (1929), Ranke (1931, 1950), and Zwislocki 1948, 1950).*

Obviously none of the models replicates *all* the properties of the original structure. However, since the structural properties of an actual cochlea cannot be varied systematically, and since the cochlear make-up is so complicated, a model is an excellent research tool. From the standpoint of easy variability, the abstract mathematical and the computer models are probably the best. However, owing to the complexity of the mathematical formulations and derivations, the factors relevant to a given event are often hard to see. The difficulties become formidable when fluid and membrane displacements are represented together, and when nonlinear events are described. Essentially, the same criticism applies to the electrical-network models. The advantage of these models is that none of them require dimensional analysis, and that electrical networks, for example, can be built in dimensions equivalent to those of an actual cochlea by using exact electrical equivalents of mechanical elements. However, electrical networks are made up of discrete components so that, for example, the smooth stiffness gradient of the partition must be replicated by a finite number of capacitors.

Enlarged mechanical models require dimensional analysis for the quantitative evaluation of observed data; therefore, determinations of the precise location or absolute magnitude of a given event within a real cochlea are not their forte. However, they are the least abstract of all the models, and thus facilitate observations of dynamic phenomena. Later, these phenomena can be verified and studied quantitatively either in other models, or, if possible, in the cochlea itself.

III. RESPONSES OF MECHANICAL COCHLEAR MODELS

In this chapter, the events taking place in mechanical cochlear models are described in detail because most of my experience has been with that type of model. My cochlear studies began with a comparison between the activities within the cochlea and those occurring in surf on sloping beaches (Tonndorf, 1956). There are some striking

---

*A good summary in English of Zwislocki's 1948 paper is contained in Zwislocki (1965).

similarities between these two events, and the observation of the latter has raised some pertinent questions concerning the fluid dynamics of the cochlear models.

A. Sine Wave Response

One can view movements of the fluid in a model by suspending aluminum dust particles in it. The stability of such suspensions is good because of the high viscosity of the fluid required to produce adequate damping in the enlarged model. Figure 4 shows the typical pattern of fluid motion in response to a sinusoidal signal. The composite drawing indicates that, although particles in the vicinity of the

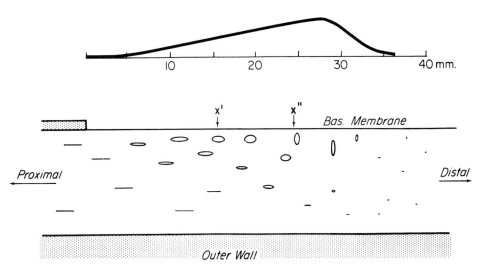

Figure 4 Particle motion in the fluids of *scala vestibuli* of a cochlear model in response to a 50-Hz signal. This drawing gives the type and relative magnitude of displacements in various locations: one-dimensional (longitudinal) in the vicinity of the window and along the outer wall; and two-dimensional (elliptical or circular) along the partition. Magnitudes are overstated for the sake of illustration. Each particle completes its pathway once each period; in the present example the rate was 50 per sec. Such two-dimensional motion is known as *trochoidal*. Implied in the present drawing is the notion that the trochoidal fluid motion forms an orthogonal vectorial field with respect to the partition at rest. This notion (although correct for freely progressing surface waves) represents an oversimplification. The magnitude of displacement in the vertical direction of the two-dimensional, trochoidal pathways in close vicinity of the partition is shown in the curve at the top of the figure. It is identical to the envelope over the traveling waves along the partition itself. (Tonndorf, 1959b. By permission from *Acta Oto Laryngologica*.)

windows move simply to and fro longitudinally under the effect of the window displacement, the pattern differs along the partition. There, each particle moves along a cyclic or elliptical pathway. This fluid motion, typical of waves along any fluid surface, is called *trochoidal*. Its mechanism is illustrated in Fig. 5. Assume two vectors—a longitudinal one in the direction of the original window displacement, and a vertical one in the direction of the up-and-down displacement of the elastic partition. Then the pathways represent *Lissajous* figures, and it is known that the patterns of Figs. 4 and 5 indicate either a 90° or a 270° phase relation between the two vectors. That is, one of them must lead the other by a phase angle of 90°. One way to determine the leading vector is to observe the direction of revolution of a given particle. It turns out that individual particles in both scalae invariably move in a distal direction while close to the membrane, and in a proximal direction while away from it (described by a clockwise rotation in Fig. 4). Considering the longitudinal movement away from the window and the vertical displacement of the partition toward the opposite scala both as a positive, then the vertical vector leads the longitudinal one by a phase angle of 90°.

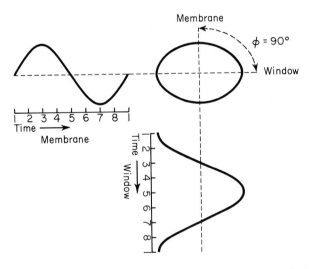

Figure 5 Trochoidal fluid motion. Each particle is under the effect of (*a*) the original window motion and (*b*) the displacement of the basilar membrane, and thus moves according to the resultant of these two vectors. The circular (or elliptical) pathways of this figure (and of Fig. 4) indicate a phase difference of 90° between vectors. The actual shape of each pathway is determined by the relative magnitudes of the two vectors; e.g., in the proximal portion, where there is no basilar membrane displacement, the vertical vector is zero, and simple longitudinal motion results.

Inspection of a layer of particles parallel to the partition indicates that the longitudinal vectors diminish gradually with distance, but that the vertical ones change in proportion to the amplitudes of the envelope over the traveling waves. One can also note that when the driving frequency is high enough, there is no fluid motion within the helicotrema (Fig. 4). Inspection of a series of particles extending from the partition to the outer wall shows that the vertical vector gradually approaches zero, but the longitudinal one remains unchanged.

These three observations — (a) the trochoidal fluid motion, (b) the similarity of the wave pattern along the partition to that within the underlying fluid, and (c) the change of the vertical vector with depth — indicate that the cochlear fluid motion and the associated displacement of the partition indeed represent a system of surface waves.* The "surface" in this case is the partition — an *interface* between two separate bodies of fluid.

Surface waves, depending upon their inherent restoring forces, are classed as *capillary* and *gravity* waves. Capillary waves are controlled by surface tension and are usually short; gravity waves (e.g., ocean waves) are much longer. In gravity waves, the group or particle velocity is less than the wave velocity, and in capillary waves this relation is reversed. A comparison of the wave- and group-velocities within the model (Tonndorf, 1960b) indicates that the cochlear waves are capillary, an understandable situation in view of the relatively strong restoring force represented by the compliance of the partition. This finding means that the cochlear traveling-wave event is not affected by gravity and hence is independent of the position of the organ in space.

Surface waves may be further classed as *deep-* and *shallow-water* waves. In deep-water waves, both the longitudinal and the vertical vectors diminish with depth, and finally approach zero. But in the cochlea, only the vertical vectors diminish with depth (Fig. 4), as in shallow-water waves.

Remember that the vertical vector of particle motion always leads the longitudinal one by 90°. That is, the *vertical vector* (associated with the displacement of the partition) is the *first time-derivative of the longitudinal vector*, which, in essence, is associated with the original displacement of the window. This relation between vectors in trochoidal wave motion is invariant, and its proper understanding is essential for analyzing the cochlear response to transient signals.

---

*The classical treatise on surface-wave phenomena is that of H. Lamb (1879).

With sinusoidal signals, derivatives are represented simply by phase shifts, but with transients, there are changes in shape as well.

B. Transient Response

Consider the response of the cochlear partition to a step function, the simplest transient signal. A comparison of the main drawing with the insert in Fig. 6 reveals that, at short distances from the windows, the early, synchronized portion of the response is pulse-shaped, once more indicating that the displacement of the partition, at least near the windows, is the first derivative of the stapedial displacement. *Thus, the cochlear partition is essentially a velocity receiver.* This conclusion is strengthened by the fact that the amplitude of maximal displacement for constant input decreases with frequency at a rate of 6 dB per octave.

Figure 6 further indicates that the "traveling bulge" (Békésy, 1928) is not a single crest. In the time domain, it looks more like a short, decaying wave *train*. So the cochlear response is essentially an *after-*

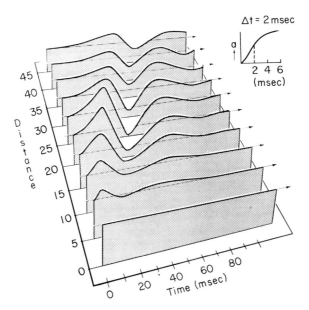

Figure 6 Traveling bulge. A three-dimensional representation (time-distance-amplitude) of the response of the partition of a cochlear model to a step-function (shown in the insert). Note that the duration of half-waves becomes longer with time and rank order for a given position as well as with distance along the partition. (Tonndorf, 1962b. By permission from *Journal of the Acoustical Society of America.*)

effect, a plausible finding because the model — like the actual ear — is less than critically damped. However, the condition of continuity of the incompressible cochlear fluids demands that, after both windows have come to rest at the termination of the signal, the *sum of all displacements along the partition always be zero.* Furthermore, although the stapedial and the associated longitudinal fluid displacements originally drive the partition, later on and farther distally, partition and fluid move as an integrated system. It is only thus that the constant phase relation of 90° between the partition and the longitudinal fluid motion at *all places of observation* (Fig. 4) can be reconciled with the fact that a phase delay of considerable magnitude develops along the partition. The phase delay within the incompressible fluids is made possible by the trochoidal mode of wave motion.

Close inspection of Fig. 6 indicates that the first crest, which represents the direct response to the signal, is not only delayed in its travel along the partition, but is also longer in duration than the signal. Figure 7 gives a plot, derived from the same data as in Fig. 6, of the ratio of amplitude (A) to duration (τ) of the first crest — a measure of its shape. Initially, when the first crest grows in amplitude (Fig. 6), it

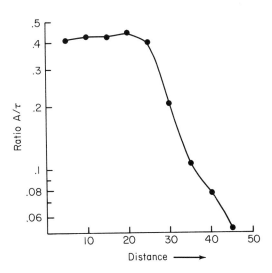

Figure 7 Alteration of shape of the first half-wave of a traveling bulge progressing along the partition, expressed as the ratio between displacement amplitude and duration (A/τ) at any given point. (Tonndorf, 1962b. By permission from *Journal of the Acoustical Society of America.*)

retains its shape. However, as soon as the point of maximal amplitude is passed, it changes rapidly. The crest becomes lower in amplitude and longer in time. Such "time smear" and amplitude loss of pulse-shaped signals occur typically when the bandwidth of a transmission system becomes narrower than that of the signal being transmitted (Goldman, 1948). The continuous downward slope of the curve of Fig. 7, in conjunction with the frequency distribution of Fig. 3, indicates that the partition is a spatially distributed, but stepless, series of low-pass filters. To engineers, such systems are known as *delay lines*. One electrical form consists of a network of capacitors gradually increasing in value with rank order (Fig. 8). The electrical-network models of the cochlea are built in just this way. The time smear makes it somewhat difficult for an observer to recognize that the displacement of the partition originally constituted the first derivative of the stapedial displacement, especially when he records the displacement of the partition (or the cochlear-microphonic response) at a rather distal point, where there is also a sizeable phase delay.

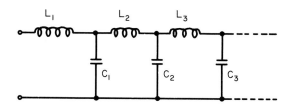

Figure 8 Electrical delay line. The size of the capacitors (C) increases with rank order. Since each LC link is recognized as a low-pass filter, it is clear that the bandwidth must decrease with rank order. In a cochlear model of this kind, resistors must be added in series with each inductor in order to simulate the frictional effects, which are mainly due to fluid viscosity.

In Fig. 9, data similar to those of Fig. 6 are plotted as the instantaneous displacement pattern for various times after signal onset, a form of presentation that emphasizes the spatial aspects of the traveling bulge pattern. In contrast to the steady-state pattern (Fig. 2), the envelope varies with each positive and negative crest; that is, the location of the point of maximal displacement migrates gradually toward the helicotrema.

From results such as those of Fig. 9, the propagation velocity of the traveling bulge along the partition can be calculated: it decreases exponentially with distance (Békésy, 1943). At a given point, it varies with the logarithm of the inverse time constant. In my original paper on this subject (Tonndorf, 1960c), I said that velocity also varies with the logarithm of signal amplitude, a statement that is only partially correct. Variations with amplitude occur only when the model is being overdriven so that its response becomes nonlinear. These earlier measurements were carried out at amplitude levels at which nonlinearity begins to play a noticeable role. At lower levels, *propagation velocity is independent of amplitude.*

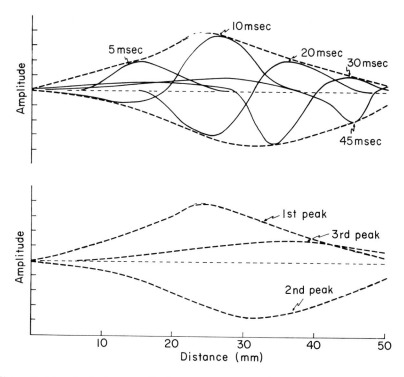

Figure 9 Top: Instantaneous displacement patterns of a traveling bulge at various times after signal onset in response to a step-function signal (time constant: 4.5 msec). Bottom: Consecutive envelopes for the first to third peaks of the same patterns (Tonndorf, 1960c. By permission from *Journal of the Acoustical Society of America*.)

C. Basic Mechanism of the Traveling Wave

One particular property of the Békésy model is responsible for the characteristic build-up and decay of the traveling bulge (or wave) along the partition – the stiffness gradient along the partition. This fact is easily demonstrated by constructing a model with a partition of uniform stiffness. In such models there may also be wave travel, provided the stiffness is not too high, but amplitude is simply attenuated with distance, and the envelope always has its highest point at the basal end. Recall that a model with a stiffness gradient, in first approximation, represents a *delay line* equivalent to the electrical one of Fig. 8. Then in the case of a mechanical or electrical model, the delay line is constituted by an increasing compliance or capacitance. In the surf analogy (Tonndorf, 1956), however, it is given by a negative gradient of mass (the decreasing amount of water upon the sloping beach). Since for each section of a delay line,

$$\frac{dM}{dC} = Z \qquad (6\text{-}5)$$

(M = mass or inductance; C = compliance or capacitance; Z = outgoing impedance), it is clear that the essential property is an *impedance gradient* in which the mass, the compliance, or both may be varied.

The characteristic shape of the envelope over the traveling-wave event results from two competing causes. Initially, the displacement amplitude must increase with distance along the partition as the opposing force, the stiffness, decreases. However, after the point is exceeded at which the passband of the partition becomes too restricted to include the signal frequency, the displacement amplitude must decrease once more. This relation is depicted in Fig. 10. Figure 10 neglects the effect of *friction*, which is mainly due to the fluid viscosity. Since the latter effect accumulates with distance, it is easily seen that its inclusion in Fig. 10 would have given the envelope its characteristic skewed shape. (Zwislocki, 1948).

When the stiffness gradient is made linear, the distribution of frequency maxima (in the sense of Fig. 3) becomes a linear function of frequency. With an exponential gradient, this distribution is a function of *log* frequency—i.e., octave intervals occupy constant distances along the partition, at least within its center portion. At both ends, the relation becomes nonlinear: (*a*) at the windows, because of the fixation of the partition at its basal end, and (*b*) apically, because of the helicotrema. In a given case, the distance occupied by an octave interval depends upon the stiffness gradient, or, in the case of an exponential gradient, upon the slope of its semilogarithmic plot. When the

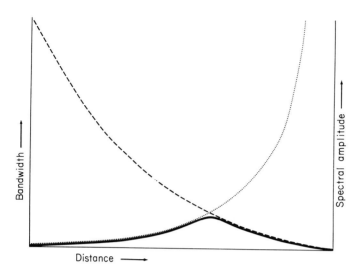

Figure 10 Composition of the envelope over the first half-wave of a traveling bulge. In first approximation, the envelope is the product of the decreasing bandwidth and increasing compliance of the partition with distance. This presentation neglects the effect of fluid viscosity. (Tonndorf, 1962b. By permission from *Journal of the Acoustical Society of America.*)

gradient is steep, octave intervals are crowded together; when it is less steep they lie farther apart (Tonndorf, 1957a).

In order to demonstrate the importance of the stiffness properties of cochlear models, Békésy (1956) made several models to obey his own concepts and those of Helmholtz, Ewald, and Rutherford by subtle alterations of the stiffness properties of the partition. Needless to say, the salient feature of his own model was the exponential stiffness gradient that he had actually observed and measured in 1928 and in 1942.

Tensing the partition shifts the operating point of the partition. Such experiments were carried out in models equipped with a "basilar membrane" and a "Reissner's membrane" (Tonndorf, 1957b). The partition was put under tension by changing the fluid volume of the "cochlear duct." Effects were largely limited to the apical end, (i.e., to places where the stiffness is low, and tension, consequently, has a relatively greater effect). Three phenomena were observed: (*a*) a loss of sensitivity with inverse frequency, (*b*) a shift of the point of maximal displacement in the direction of the base of the cochlea (once more, the degree of the shift varies with inverse frequency)*, and (c) even-harmonic distortion appearing at signal amplitudes that are low relative to the sensitivity loss encountered (also, the distorted waveform shifts in phase as a function of whether the "endolymphatic" fluid volume is larger or smaller than normal). All three phenomena vary in proportion to the change in fluid volume.

These three changes are equivalent to symptoms seen clinically in Ménière's disease, which is due to paroxysmal increases of fluid volume within the endolymphatic space (*endolymphatic hydrops*). The equivalent clinical symptoms are (a) low-frequency hearing loss, (b) diplacusis, (c) relatively early onset of even-harmonic distortion. In the early stages of the disease, the cause of which is not known, the low-frequency hearing loss fluctuates markedly over short periods of time, perhaps because of changes in endolymphatic fluid pressure.

In 1952, Wever and Lawrence performed a series of experiments that at first sight seem to refute the traveling-wave concept. They applied the same signal simultaneously to a cat's inner ear by two different routes: (a) via the stapes, and (b) via a hole drilled near the apex. The cochlear response was measured by registration of cochlear microphonics. They argued that if the traveling-wave concept were correct, it should be possible to produce two trains of waves traveling in opposite directions, and, provided damping were not too high, establish a system of standing waves by proper adjustment of amplitude and phase relations. They found evidence for stimulation of hair cells located basally by signals applied apically. However, they were unable to bring the two signals to cancellation, a finding they interpreted as evidence against the entire concept of cochlear wave travel.

Békésy (1955) then solved the apparent dilemma by demonstrating that, regardless of the point of signal input, *wave travel along the cochlear partition is invariably directed toward the helicotrema.* This finding can be explained in a manner that was first used to describe compressional bone conduction (Tonndorf, 1962a). Since the cochlear partition represents a series of low-pass filters, decreasing in bandwidth from base to apex, a high-frequency signal applied to the apical region of *scala vestibuli,* for example, cannot be transmitted directly through the partition into *scala tympani.* Its frequency is outside the passband of the partition in this region. The signal must seek a place

---

*That the point of maximal displacement shifts toward the cochlear base indicates that the shift is caused by the increase in *mass* (due to the accumulation of endolymphatic fluids), but not by the increase in *tension.* From a clinical standpoint (e.g., Ménière's disease), both stiffness- and mass-induced shifts may be incurred (Tonndorf, 1969).

along the partition where it can be admitted — where the passband is wide enough. Wherever the signal is transmitted into *scala tympani*, the partition is displaced and acquires potential energy by virtue of its displacement. (The fluid displacement in *scala tympani* must obviously continue all the way to the round window.) The resultant bulge is propelled along the partition toward places of lesser impedance (i.e., toward the cochlear apex) in order to restore the equilibrium of the system. Thus, wave travel from base to apex is initiated. From Eq. (6-5) it is clear that the impedance is highest basally, where the stiffness is high, and minimal within the helicotrema, where the stiffness is zero, and the impedance is purely resistive. These descriptions are wholly compatible with Zwislocki's (1953) mathematical account of the cochlear response to bone-conducted sounds. Temporally, the traveling wave is an afterevent. It serves to restore the equilibrium of the cochlear membrane-and-fluid system.

D. Shearing Motion within the Cochlear Duct

The notion had been held, even before Békésy, that hair-cell stimulation ought to result, directly or indirectly, from the displacement of the basilar membrane. Some assumed that these cells might be alternately compressed and stretched along their long axes during the up-and-down motion of the partition. However, von Holst (1950) and others demonstrated that, in other related organs that are also equipped with hair cells (such as the lateral-line organ of certain fishes, and the vestibular organ), the adequate stimulus consists invariably of a *tangential shear motion* between the organ and its covering structure — a motion that bends (or displaces[*]) the sensory hairs.

The true position of the tectorial membrane, as shown schematically in Fig. 14, was demonstrated by de Vries (1949) and confirmed by A. Hilding (1952). Later, Kimura (1966) was able to show, with the electron microscope, that the sensory hairs are pegged into suitable, but quite shallow indentations on the undersurface of the tectorial membrane.

---

[*]Engström (personal communication), when employing his microscopic "surface preparation," noted that the sensory hairs are quite brittle. The pressure exerted by a cover slide often breaks them off like matchsticks. He suggested that the tuft of hairs and the cuticular layer in which they are firmly rooted are displaced *in toto*. The fact that the cuticular layer sits in the top part of the hair cell like a stopper in a bottle, but leaves a small gap laterally, makes this notion quite plausible.

224   JUERGEN TONNDORF

A. Hilding (1953), in further pursuit of his anatomical studies, also proposed a shearing mechanism between the organ of Corti and the tectorial membrane, thus reviving Hurst's (1895) and ter Kuile's (1900) older suggestions. Independently, and at the same time, Békésy (1953a) became interested in the same question, starting from the general notion that tangential shear stresses develop between the various layers of nonhomogeneous structures that are being bent. Since the basilar membrane, the organ of Corti, and the tectorial membrane comprise such layers, he looked for and indeed found shearing displacements that take place between the tectorial membrane and the organ of Corti of living guinea pigs. Somewhat unexpectedly, he found *two* modes of shear (Fig. 11): proximal to the place of maximal vertical displacement, he saw *radial* shear, and farther distal, *longitudinal* shear. The zones were separated by a small region in which there appeared to be nothing but vertical displacement. Tonndorf (1960a) then measured the relative amplitude distribution of the three modes of motion in cochlear models. First of all, it turned out (Fig. 12) that the area between the two modes of shear apparent in Fig. 11 is not real, but is simply due to the limited optical resolution of the experimental arrangement Békésy employed.

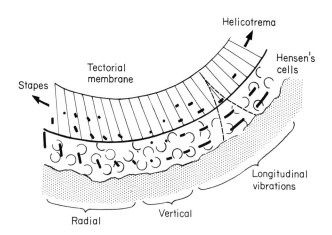

Figure 11 Distribution of radial and longitudinal shear motions along the organ of Corti of a guinea pig (schematic view from above, through Reissner's membrane), in response to a sinusoidal signal. (Békésy, 1953a. By permission from *Journal of the Acoustical Society of America*.)

Figure 12 shows further that the amplitude of the shearing displacement is smaller, by 15 to 20 dB, than that of the original displacement of the partition. As Békésy (1953a) pointed out, this reduction in
amplitude is the manifestation of a second transformer action within
the ear – the first one being that of the middle ear. This second force
transformation is needed because the work the shearing force must
perform consists of bending (or displacing) thousands of sensory hairs
within a relatively small area (there are approximately 80 hairs per
individual cell).

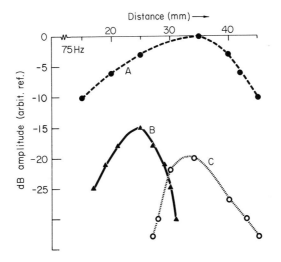

Figure 12   Envelopes of the three modes of motion in a cochlear model: (A) traveling-
wave; (B) radial shear; (C) longitudinal shear. The maximal amplitude of the traveling-
wave pattern is arbitrarily set at unity. The ordinate is given in log units to show the
change of slope in the transformation of the traveling-wave event into shear motion.
Note that, in this transformation, amplitude is reduced by a factor of 15 to 20 dB.
(Tonndorf, 1960a. By permission from *Journal of the Acoustical Society of America.*)

The model's findings revealed *why* there are two modes of shear
motion perpendicular to each other. Shearing stresses are known to
develop both in the direction of, and in proportion to, the curvature
of the structure being bent. One often tends to forget that the basilar
membrane is not a vibrating ribbon of the sort shown in Fig. 13A. In
reality, it is restricted along both lateral rims so that Fig. 13B is a more
exact representation of its instantaneous displacement pattern. Thus,
in the region proximal to the maximal vertical displacement, where

the length of half-waves is large, the dominant curvature is in the radial direction, and the resultant shear motion is likewise directed radially. However, as soon as the region of shorter half-waves is reached, especially beyond the point of maximal amplitude (where the vertical amplitude is quite small), the radial curvature becomes negligible, and the longitudinal one begins to dominate. Consequently, in this region the resultant shear motion is in the longitudinal direction.

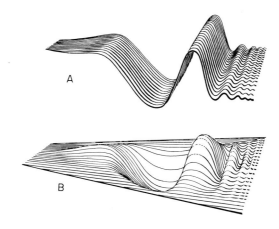

Figure 13 Traveling-wave patterns: (*a*) executed by a hypothetical ribbon-like partition; (*b*) observed along the single-layer partition of a cochlear model. Scales are arbitrary in both drawings, and magnitudes are exaggerated. (Tonndorf, 1960a. By permission from *Journal of the Acoustical Society of America*.)

The transition between the two modes is clearly seen when one inspects a traveling-wave pattern by looking straight down upon the partition with the light adjusted so as to throw long shadows of the displaced portions. Initially, the wavecrests are quite long and pear-shaped—the longitudinal curvature is much smaller than the radial one. In the region of maximal vertical displacement, the wavecrests grow gradually shorter, finally becoming radially-oriented ridges with strong longitudinal, but negligible, radial curvatures. Figure 13B shows both of these features.

Johnstone and Johnstone (1966), in a paper on the origin of the summating potential, came to a different conclusion concerning the *mechanical* displacement of the pad that consists of the basilar membrane, the organ of Corti, and the tectorial membrane. They thought that the organ is completely rigid in the radial direction and should be displaced like the stapes footplate within the oval window, with the necessary yielding provided for by the marginal portions of the basilar membrane—as it is by the annular ligament around the stapes. This concept was based upon what appears to be a misunderstanding of some of Békésy's published findings, an example of which is presented in Fig. 14A. This drawing gives compliance, in *cm per dyne*, of the main structures of the cochlear duct. Tests were made by applying a point-shaped constant force sequentially to a number of places that are distributed in the radial direction. On first glance, it seems indeed as if the reticular membrane and Reissner's membrane were rigid structures. The latter conclusion shows the fallacy of the argument. The findings concerning Reissner's membrane and the reticular membrane are typical for high-compliance structures for which (when a point-shaped force is applied sequentially to a number of places)

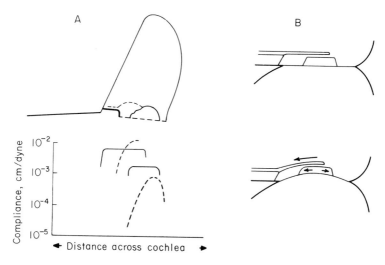

Figure 14   (A) Elastic properties of cochlear structures for a position 20 mm from the stapes, according to measurements by Békésy in a human cadaver specimen. A schematized cross section of the cochlear turn is given above (with Reissner's membrane facing left). The data below resulted from application of a point-shaped constant force sequentially to various places along the cross section. The key to the lower drawing is given in the upper drawing. (Békésy, 1947. By permission from *Journal of the Acoustical Society of America.*) (B) Interpretation of the results of (A) to the situation in which a hydro-static force is applied that acts uniformly over the entire cross section. The basilar membrane, the organ of Corti, and the tectorial membrane are shown in a highly schematic cross section. Top: organ at rest; bottom: organ displaced upward. Note that, in this displacement, the organ is stretched wider and, consequently, must become a little flatter in order to maintain a constant volume.

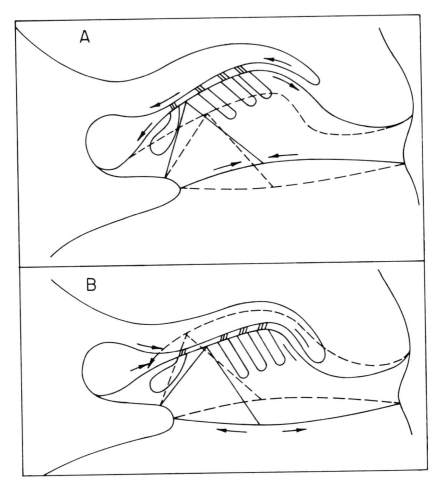

Figure 15 Schematic cross sections of the organ of Corti, illustrating the shearing displacements between the organ of Corti and the tectorial membrane. In (A), the basilar membrane is displaced upward; in (B), downward. In both instances, the opposite positions of the basilar membrane and of the organ are shown as shaded outlines. The directions of shearing stresses are indicated by arrows.

The directions of radial shear within the reticular membrane (i.e., the upper surface of the organ of Corti) and within the basilar membrane oppose each other, since these two membranes form the upper- and lowermost layers of an inhomogeneous structure. Note too that, on both sides of the center line, shearing stresses occur in opposite directions, which is due to the bilateral fixation of the whole structure.

By contrast, the tectorial membrane is fastened along its medial rim only. Therefore, radial shearing stresses have the same direction over the entire cross section. Consequently, only in the region of the *outer* hair cells are relative displacements (in the

the effect of their lateral fixation is negligible. However, the shapes of the curves for the basilar membrane and for the tectorial membrane under the same condition are typical for structures of lower compliance. The difference between them is that the basilar membrane is fixed along both of its rims, whereas the tectorial membrane is fixed only along its medial rim.

When the combined structure is displaced by a *hydrostatic* force (the effect of which is distributed over the whole cross-section) the results look very different (Fig. 14B)—consider the ballooning out of Reissner's membrane in endolymphatic hydrops. The soft pad that represents the organ follows the displacement of the (stiffer) basilar membrane and is slightly stretched in the process. The tectorial membrane slides to and fro, mainly in the radial direction. Thus, it turns out that the compliance measurements Békésy made in actual cochleae (Fig. 14A) are in complete accord with the notions underlying the construction of the model from which the results of Fig. 12 were obtained, and with their interpretation in Fig. 13.

How do the hair cells respond to the two modes of shear shown in Figs. 11 and 12? In another study, Békésy (1953b) obtained results that suggested that the outer hair cells might respond to *radial* shear, and the inner ones respond to longitudinal shear. This apparent directional selectivity of the two types of hair cells raises the further question of whether the property is built into the hair cells themselves, or whether it has mechanical causes.

Kharina (personal communication) noted that the radial shear motions on the two sides of the center line of the partition are in phase opposition (Tonndorf, 1960a). He suggested that, because of its unilateral fixation, the tectorial membrane moves in phase with the underlying organ in the region of the inner hair cells, and in phase opposition in the region of the outer hair cells (Fig. 15). Consequently, a shearing motion is brought about only in the region of the outer hair cells; the inner hair cells remain unaffected.

A similar argument can be made with respect to the longitudinal shear. Because of the cochlear coiling, the innermost portion of the

---

radial direction) brought about between the tectorial membrane and the underlying organ of Corti—the shearing stresses in the two structures are opposite. However, in the region of the inner hair cells, where the shearing stresses in both structures are in the same direction, there can be little or no relative displacement between the tectorial membrane and the organ of Corti. Note that the displacements of the hairs on the outer hair cells are confined to one side of the cell axis. This "half-wave" rectification is due to the slanted position of the outer hair cells as was first postulated by de Vries (1949).

tectorial membrane might be more rigidly supported by the spiral limbus and therefore be relatively stiff. Then there would be longitudinal displacement only between the tectorial membrane and the inner hair cells, under the effect of longitudinal shear. In contrast, the lateral free rim of the tectorial membrane would lie more loosely upon the organ, and thus be able to follow the displacement more closely, thereby cancelling any longitudinal shear motion in this region.

Békésy (1951) showed that the hair cells are *displacement* receivers. De Vries (1952) found that the sensory cells of the lateral-line organ generate microphonic potentials upon displacement of their hairs in either direction. Thus, the lateral-line organ responds (to a sinusoidal signal) with twice the original frequency. Since the cochlea obviously does not, de Vries postulated a *mechanical* bias of the cochlear hair cells, and, for the outer hair cells, he attributed it to their slanted position. Figure 15 shows clearly that the displacement of the sensory hairs occurs only on one side of the axis of each cell (to the right, in the figure). Van Bergeijk and Speeth (1960) extended this principle to the inner hair cells and postulated a slant of these cells in the longitudinal direction. Tonndorf *et al.* (1962) demonstrated by vital staining that the inner hair cells are indeed slightly slanted, with their hair-bearing ends pointing slightly toward the cochlear apex.

Electron microscopy (Engström *et al.*, 1962; Flock *et al.*, 1962) confirms Held's (1902) finding that the hairs of the sensory cells are oriented in a regular manner. Those of the outer hair cells (in guinea pigs) are grouped in three rows and show a **W**-shaped distribution, with the bottom of the **W** pointing laterally; those of the inner hair cells are grouped in two rather flat rows also facing laterally.

In both types of cells, the so-called *centriole* lies lateral to the rows of hairs. It is the movement of the hairs *toward* the centriole that causes electrical depolarisation of a given cell (Löwenstein and Wersäll, 1959). Thus, the electron-microscopic findings suggest that *both* types of cells are sensitive to shear motion in the radial direction, and only to that. This conclusion does not completely refute all of the observations concerning the effects of *mechanical* causes.* It only throws doubt upon the effect of longitudinal shear in eliciting hair-cell responses, and upon Békésy's interpretation of his own experimental

---

*De Vries's (1952) finding that there is frequency-doubling in the lateral-line organ is explained by the fact that those hair cells are not all aligned in one direction — about 50 percent face forward and 50 percent backward. His view of the mechanical bias as expressed in Fig. 15 may still be correct.

findings concerning the directional sensitivity of the inner and outer hair cells. Clearly, further experimental evidence is needed. What is clear at this time is that *shearing motion presents the ultimate mode of mechanical input to the hair cells.*

E. Mechanical Sharpening of the Response

Although Békésy's traveling-wave concept became gradually accepted, some writers saw difficulties in reconciling the extent of the measured envelopes (Fig. 3) with the sharp frequency discrimination of the ear. For example, the envelopes for 1000 Hz and 1010 Hz, two frequencies the human ear can easily differentiate, overlap each other almost completely. Since the restriction of the envelope due to the shear-wave transformation (Fig. 12) was not known then, and the displacements of the basilar membrane were considered the ultimate stimulus to the hair cells, "neural sharpening" became the watchword.

However, some writers had second thoughts. Huggins and Licklider (1951) proposed a "beam" hypothesis that assumed that the tectorial membrane lies on top of the organ like a stiff beam, and that the hair cells are pressed against this beam during the upward displacement of the basilar membrane. Mathematically, they showed that, under such conditions, forces are developed that are proportional to the fourth derivative of the displacement pattern of the partition. Each consecutive derivative of the instantaneous displacement pattern becomes more sharply peaked around the place of maximal amplitude (Békésy, 1953a). Thus, the envelope over the fourth derivative is much more restricted than that over the original displacement pattern.

The results of the shearing experiments (Figs. 11 and 12) confirmed the soundness of the general concept of Huggins and Licklider that the sharpening may be mechanical, although the underlying mechanism turned out to be a different one. In Fig. 12, note that in the transformation from vertical displacement to either mode of shear motion, the proximal slope of the envelope becomes approximately as steep as the distal one (which hardly changes at all). Thus, some sharpening has indeed occurred in the shear-wave transformation. This finding is interesting from the standpoint of signal coding within the first-order neuron of the cochlear nerve. Reference has been made repeatedly to the wide discrepancy between the mechanical tuning curves of the basilar membrane, as measured by Békésy (1942, 1944), and those of single fibers of the first-order neuron, as measured by Katsuki *et al.* (1962) and by Kiang *et al.* (1965) with respect to their

Q–factors (a measure of peakedness). The implication was that the much narrower tuning of the neural curves must have been brought about *beyond* the mechanical events of the cochlea. The results shown in Figs. 11 and 12 throw a new light upon this issue. It is clear too that what occurs in the spatial domain of Figs. 11 and 12 applies also to the frequency domain.

There had been a second difficulty: all of Békésy's mechanical tuning curves were measured, for technical reasons, in the apical sections of the cochlea (i.e., for low frequencies), whereas most of the neural tuning curves were measured for higher frequencies. This difficulty was removed by Johnstone and Boyle (1967), who measured tuning curves at a point 1.4 mm from the stapes in guinea pigs. A comparison of their data and those of Békésy shows, at least for the case of guinea pigs, that the Q-factor of the mechanical tuning curves of the basilar membrane increases with frequency in what appears to be a linear manner (Tonndorf and Khanna, 1968). The Q-factor of the neural tuning curves (first-order neuron) also increases with frequency, although the relation does not appear to be linear (Kiang *et al.*, 1965). But then, the latter data were obtained in cats. Preliminary calculations by my associate, S. Khanna (personal communication), have taken these findings and conditions into account, and indicate that it is most likely the shearing transformation that contributes most if not all of the increase in sharpening displayed by the tuning curves of single fibers of the first-order neuron of the cochlear nerve. It is certainly not my intent to deny the existence of neural sharpening. However, the data at hand appear to indicate that such a property may belong only to higher stations of the central auditory system.

F.   Cochlear Analysis

Ohm's Acoustic Law states that the cochlea executes a Fourier analysis of the incoming sound, a concept that leaves many psychological observations unexplained, including the evidence for the detection of envelope or periodicity pitch (Seebeck, 1841; Schouten, 1938; de Boer, 1956; Small, 1955; Schouten *et al.*, 1962; and others). Some of this evidence makes it unlikely that the time analysis required for periodicity detection takes place within the peripheral ear. Schouten, for one, postulated a central mechanism.

Let us look at the type of analysis performed by a cochlear model. According to neurophysiological evidence (Tunturi, 1944; Galambos,

1954), the place of maximal excitation of the hair cells determines the pitch perception associated with an applied frequency.* When a cochlear model is driven by a complex signal of simple configuration (e.g., one composed of first and second harmonics; first and third harmonics; or first, second and third harmonics), the depth of penetration of the various harmonics into the model is in inverse proportion to their frequency. Figure 16 is a composite drawing of the fluid-motion pattern under such a condition. Actually, this response is to be expected because of the low-pass filter properties of the model. The phase relations between the harmonics of Fig. 16 never alter — another characteristic of shallow-water waves. (In deep water, the propagation velocity is in inverse proportion to frequency: long, low-frequency waves are constantly overtaking short, high-frequency waves.)

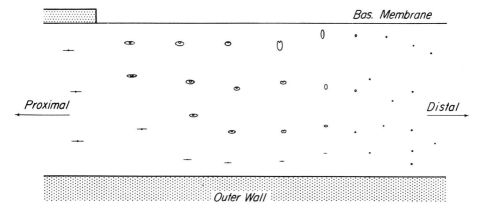

Figure 16   Perilymphatic fluid motion in one scala of a cochlear model in response to a complex harmonic signal consisting of two partials (50 Hz and 100 Hz). In principle, the distribution of vectorial amplitudes is not unlike that shown in Fig. 4. However, individual particle pathways are now complex Lissajous figures characteristic of a 1:2 frequency relation. With distance, the particle pathways loose their complexity and become simple. Note that the interharmonic phase, indicated by the relative position of the inner loops in each particle pathway, never alters along the partition. (Tonndorf, 1962b. By permission from *Journal of the Acoustical Society of America.*)

---

*According to the findings presented in connection with Figs. 11–15, this place is where the shearing envelope reaches its maximum, although the envelope, which is only a construct, obviously cannot stimulate cells itself. For the sake of simplicity, the discussion considers only the displacement pattern of the basilar membrane.

Figure 17 indicates that, in the case of a harmonic signal of simple configuration, the envelope along the partition becomes definitely multi-modal, with the maxima distributed correctly. Thus, there is evidence for the execution of a Fourier analysis within the model, at least for complex tones of simple configuration. Matters become very different with pulse trains, though.

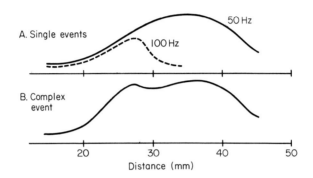

Figure 17 Envelopes over traveling waves in a cochlear model in response to steady-state signals. (A) Two individual sinusoidal events (50 Hz and 100 Hz). (B) Complex event, composed of the same two frequencies as in (A). (Tonndorf, 1962b. By permission from *Journal of the Acoustical Society of America.*)

The model's transient response (Figs. 6 and 10) shows no evidence of a Fourier analysis. The Fourier spectrum of the signal is continuous and hyperbola-shaped; amplitude is infinitely high at zero frequency, and decreases with frequency thereafter. However, in the model, the response maximum does not occur at the helicotrema ($f = 0$), but at a definite place along the partition. Systematic variation of the applied signal revealed that the location is a function of the time constant of the *waveform* (Fig. 18), a finding compatible with Gabor's (1946) mathematical concepts. He combined time and frequency in a simple diagram with a sine wave representing one extreme (a line of infinite length parallel to the time axis), and a pulse of zero duration the other (a line of infinite length parallel to the frequency axis) (Fig. 19). Gabor described his diagram by

$$\Delta f \cdot \Delta t \geqslant \tfrac{1}{2}. \tag{6-6}$$

With the exception of the sine wave and the pulse (which are uni-

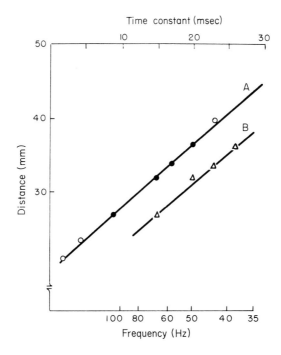

Figure 18 Position of maximal amplitudes along the partition of a cochlear model. (A) Of the first half-waves of traveling bulges (transient events) of varying time constants (Δt). (B) Of traveling waves (steady-state events) for sinusoidal signals of frequencies corresponding to the inverse time constants ($1/\Delta t$) of curve A. (Tonndorf, 1962b. By permission from *Journal of the Acoustical Society of America*.)

dimensional), all acoustic signals occupy *areas* within the diagram made up of $\Delta f \cdot \Delta t$ rectangles.[*]

Figure 18 shows that the model follows Gabor's equation. The points along curve A (transient responses) have amplitude maxima that depend upon the time constants; for curve B (the sine-wave responses), they depend upon frequency. The two curves do not coincide, and their distance is given by

$$\Delta f \cdot \Delta t = 3/2, \qquad (6\text{-}7)$$

a result that fits Eq. (6-6).

---

[*]The interesting similarity between Gabor's equation and Heisenberg's uncertainty principle is detailed in Licklider, 1951.

Responses to all other types of signals—amplitude- or frequency-modulated, beating, etc.—fall between the extremes of Fig. 19. They undergo frequency as well as time analyses. A beating signal (Tonndorf, 1959a), for example, results in a traveling-wave whose place of maximal amplitude corresponds to the so-called intertone: $(f_1 + f_2)/2$. The two spectral components (f_1 and f_2) are nowhere in evidence in the traveling-wave pattern. The amplitude waxes and wanes with the beat rate $(f_1 - f_2)$. If the amplitude of one component is larger than that of the other, an additional small frequency modulation becomes evident: the place of maximal amplitude shifts slightly up and down the partition.

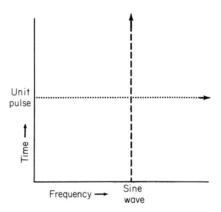

Figure 19 Time/frequency diagram after Gabor. In this form of presentation, a unit pulse is represented by a horizontal line, and a sine wave by a vertical line. All other signals are given as *areas* of various shapes. (Gabor, 1946. By permission from *J. Inst. Elect. Engrs.*)

The beat rate itself is also detected in the model, and when high enough in frequency, forms its own traveling wave. The latter extends much farther into the model than that due to the higher primary frequencies that are filtered out more basally.

That the detection of the beat rate is not simply the same nonlinear effect that produces a difference tone is demonstrated by using beats of mistuned consonances. For example, for the two primaries, 50 Hz and 104 Hz, the model detects 4 Hz—the beat rate—but the difference tone is 54 Hz. It is clearly a form of envelope detection or demodulation.

G.   Intracochlear Demodulation of Hydrodynamic Origin

The envelope detection just described is only observed in mechanical cochlear models (it is not seen in electrical ones because the required properties have not been built into them). The detection occurs because (*a*) the displacement of the cochlear fluids (and of the partition) is asymmetrical (so, in response to beating signals, energy is made to appear at the frequency of the envelope, i.e., the beat rate); and (*b*) the low-pass filter action of the model lets the wave representing the newly introduced low-frequency energy travel farther in the apical direction than that due to the primary frequencies. The demodulated waveform shows all the properties of a traveling wave—a fact that is best recognized with rapid beat rates and high-frequency primaries.

Although the ultimate cause of the underlying distortion process is not properly understood, there is a sufficient number of detailed observations to permit pinpointing the region of its origin (Tonndorf, 1959a; 1962b; 1969). The asymmetry is invariably directed away from the input at the oval window (see Fig. 20). In the fluid motion of *scala vestibuli,* larger amplitudes occur toward the helicotrema (horizontal vector) and toward the partition (vertical vector). Opposite directions prevail in *scala tympani.* Consequently, the displacement of the partition is larger toward *scala tympani* than toward *scala vestibuli.*

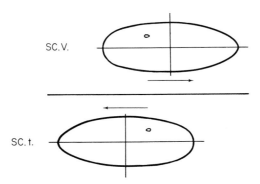

Figure 20 Modulated response of two fluid particles, adjacent to each other across the cochlear position, in response to a beat signal (schematic). Location: basal region. Shown are the Lissajous figures at minimal (small ovals) and maximal amplitudes (large ovals). They are not symmetrically modulated around their respective centers, but are asymmetrical in both the longitudinal and the transverse direction. (Adapted from Tonndorf, 1959a. By permission from *Journal of the Acoustical Society of America.*)

When the stiffness of the partition is varied linearly with distance ("linear stiffness gradient") the degree of asymmetrical displacement, for a constant beat rate, is practically independent of the range of the primary frequencies, though only for primaries that are sufficiently high in frequency so that the resulting traveling wave does not involve the helicotrema. For primary frequencies below this limit, the degree of asymmetrical displacement decreases rapidly with inverse frequency. In contrast, with the usual exponential stiffness gradient, the degree of asymmetrical motion increases monotonically with the range of primary frequencies (for a constant beat rate). These observations show that the generation of asymmetry depends upon some local value of the stiffness gradient; i.e., it is a *localized phenomenon*.

Neither the windows nor the helicotrema (except for the special case just mentioned) are primarily involved in the generation of asymmetrical motion. The source of asymmetry, then, might be the region of the partition that shows an amplitude maximum in response to a given pair of primaries. This conclusion is further supported by the observation that the asymmetry varies with the steepness of the (linear) stiffness gradient. For a given pair of primary frequencies (or for a single frequency, for that matter), an increase in the steepness of the stiffness gradient renders the traveling-wave envelope more peaked as the filter action per unit length of the partition is being increased. In other words, the asymmetry depends upon the peakedness of the envelope over the traveling waves. Significantly, when the stiffness gradient is zero, waves simply attenuate with distance — there is no Békésy-type envelope, and no asymmetrical displacement either.

The degree of asymmetry is independent of the amplitude of the beating signals. This observation indicates that the asymmetry is most likely caused *hydrodynamically*. In solid structures, the force opposing displacement is elastic, and elastic properties, as they approach their limiting values, vary nonlinearly with amplitude. Therefore, distortion in such structures usually varies with higher powers of the signal amplitude. In incompressible and viscous fluids, however, the opposing force is viscous, and such properties do not possess any limiting value. Thus, in hydrodynamic systems, more often than not, waveform distortion varies linearly with the signal amplitude, a fact that was apparently first recognized and expressed mathematically by Schaefer (1910).

Figure 21 shows that the degree of asymmetry increases with inverse viscosity. This fact suggests that the underlying phenomenon might be a *boundary-layer* effect. According to Prandtl and Tietjens

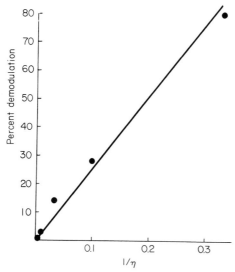

Figure 21 Percent demodulation vs. inverse viscosity determined for one pair of primaries of 50 Hz and 55 Hz in a mechanical cochlear model. The magnitude of the beat rate (5 Hz) was measured within the helicotrema, and that of the resultant of the two primaries, in the region of their maximal amplitude. (Tonndorf, 1969.)

(1934), who first defined such layers and their effects, the boundary layer at a fluid-to-solid interface is the thin layer of a viscous fluid that adheres to the solid surface due to the mutual attraction of molecules across the interface. For example, when a dc stream of fluid moves along a solid wall, a gradient of velocity is set up; i.e., velocity varies from zero at the interface itself to the value of the "free" stream some distance away from it. This gradient sets up shearing stresses. The thickness of boundary layers varies with viscosity, so, for low viscosities, the boundary layer is very thin, the velocity gradient is steep, the shearing stresses are strong; and vice versa.

There is no interface within the helicotrema of a cochlear model and no boundary layers exist there. This limitation may explain why the traveling waves that reach the helicotrema (in the case of low-frequency primaries) show lesser degrees of asymmetrical motion.

Waves traveling along free surfaces are inherently and strongly nonlinear. Intuitively, one should expect that such nonlinearities would be cancelled out when waves occur along an interface separating two bodies of otherwise identical fluids. It is especially difficult to see how an asymmetry could develop in this situation. There is one more observation that might at least shed some light upon the problem. To discuss it, we have to return to the trochoidal form of fluid motion underlying wave motion along the cochlear partition. In waves progressing along free fluid surfaces, the two axes of individual particle orbits form an orthogonal field with respect to the resting surface. The presentation in Fig. 4 is based upon such a premise. Figure 22 indicates, however, that this assumption is correct only as a first-order approximation. The figure shows that, close to the partition, and especially around the place of maximal displacement, the particle orbits appear slightly inclined. This inclination changes direction at the place of maximal displacement so that the vertical axes appear to point approximately toward the maximum. The lower the viscosity of the fluid, the more the orbits are inclined, revealing this phenomenon to be a boundary-layer effect.

In 1962, I thought that the apparent inclination might be due to a localized alteration of the normal 90° phase relation between the two vectors of fluid motion, and thus called it a "vectorial phase distortion." Later, I learned that in 1951 Biesel (Kinsman, 1965) had made the same observation in surf; at least he found the backward inclination of orbits in the region proximal to the place of maximal amplitude. According to Biesel, the orbits are tilted *in toto*, i.e., both the major axes and the minor ones are inclined by the same amount. If we accept his viewpoint, we must agree that the fluid motion has ceased to be laminar, and that vortex motion has ensued. Vorticity, by definition, means the introduction of nonlinear factors. This explanation would also account for the fact, seen in Fig. 22, that the inclination of particle orbits extends over a much wider area than that of the boundary layer in which it was supposed to originate. Vorticity is known to spread into adjacent fluid layers by advection (Batchelor, 1967).

In summary, the present results support the hypothesis that the asymmetrical displacement of the partition and the subsequent envelope detection arises as a boundary-layer effect in the region of the displacement maximum formed by the traveling waves. It should be mentioned that the asymmetrical displacement as described here was observed (*a*) in the trochoidal fluid motion, (*b*) in the displacement pattern of the cochlear partition, and (*c*) in both modes of shear motion (Tonndorf, 1960c).

With specific reference to beats, their *visual* detection in the model varies with their complexity in the same order as found by Helmholtz (1954) for their *auditory* detection: imperfect unison 1:1, then the mistuned consonances 1:2, 1:3, 1:4, 2:3, and so on (Tonndorf, 1959a). It is proportional to the degree of variation of the envelope,

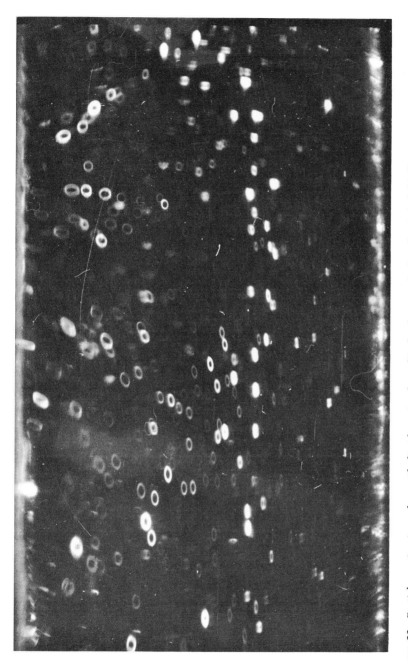

Figure 22   Particle motion in *scala vestibuli* at low signal amplitude photographed under dark-field illumination. The outer wall runs along the bottom, and the partition along the top of the picture. The window is toward the left; the helicotrema is toward the right. The place of maximal displacement due to the traveling wave is slightly to the right of the center. Note the leaning-over of the individual particle orbits, first toward the right, and later toward the left. (Tonndorf, 1962b. By permission from *Journal of the Acoustical Society of America*.)

supporting the hypothesis that we are dealing with a process of *enve-lope detection.*[*]

H.   Cochlear Eddies – Intracochlear Harmonic Distortion

The first phenomenon one notices in a cochlear model, driven by a steady-state signal, is the pair of eddies (Fig. 23) on either side of the partition (Békésy, 1928). The eddy currents do not revolve at a uniform speed (Tonndorf, 1958a). As indicated by the lengths of the arrows in Fig. 23, there is a fast increasing acceleration along the partition, with the highest velocity being reached precisely at the point where the eddies turn away from the partition. Then, there is a sudden and sharp reversal of acceleration. Negative acceleration continues all along the return path, with the velocity becoming slower and slower. Because of the condition of continuity, the same amount of fluid must be moved through every section of each eddy per unit time. Hence, the change in acceleration must be accompanied by a reciprocal change in the *width* of the eddies' channels, as indicated in Fig. 23. At the point of highest velocity (distal end), the channel is very narrow and the eddy jets through. Along the return path, the channel is much wider.

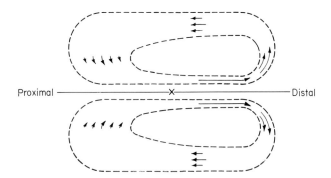

Figure 23   Pattern of eddy motion in both perilymphatic scalae (schematic). The (x) denotes the locus of maximal displacement along the cochlear partition. Note the reciprocal relation between the diameter of the eddies' channels and their velocity (length of arrows). In reality, there is no static center as is indicated here for the sake of illustration. (Tonndorf, 1958. By permission from *Journal of the Acoustical Society of America.*)

---

[*]A finding of Goldstein (1967) concerning the *audible* appearance of the combination tone $2f_1-f_2$ has been corroborated electrophysiologically by Kiang (personal communication). Kiang's observations suggest an intracochlear origin of this component.

With an increase in *frequency* of the driving signal, the eddies become smaller in both dimensions (thus staying closer to the partition). In response to low-frequency signals, they fill almost all of the available perilymphatic spaces. Invariably, however, they are centered approximately on the place of maximal amplitude of the traveling wave in response to a given frequency. (Actually, there are no dead centers within the eddies; they were included in Fig. 23 just to illustrate the change in channel width.)

With increasing *amplitude,* the eddies grow in size (in both dimensions), and their velocity at a given point (e.g., in the region of maximal amplitude of the traveling wave) increases. Measurements over a limited range of 24 dB indicate that the eddy velocity varies approximately with the *square* of the driving amplitude — that is, it is proportional to the driving power. This relation was predicted by Zwislocki (1948) on theoretical grounds.

The eddies are of course another hydro-dynamic phenomenon. For constant signal amplitude, they also vary with inverse viscosity — as best as can be determined with its *square* (Tonndorf, 1957a). Under the same condition, the displacement amplitude of the partition varies *linearly* with inverse viscosity, indicating that signal transmission through the cochlear fluids is affected by its resistive properties. These two facts have a practical application for model experimentation. By making viscosity very high, one can obtain a model that produces no noticeable eddy motion, even at high input values; yet it will display relatively large displacement amplitudes of the trochoidal fluid motion and of the partition.

The eddy currents are another boundary-layer phenomenon. The equivalent in surf is the undertow (Tonndorf, 1956). Recall that the partition and the surrounding fluids are coupled together. As soon as the wave motion along the partition reaches a certain critical amplitude, it begins to propel some fluid particles in its immediate vicinity (i.e., within the boundary layer), much in the same manner as a wave crest propels a surf board. The higher the viscosity of the fluids, the wider the boundary layer, and the larger its resistance to this propagating force. In contrast to the traveling-wave motion, which *de*celerates as it progresses, the eddy currents *ac*celerate while moving in the same direction. There are two facts to explain this seeming paradox: (*a*) driving the fluid becomes more effective as the wave-like displacement of the partition becomes steeper (Fig. 2); and (*b*) the effect of this driving force accumulates with time and distance. Because of the inverse relation between eddy speed and traveling-wave speed, one could imagine a point beyond which the eddy speed would exceed that of the wave—a phenomenon that cannot occur. The fluids in the distal sections of the model, not being propelled by the partition at any appreciable rate, nor by large waves at all, stand in the way of the onrushing eddy currents. Thus, the eddies begin to pile over the stagnant distal fluids, leave the partition, and initiate their return movement, which is necessary in order to preserve the continuity of the fluid.

At one time, the eddies were thought to represent the ultimate mechanical stimulus to the hair cells of the organ of Corti, a notion that Zwislocki (1948) dispelled by demonstrating mathematically that their inherent power is much too small for such a task, especially in view of the fact that they occur outside of the cochlear duct. However, this hydro-dynamic by-product of wave motion along the partition does have significance in cochlear function. It introduces harmonic distortion (Tonndorf, 1958a). By definition, the eddies themselves, being *rectified* events, must be considered nonlinear phenomena. The interaction between the eddy current accelerating along the partition and the trochoidal fluid motion is best observed in the pathways of individual fluid particles. Their mode of motion changes from purely trochoidal to *accelerating epicycloids,* and that results in peak-clipped waveforms (Fig. 24).

The argument that the peak-clipping might have been caused by the partition exceeding its elastic limits is easily countered by varying the viscosity of the cochlear fluids. The onset of distortion does not depend upon a fixed value of the displacement amplitude of the traveling-wave response, but solely upon the appearance of the eddy currents. Furthermore, when eddy currents are induced artificially by producing fluid circulation within the model from an external source, essentially the same distortion of trochoidal fluid motion is observed as that shown in Fig. 24 (Tonndorf, 1958a).

If, in a standard model, the input signal is increased beyond the point where eddies first appear, small *subeddies* form within the gradually growing original eddy, mainly at places proximal to that of maximal displacement. Each of these subeddies corresponds in place to a higher harmonic. Their appearance may be explained by the fact that the high-frequency energy they represent cannot penetrate too far apically because of the model's band-pass limitations.

Stroboscopic examination shows that, in addition, each harmonic forms a small, but clearly recognizable, amplitude maximum of its own at its proper place along the partition. (Although it shows the

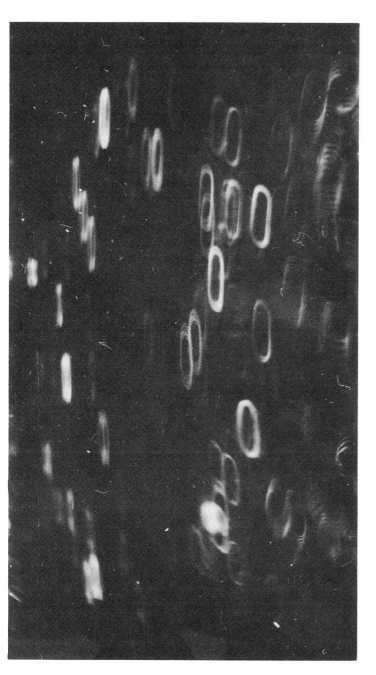

Figure 24 Particle pathways within the perilymphatic fluids of a cochlear model in response to a sinusoidal signal, and in the presence of strong eddy motion (photographed under dark-field illumination). The basilar membrane is on top, and the cochlear base is toward the left; the eddy moves clockwise. The presence of the eddy is indicated by the fact that, along the partition, where its velocity is high, the particle pathways are expanded into helical figures. The particle pathways are flattened on top and bottom and their upper right-hand corners are drawn out. An analysis of such pathways indicates that the displacement of the partition is both peak-clipped and asymmetrical, with the larger amplitude directed toward *scala tympani*. Note the slight inclination (top left) of the helical figures, in correspondence with Fig. 22. (Tondorf, 1958. By permission from *Journal of the Acoustical Society of America*.)

response to an externally-applied harmonic signal, Fig. 17 depicts a situation that is basically similar.) The order of visual appearance of higher harmonics vs. frequency of the fundamental in the model is essentially the same as that first described by Fletcher (1929) for their *audible* detection (Tonndorf, 1958a). As demonstrated here, the *hydro-dynamic, endochochlear, harmonic distortion produces responses in accord with the place principle.*

The harmonic distortion due to the eddy currents varies with the square of the driving signal (and also of fluid viscosity). In contrast, the demodulation process and its underlying mechanism varies as a *linear* function of these two parameters. This fact clearly differentiates these two phenomena from each other. Yet there is some interaction between these processes. (*a*) The change in particle motion shown in Fig. 24 not only entails peak clipping, but also an *asymmetrical* motion whose polarity is identical to that induced by the mechanism underlying demodulation. (*b*) When eddy currents interact with a modulated trochoidal fluid motion, the eddies themselves become modulated; they stop and go in synchrony with the rate of modulation (Tonndorf, 1959a). In this case, the onset of eddy motion is accompanied by a sharp increase in the relative magnitude of the f_1–f_2 component which becomes approximately proportional to the square of the amplitude of the driving signal. This sudden change, indicating the appearance of the *first order difference tone,* may once more be related to the peakedness of the traveling-wave envelope. For the envelope becomes more peaked (at the expense of its distal slope) in some proportion to the velocity of the eddy currents. At levels below the eddy onset, envelopes simply grow in size with an increase in signal amplitude, but retain their shape (Tonndorf, 1958a).

It is thus shown that the eddies introduce harmonic distortion by their interaction with the trochoidal fluid motion, but also that they act as feed-back loops carrying the energy contained in the newly-generated waveform distortion back to more basal sections of the model so that the various components can be resolved along the partition in the usual manner.

IV. CONCLUDING REMARKS

By and large, I have confined my discussion to the responses of mechanical cochlear models, and you may wonder about the applicability of these findings to the function of an actual cochlea. First and important steps have been taken in this regard. Békésy (1942) and Perlman (1950) observed the traveling-wave pattern in living guinea pigs. Moreover, Békésy (1944, 1947) measured envelopes and tuning curves in a variety of animals and fresh cadavers, including human temporal bones. Admittedly all these observations were carried out at very high signal levels required by the limited resolving power of optical microscopes. The high-frequency tuning curves meas-ured by Johnstone and Boyle (1967) were actually measured at lower levels. Tasaki *et al.* (1952) and Teas *et al.* (1962) avoided that problem. They recorded microphonic responses at physiological signal levels from multiple pick-up points along the cochleae of guinea pigs. The traveling waves implicit in their data were similar to those occurring in the mechanical model both for sine waves (1952) and for transient signals (1962). In particular, inspection of the Teas *et al.* data makes it clear that, like the mechanical displacement of the partition, the microphonic response of the cochlea represents the first (time) derivative of the signal applied to the stapes.

Experiments in guinea pigs, employing cochlear microphonic measurements (Leibbrandt, 1966; Tonndorf; 1958a, 1969) have sup-ported the notions (*a*) that indeed demodulation takes place in the cochlea, (*b*) that it leads to apical detection of the involved low fre-quency, (*c*) that the underlying process takes its origin from the region of the maximum in response to the applied primary signals, and (*d*) that the input/output function is linear, at least at lower amplitudes.

Dallos and Sweetman (1967) reached different results. They used high-frequency primaries and high-frequency beats ($f_1 - f_2 = 1050$ Hz). They observed appropriate cochlear microphonics, but failed to find an increase in the magnitude of the beat-frequency response between turns 1 and 3. Although the difference between their results and those of Leibbrandt and of Tonndorf appears to lie in their use of a high beat rate, I do not know of any real explanation for this difference. Furthermore, Dallos and Sweetman were unable to cancel the beat response simultaneously in both turns by applying the same signal via bone conduction. To be sure, they could cancel for each place of observation separately at a given time. This finding is easy to accept (although not so easy to explain) because I made the same observa-tion in models (Tonndorf, 1959a). However, such cancellations were possible when I used a partition with a *linear* stiffness gradient, in-stead of the usual *exponential* one. This observation shows that, when there is an exponential stiffness gradient, the traveling wave in response to a beat rate, and derived internally, cannot be precisely the same as that for a signal applied externally. Since it is the value of the stiffness gradient that determines the degree of demodulation, the contribution of various places within the (narrow) region of origin must vary with the changing slope of the gradient. Hence, although the apparent traveling wave is the resultant of these various contributions, one can achieve cancellation by applying an external signal only for very limited areas along the partition.

The asymmetrical displacement of the partition* (or of the shearing displacement for that matter) is similar to the negative electrical summating potential (Tonndorf, 1958a, 1960a). The polarities are identical. Of late, several authors have weighed the possibility that the summating potential may be of mechanical origin. This notion is supported by an observation of Allen and Habibi (1962), who found (in cats) a temporary reversal of polarity of the summating potential with increases in perilymphatic pressure. Whitfield and Ross (1965), Johnstone and Johnstone (1966), and Engebretson and Eldredge (1967) developed various concepts in this regard. The results of Tonndorf (1958b, 1969) are compatible with the notion that the negative summating potential might actually be the result of a mechanical demodulation process. And then again, Kupperman (1966) and Johnstone (personal communication) found evidence for a dual origin of the summating potential (its positive and negative components), one of which may be mechanical, the other electrical in nature.

Originally, the summating potential was described as being proportional to the square of the input amplitude (Davis et al., 1958). More recent investigators (Honrubia and Ward, 1967) maintained that the relation is a *linear* one. The apparent conflict may be resolved by referring to the transition of the initially linear demodulation process into a nonlinear one as soon as the eddies get under way.

Envelope detection appears to be used to analyze modulated signals. Winckel (1959) and Voots (1962) independently demonstrated that human subjects with steep high-frequency hearing losses are able to detect the periodicity of a high-frequency complex at a level lower than that at which they can hear the complex itself. In addition,

---

*In this respect, an observation by J. E. Hind (pers. comm.) is of great interest. When Hind participated in Perlman's (1950) direct observations in guinea pig cochleae, he was intrigued by a visible dc shift of the partition towards *scala tympani* as soon as the signal was switched on. The polarity was identical to that observed here.

Voots showed that, in such subjects, the periodicity sensation can be masked by an appropriate low-frequency sound. Once more, these observations are compatible with the model findings. However, the suggestion of Schouten (1938) — and of others — that the detection of time properties by normal-hearing listeners is most likely a central (i.e., an extracochlear) function was made because (a) the periodicity pitch does not beat with signals of nearby frequencies, and because (b) masking is due to components of the original high-frequency complex. It appears therefore, as Békésy pointed out, that the auditory system may have two mechanisms — one of them cochlear, the other central — by which it is able to detect time properties of acoustic signals. Such dual effects serving the same end are by no means rare in biological systems.

The model experiments suggested a study to confirm the multilocal reception of harmonics generated by intracochlear distortion. It was carried out in guinea pigs with the aid of cochlear microphonics recorded from a number of differential electrodes placed along the cochlea (Tonndorf, 1958b). Each component frequency is reduced in amplitude past its estimated point of maximal response, in a manner similar to that of Fig. 18. However, interharmonic phase relations in the response waveform changed with distance along the partition — something not observed in the model. This discrepancy is most likely due to a shortcoming of the cochlear microphonic recording technique. Differential electrodes are not as immune to remote pick-up as believed hitherto (Dallos, 1969). Dallos and Sweetman (1969) duplicated Tonndorf's earlier experiments in the guinea pig, but could confirm his findings only at higher signal levels. At lower levels, they found no evidence for a multilocal distribution of harmonics pro-duced intracochlearly. And then again, Beck and Michler (1960), in their studies on cyto-chemical changes in hair cells of guinea pigs following exposure to sound, noted that at high exposure levels changes were not confined to the place of the signal frequency, but occurred also at those corresponding to its higher harmonics that had not been part of the original signal. At lower levels of exposure, the changes were limited to the place of signal frequency. These observations are compatible with the model findings in which intra-cochlear distortion had also led to a multilocal distribution of the harmonics as soon as eddy currents had established themselves.

It is certainly not my contention that *all* distortion is caused in the same manner. There are other potential causes. However, the results of hydro-dynamic distortion and the phenomena observed in actual cochleae correlate very well, justifying the conclusion that hydro-dynamic distortion may well be the leading cause of intracochlear distortion.

V. SUMMARY

In this chapter, I have discussed the mechanical and hydro-dynamic events taking place in a cochlear model, given a brief account of Békésy's classical traveling-wave concept, and attempted a more detailed description of several associated phenomena observable in cochlear models: the nature of fluid motion, sine-wave and transient responses and their respective mechanisms, shearing motions within the cochlear duct and their contribution to a mechanical sharpening of the response, the mode of signal analysis performed by a mechanical cochlear model, the mechanism of demodulation that occurs in such models, and, finally, Békésy's eddies and their significance for intracochlear harmonic distortion. Results of observations in experimental animals, generally, are in good agreement with the model findings, although some gaps remain to be filled.

REFERENCES

Allen, G. W. and Habibi, M. (1962). The effect of increasing the cerebrospinal fluid pressure upon the cochlear microphonics. *Laryngoscope*, **72**, 423–434.

Batchelor, G. K. (1967). *An introduction to fluid dynamics.* Cambridge Univ. Press, Cambridge, England.

Beck, C. and Michler, H. (1960). Feinstrukturelle und histochemische Veränderungen an den Strukturen der Cochlea beim Meerschweinchen nach dosierter Reintonbeschallung. *Arch. Ohr.-Nas. -u.KeihkHeilk.*, **174**, 496–567.

von Békésy, G. (1928). Zur Theorie des Hörens. *Phys. Z.*, **29**, 793–810.

von Békésy, G. (1941). Über die Elastizität der Schneckentrennwand des Ohres. *Akust. Z.*, **6**, 265–278.

von Békésy, G. (1942). Über die Schwingungen der Schneckentrennwand beim Präparat und Ohrenmodell. *Akust. Z.*, **7**, 173–186.

von Békésy, G. (1943). Über die Resonanzkurve und die Abklingzeit der verschiedenen Stellen der Schneckentrennwand. *Akust. Z.*, **8**, 66–76.

von Békésy, G. (1944). Über die mechanische Frequenzanalyse in der Schnecke verschiedener Tiere. *Akust. Z.*, **9**, 3–11.

von Békésy, G. (1947). The variation of phase along the basilar membrane with sinusoidal vibrations. *J. Acoust. Soc. Am.*, **19**, 452–460.

von Békésy, G. (1951). DC potentials and energy balance of the cochlear partition. *J. Acoust. Soc. Am.*, **23**, 576–582.

von Békésy, G. (1953a). Description of some mechanical properties of the organ of Corti. *J. Acoust. Soc. Am.*, **25**, 770–785.

von Békésy, G. (1953b). Shearing microphonics produced by vibrations near the inner and outer hair cells. *J. Acoust. Soc. Am.*, **25**, 786–790.

von Békésy, G. (1955). Paradoxical direction of wave travel along the cochlear partition. *J. Acoust. Soc. Am.*, **27**, 137–145.

von Békésy, G. (1956). Current status of theories of hearing. *Science*, **123**, 779–783.

von Békésy, G. (1960). *Experiments in hearing*. McGraw-Hill, New York.

von Békésy, G. (1962). Concerning the pleasures of observing, and the mechanics of the inner ear. *Prix Nobel, 1961*. Norstedt Söner, Stockholm.

von Békésy, G. and Rosenblith, W. A. (1951). The mechanical properties of the ear. In S. S. Stevens (Ed.) *Handbook of experimental psychology*. Pp. 1075–1115. Wiley, New York.

van Bergeijk, W. A. and Speeth, S. A. (1960). Slant of hair cells in the cochlea. *J. Acoust. Soc. Am.*, **32**, 1494 (A).

de Boer, E. (1956). On the "residue" in hearing. Unpublished doctoral dissertation, University of Amsterdam.

Brecher, G. A. (1934). Die untere Hör- und Tongrenze. *Pflügers Arch. Ges. Physiol.*, **234**, 380–393.

Bridgman, P. W. (1922). *Dimensional analysis*. Yale Univ. Press, New Haven, Connecticut.

Carslaw, H. S. (1950). *Introduction to the theory of Fourier series and integrals*. (Reprinted) Dover, New York.

Dallos, P. (1969). Comments on the differential-electrode technique. *J. Acoust. Soc. Am.*, **45**, 999–1007.

Dallos, P. and Sweetman, R. H. (1969). Distribution pattern of cochlear harmonics. *J. Acoust. Soc. Am.*, **45**, 37–46.

Davis, H., Deatherage, B. H., Eldredge, D. H., and Smith, C. A. (1958). Summating potentials of the cochlea. *Am. J. Physiol.*, **195**, 251–261.

Diestel, H.-G. (1954). Akustische Messungen an einem mechanischen Modell des Innenohres. *Acustica*, **4**, 489–499.

Engebretson, A. M. and Eldredge, D. H. (1968). Model for the nonlinear characteristics of cochlear potentials. *J. Acoust. Soc. Am.*, **44**, 548–554.

Engström, H., Ades, H. W., and Hawkins, J. E., Jr. (1962). Structure and functions of the sensory hairs of the inner ear. *J. Acoust. Soc. Am.*, **34**, 1356–1363.

Ewald, J. R. (1899). Zur Physiologie des Labyrinths. VI. Mittheilung. Eine neue Hörtheorie. *Pflügers Arch. Ges. Physiol.*, **76**, 147–188.

Ewald, J. R. (1903). Zur Physiologie des Labyrinths. VII. Mittheilung. Die Erzeugung von Schallbildern in der Camera acustica. *Pflügers Arch. Ges. Physiol.*, **93**, 485–500.

Flanagan, J. L. (1962). Computational model for basilar-membrane displacement. *J. Acoust. Soc. Am.*, **34**, 1370–1376.

Fletcher, H. (1929). *Speech and hearing*. Van Nostrand, New York.

Flock, Å., Kimura, R. S., Lundquist, P.-G., and Wersäll, J. (1962). Morphological basis of directional sensitivity of the outer hair cells in the organ of Corti. *J. Acoust. Soc. Am.*, **34**, 1351–1355.

Fourier, J. B. J. (1824). Théorie du Mouvement de la Chauleur dans les Corps Solides. *Mem. Acad. Sci. Inst. Fr.*, **4**, ser. 2, 185–525.

Gabor, D. (1946). Theory of communication. *J. Instn Elect. Engrs*, **93** (3), 429–457.

Galambos, R. (1954). Neural mechanisms of audition. *Physiol. Rev.*, **34**, 497–528.

Gisselsson, L. (1950). Experimental investigations into the problem of humoral transmissions in the cochlea. *Acta Oto-Lar., Suppl.* **82.**

Goldman, S. (1948). *Frequency analysis, modulation and noise.* McGraw-Hill, New York.

Goldstein, J. L. (1967). Auditory nonlinearity. *J. Acoust. Soc. Am.*, **41**, 676–689.

Hauser, H. (1961). Beitrag zur Theorie der Schwingungsmechanik des Innenohrs. *Proc. III Int. Congr. Acoust.* **1**, 40–44. Elsevier, Amsterdam.

Held, H. (1902). Untersuchungen über den feineren Bau des Gehörorgans der Wirbeltiere. *Abh. sächs. Akad. Wiss. Leipzig, Math-Phys. Kl., Abh. I.*, **28**, 1–74.

von Helmholtz, H. (1863). *On the sensation of tone as a physiological basis for the theory of music.* (First American ed. of the second English ed. of the fourth German ed.) Dover, New York, 1954.

Hilding, A. C. (1952). Studies on the otic labyrinth. *Ann. Otol. Rhinol. Lar.*, **61**, 354–370.

Hilding, A. C. (1953). The tectorial membrane in the theory of hearing. *Ann. Otol. Rhinol. Lar.*, **62**, 757–769.

von Holst, E. (1950). Die Arbeitsweise des Statolithenapparates bei Fischen. *Z. Vergl. Physiol.*, **32**, 60–120.

Honrubia, V. and Ward, P. H. (1967). Interdependence of the cochlear microphonics and summating potentials upon the endocochlear potential. *J. Acoust. Soc. Am.*, **42**, 1157 (A).

Huggins, W. H. and Licklider, J. C. R. (1951). Place mechanisms of auditory frequency analysis. *J. Acoust. Soc. Am.*, **23**, 290–299.

Hurst, C. H. (1895). A new theory of hearing. *Trans. Liverpool Biol. Soc.* **9**, 321–353.

Johnstone, B. M. and Boyle, A. J. F. (1967). Basilar membrane vibration examined with the Mössbauer technique. *Science*, **158**, 389–390.

Johnstone, J. R. and Johnstone, B. M. (1966). Origin of summating potential. *J. Acoust. Soc. Am.*, **40**, 1405–1413.

Katsuki, Y., Suga, N., and Kanno, Y. (1962). Neural mechanism of the peripheral and central auditory system in monkeys. *J. Acoust. Soc. Am.*, **34**, 1396–1410.

Khanna, S. M., Sears, R. E., and Tonndorf, J. (1968). Some properties of longitudinal shear waves. *J. Acoust. Soc. Am.*, **43**, 1077–1084.

Kiang, N. Y-s., Watanabe, T., Thomas, E. C., and Clark. L. F. (1965). Discharge patterns of single fibers in the cat's auditory nerve. *M.I.T. Res. Lab. Electron. Tech. Rep.* **13.**

Kimura, R. S. (1966). Hairs of the cochlear sensory cells and their attachment to the tectorial membrane. *Acta Oto-Lar.*, **61**, 55–72.

ter Kuile, E. (1900). Die Übertrangung der Energie von der Grundmembran auf die

Kinsman, B. (1965). Wind waves, their generation and propagation on the ocean surface. Prentice Hall, Englewood-Cliffs, New Jersey.

Haarzellen. *Pflügers Arch. Ges. Physiol.*, **79**, 146–157.

Kupperman, R. (1966). The dynamic DC potential in the cochlea of the guinea pig (summating potential). *Acta Oto-Lar.*, **62**, 465–480.

Lamb, H. (1879). *Hydrodynamics.* (First American ed. of the sixth English ed.) Dover, New York, 1945.

Leibbrandt, C. C. (1966). Periodicity analysis in the guinea pig cochlea. *Acta Oto-Lar.*, **61**, 413–422.

Licklider, J. C. R. (1951). Basic correlates of the auditory stimulus. In S. S. Stevens (Ed.) *Handbook of experimental psychology.* pp. 985–1013. Wiley, New York.

Löwenstein, O. and Wersäll, J. (1959). A fundamental interpretation of the electron-microscopic structure of the sensory hairs in the cristae of the elasmobranch Raja Clavata in terms of directional sensitivity. *Nature*, **184**, 1807–1808.

Meyer, M. F. (1928). The hydraulic principles governing the function of the cochlea. *J. Gen. Psychol.*, **1**, 239–265.

Ohm, G. S. (1843). Über die Definition des Tones, nebst daran geknüpfter Theorie der Sirene und ähnlicher tonbildender Vorrichtungen. *Poggendorff's Annln Phys. Chem.*, **59**, *ser. 2*, 497–565.

Perlman, H. B. (1950). Observations through cochlear fenestra. *Laryngoscope*, **60**, 77–96.

Peterson, L. C. and Bogert, B. P. (1950). A dynamic theory of the cochlea. *J. Acoust. Soc. Am.*, **22**, 369–381.

Prandtl, L. and Tietjens, O. G. (1934). *Fundamentals of hydro- and aeromechanics.* McGraw-Hill, New York. (Reprinted, Dover, New York, 1954.)

Ranke, O. F. (1931). *Die Gleichrichter-Resonanztheorie.* Lehmann, Munich.

Ranke, O. F. (1950). Theory of operation of the cochlea. *J. Acoust. Soc. Am.*, **22**, 772–777.

Rutherford, W. (1886). A new theory of hearing. *J. Anat. Physiol., Lond.*, **21**, 166–168.

Schaefer, C. (1910). Über mögliche Erweiterungen der Helmholtzschen Theorie der Kombinationstöne. *Annln Phys.*, **33**, *ser. 4*, 1216–1226.

Schouten, J. F. (1938). The perception of subjective tones. *Proc. K. Ned. Akad. Wet.*, **41**, 1086–1093.

Schouten, J. F. (1940a). The perception of pitch. *Philips Tech. Rev.*, **5**, 286–294.

Schouten, J. F. (1940b). The residue, a new component in subjective sound analysis. *Proc. K. Ned. Akad. Wet.*, **43**, 356–365.

Schouten, J. F., Ritsma, R. J., and Lopes Cardozo, B. (1962). Pitch of the residue. *J. Acoust. Soc. Am.*, **34**, 1418–1424.

Seebeck, A. (1841). Beobachtungen über einige Bedingungen der Entstehung von Tönen. *Annln Phys.*, **53**, *ser. 2*, 417–436.

Seebeck, A. (1843). Ueber die Sirene. *Annln Phys.*, **60**, *ser. 2*, 449–481.

Small, A. M. (1955). Some parameters influencing the pitch of amplitude modulated signals. *J. Acoust. Soc. Am.*, **27**, 751–760.

Tasaki, I., Davis, H., and Legouix, J.-P. (1952). The space-time pattern of the cochlear microphonics (guinea pig), as recorded by differential electrodes. *J. Acoust. Soc. Am.*, **24**, 502–519.

Teas, D. C., Eldredge, D. H., and Davis, H. (1962). Cochlear responses to acoustic transients. *J. Acoust. Soc. Am.*, **34**, 1438–1459.

Tonndorf, J. (1956). The analogy between fluid motion within the cochlea and formation of surf on sloping beaches and its significance for the mechanism of cochlear stimulation. *Ann. Otol. Rhinol. Lar.*, **65**, 488–506.

Tonndorf, J. (1957a). Fluid motion in cochlear models. *J. Acoust. Soc. Am.*, **29**, 558–568.

Tonndorf, J. (1957b). The mechanism of hearing loss in early cases of endolymphatic hydrops. *Ann. Otol. Rhinol. Lar.*, **66**, 766–784.

Tonndorf, J. (1958a). Harmonic distortion in cochlear models. *J. Acoust. Soc. Am.*, **30**, 929–937.

Tonndorf, J. (1958b). Localization of aural harmonics along the basilar membrane of guinea pigs. *J. Acoust. Soc. Am.*, **30**, 938–943.

Tonndorf, J. (1959a). Beats in cochlear models. *J. Acoust. Soc. Am.*, **31**, 608–619.

Tonndorf, J. (1959b). The transfer of energy across the cochlea. *Acta Oto-Lar.*, **50**, 171–184.

Tonndorf, J. (1960a). Dimensional analysis of cochlear models. *J. Acoust. Soc. Am.*, **32**, 493–497.

Tonndorf, J. (1960b). Response of cochlear models to aperiodic signals and to random noises. *J. Acoust. Soc. Am.*, **32**, 1344–1355.

Tonndorf, J. (1960c). Shearing motion in scala media of cochlear models. *J. Acoust. Soc. Am.*, **32**, 238–244.

Tonndorf, J. (1962a). Compressional bone conduction in cochlear models. *J. Acoust. Soc. Am.*, **34**, 1127–1131.

Tonndorf, J. (1962b). Time/frequency analysis along the partition of cochlear models. *J. Acoust. Soc. Am.*, **34**, 1337–1350.

Tonndorf, J. (1969). Nonlinearities in cochlear hydrodynamics. *J. Acoust. Soc. Am.*, **45**, 304–305.

Tonndorf, J. and Khanna, S. M. (1968). Displacement pattern of the basilar membrane. *Science*, **160**, 1139–1140.

Tonndorf, J., Duvall, A. J., III, and Reneau, J. P. (1962). Permeability of intracochlear membranes to various vital stains. *Ann. Otol. Rhinol. Lar.*, **71**, 801–841.

Tunturi, A. R. (1944). Audio frequency localization in the acoustic cortex of the dog. *Am. J. Physiol.*, **141**, 397–403.

Völz, H. (1961). Vorschlag eines elektrischen Ersatzchaltbildes für das menschliche Gehör. *Proc. III Int. Congr. Acoust.* **1**, 37–39. Elsevier, Amsterdam.

Voots, R. J. (1962). Periodicity pitch and masking in pathologic ears. *J. Acoust. Soc. Am.*, **34**, 739 (A).

de Vries, Hl. (1949). Struktur und Lage der Tektorialmembran in der Schnecke, untersucht mit neueren Hilfsmitteln. *Acta Oto-Lar.*, **37**, 334–338.

de Vries, Hl. (1952). Brownian motion and the transmission of energy in the cochlea. *J. Acoust. Soc. Am.*, **24**, 527–533.

Wever, E. G. (1962). Development of traveling-wave theories. *J. Acoust. Soc. Am.*, **34**, 1319–1324.

Wever, E. G. and Lawrence, M. (1952). Sound conduction in the cochlea. *Ann. Otol. Rhinol. Lar.*, **61**, 824–835.

Whitfield, I. C. and Ross, H. F. (1965). Cochlear-microphonics and summating potentials and the outputs of individual hair-cell generators. *J. Acoust. Soc. Am.*, **38**, 126–131.

Wien, M. (1905). Ein Bedenken gegen die Helmholtzsche Resonanztheorie des Hörens. In *Festschrift Adolph Wüllner.* pp. 28–35. B. G. Teubner, Leipzig.

Winckel, F. (1959). Der Informationsgehalt von Hörresten. *Arch. Ohr.-, Nas.- u. Kehlk-Heilk.*, **175**, 391–396.

Zwislocki, J. (1948). Theorie der Schneckenmechanik. *Acta Oto-Lar.*, *Suppl.* **72**.

Zwislocki, J. (1950). Theory of the acoustical action of the cochlea. *J. Acoust. Soc. Am.*, **22**, 778–784.

Zwislocki, J. (1953). Wave motion in the cochlea caused by bone conduction. *J. Acoust. Soc. Am.*, **25**, 986–989.

Zwislocki, J. (1965). Analysis of some auditory characteristics. In R. D. Luce, R. R. Bush, and E. Galanter (Eds.) *Handbook of mathematical psychology.* Vol. 3, pp. 1–97. Wiley, New York.

Chapter Seven

Cochlear Processes

FOREWORD

Just as the miniature mechanical systems of the inner ear are only imperfectly under-stood, so the complex electrical patterns are still incompletely analyzed. Many kinds of cochlear voltage have been recorded, yet there is no certainty about whether some of them play a necessary role in the acoustic-mechanical-electrical-neural transduction. Even the historically-most-important cochlear microphonic is sometimes questioned as to its relevance to the auditory process. Some forms of nerve potential are of uncertain function. And the fixed (dc) cochlear voltages are susceptible to all kinds of speculation regarding their purpose in the transmission of intelligence into the auditory nervous system. Don Teas's work in cochlear electrophysiology has let him bring to this chapter not only his knowledge of the structure and action of the cochlea, but also his concepts on the nature of cochlear analysis.

Cochlear Processes

Donald C. Teas*

I. INTRODUCTION

A change in the ambient pressure at the tympanum, the drumhead of the "eardrum," causes it to move – inward if the change is an increase in ambient pressure, outward if the change is a decrease. This movement of the tympanum is transmitted, via the small bones in the middle ear, to the stapes, effectively a piston. Movement of the stapes displaces a bit of fluid in one cochlear canal, the volume of which is taken up by the round window membrane working into the middle-ear cavity. If the change in ambient pressure is rapid enough, the organism may detect it through a series of events initiated in the inner ear.

To tell the story of this chain of events, we must first review the anatomy of the cochlea, and describe its electrical properties and the methods used to explore those properties. The electrophysiological method rests on the assumption that the electrical response – the sign and activity – is related to the physiological function of its generator. But the electrical sign of function depends upon the details of recording and upon anatomical characteristics. Because of this dependence, the experimental procedures for investigation of the ear are complicated. Also, our knowledge of the physiology of hearing is becoming sufficiently detailed that only studies employing exhaustive systematic variation in stimulus properties can add significant information,

*Departments of Speech, Psychology, Physiology, and Electrical Engineering, University of Florida, Gainesville, Florida.

thereby adding further complication, at the consumer's level at least, to an already difficult subject.

One serious difficulty with the cochlea is its location. In primates, the inner ear is a spiral hole deep in the temporal bone. Nerve fibers terminating within the inner ear are not easy to reach with micro-electrodes. Fortunately, not all ears are as inaccessible as those of primates, and so investigators use species that present fewer problems.

Data gathered from different experimental species show differences. We know enough about the ears of different organisms to recognize the gross variations and sometimes to use them. An example is the contrast between the data on frog and guinea pig ears. Inhibitory-like phenomena are prominent in the anatomically less complicated system of the frog; in complicated ears, such as the guinea pig's or cat's, although the phenomena may be present, they may be less prominently displayed. But differences between electrical responses from the cat and from the guinea pig are more difficult to understand; their ears are similar, and both are complicated systems. There may be second-order differences in their responses, not demonstrable with gross techniques, but which appear as the experimental techniques become more precise. This chapter will consider some of the limitations of the procedures used to sample the electrical activity of the ear as well as some of the substantive data that have been gathered.

II. ANATOMICAL ORGANIZATION

A. General Features

The complexity of the mechanism for receiving vibratory signals varies with the organism's position in the phylogenetic series. The overall response of the receptive organ to vibratory stimuli in several species has been explored by Wever and his students (Wever and Vernon, 1956; Wever and Vernon, 1960; Wever *et al.*, 1963).

The emphasis of this chapter is on function in animals such as the cat, guinea pig, chinchilla, and monkey, with some illustrative exceptions from other species. Generally speaking, these cochleae are similar to man's (Guggenheim, 1948).

Visualization. The cochleae of the animals most frequently used in experiments on the ear are in the form of a coil. The large basal coil comprises about one-half the total length of the cochlea in the guinea pig and about two-thirds in the cat. Although in primates the cochlea is *imbedded* in the temporal bone, in most species used for physiological experiments, it is contained within a bony capsule which protrudes into an air-filled cavity, the bulla. Within the bulla, the protruding cochlea is covered by a relatively thin layer of bone. Its ventral aspect can be visualized as shown in Fig. 1. For animals with an imbedded cochlea, the only aspect that can be viewed easily in the living animal is the round window, through the middle ear.

Cochlear Organization. Inside its bony capsule, the membranous labyrinth divides the cochlea into three scalae: tympani, media, and vestibuli. Scala vestibuli, containing perilymph, is bounded by the membranous lining of the bony capsule and, adjacent to scala media, by Reissner's membrane. Scala tympani, also containing perilymph, is bounded by the membranous lining and, adjacent to scala media, by the basilar membrane. Scala media lies between the other two scalae and may be referred to, along with the organ of Corti, as the cochlear partition.

Figure 2 shows a cross-section of the cochlea and the relations among the three scalae. The scala media is relatively small and uniform in cross-section compared to scala tympani and scala vestibuli (Fernández, 1951). Its outer edge is formed by the stria vascularis, a dense network of blood vessels. Within scala media, the basilar membrane becomes wider toward the apex although the osseous spiral lamina becomes narrower. Reissner's membrane is continuous with the vestibular edge of the spiral ligament at the outer limit of the scala media as well as with the limbus at the junction of the two toward the modiolus at the inner limit of scala media. The triangular cross section formed by the spiral lamina-basilar membrane, stria vascularis, and Reissner's membrane does not define scala media electrically, however.

Scala media contains endolymph. Scala vestibuli and scala tympani contain perilymph. The perilymph is similar to cerebrospinal fluid, but endolymph is similar to the inside of cells: it is high in potassium, low in sodium. The inside of cells is, of course, electrically negative. Scala media, however, is electrically positive. The electrical properties of scala media and the chemistry of endolymph are, in one sense, in opposition to each other. Searches with microelectrodes show that the electrical positivity is restricted to the region from the inner wall of Reissner's membrane to the inner wall of stria vascularis and to the reticular lamina above the hair cells

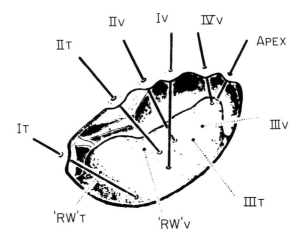

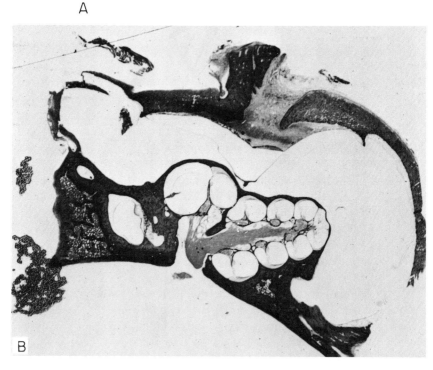

Figure 1 Visualization of the bony capsule of the cochlea as in a ventral approach to the bulla in young guinea pigs. A similar approach is used for the chinchilla, but its cochlea has fewer turns. (A) I, II, III, and IV represent turns of the guinea pig's cochlea; RW, the round window; V, the scala vestibuli; and T, the scala tympani. Cochlear microphonic responses can be sampled from more than one position in turn I. (Tasaki *et al.*,

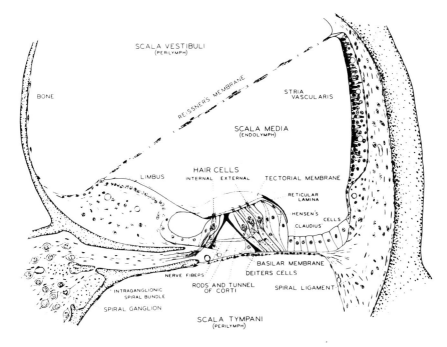

Figure 2 Cross section at turn II, guinea pig cochlea, based on camera lucida drawing. (H. Davis *et al.*, 1953. By permission from *Journal of the Acoustical Society of America*.)

(Tasaki *et al.*, 1954). Thus, the excitable tissues of the organ of Corti, below the reticular lamina, lie outside the region of high electrical positivity (and presumably of high potassium).

The organ of Corti is situated between the basilar membrane and the reticular lamina. Radially, the rods of Corti divide the single row of inner hair cells from the three rows of outer hair cells. Between the rods of Corti is the tunnel of Corti, a space, and there are also relatively large intercellular spaces among the outer hair cells.

The hairs, or cilia, on the hair cells extend above the reticular lamina. Outer hair cells show about 140 hairs. On inner hair cells, the number of hairs is 40 or so, arranged in two parallel rows (Engström *et al.*, 1962). Above the hairs is the tectorial membrane. Although

1952. By permission from *Journal of the Acoustical Society of America*.) (B) Midmodiolar section of the guinea pig's cochlea. Electrodes shown in (a) are in fluid of scalae. For turn II, the tympani electrode must pass close to the turn I vestibuli electrode. The direction of the hole drilled for the electrode is critical (D. H. Eldredge, personal communication, 1960.)

previous statements have suggested that the hairs were imbedded in the tectorial membrane, some findings question this belief (Engström *et al.*, 1962).

From their cell bodies in the spiral ganglion, nerve fibers travel to, then through small holes (habenula perforata) in the limbus. As they penetrate the basilar membrane, they are without myelin. The *radial fibers* course outward from the modiolus to end at the base of some hair cells; the *longitudinal fibers*, after radiating, turn and travel as much as one-half turn to innervate several hair cells. Figure 3 shows the innervation of internal and external hair cells. According to Fernández (1951), there is both a dominant and a secondary innervation of both inner and outer hair cells. Inner hair cells receive predominantly radial fibers, but secondarily, longitudinal fibers. Outer hair cells receive predominantly longitudinal fibers, but, secondarily, some radial fibers. Recent work with the electron microscope has

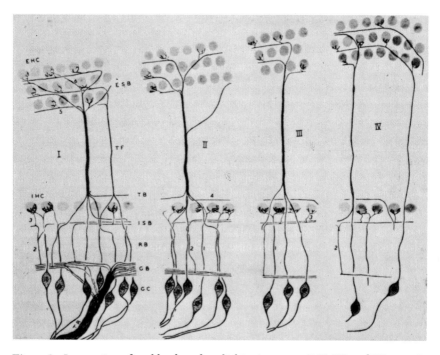

Figure 3 Innervation of cochlea based on light microscopy. I, II, III, and IV, turns in guinea pig cochlea; EHC, external hair cells; IHC, internal hair cells; ESB, external spiral bundle; TF, tunnel fiber; TB, tunnel bundle; ISB, internal spiral bundle; RB, radial bundle; GB, intraganglionic spiral bundle; and GC, ganglion of Corti. (Fernández, 1951. By permission from *Laryngoscope*.)

added much to our knowledge of the fine unmyelinated fibers and the forms of the nerve endings at the base of hair cells.

Figure 4 shows another view of the organ of Corti. The small bundles of unmyelinated nerve fibers cross the tunnel and the inter-

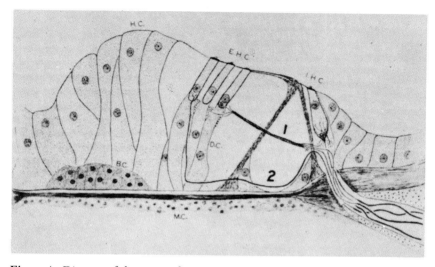

Figure 4 Diagram of the organ of Corti in cross section. HC, Hensen's cells; EHC, external hair cells; IHC, internal hair cells; BC, Boettcher's cells; MC, mesothelial cells. 1: Four nerve fibers crossing tunnel (two from habenula perforata, one from internal spiral bundle, one from tunnel spiral bundle). 2: Basilar fiber from habenula perforata. (Fernández, 1951. By permission from *Laryngoscope*.)

cellular space in order to reach the base of the hair cells. It should be clear that the problems of sampling electrical activity of these small unmyelinated fibers in response to acoustic stimulation are severe. Because of the difficulty in measuring the electrical activity at these anatomically protected locations, histochemical methods are particularly important for cochlear physiology. Churchill and Schuknecht (1956) and Schuknecht et al. (1959) compared acetylcholinesterase deposit in normal ears and in ears for which the olivocochlear bundle was cut. Staining was marked at the internal spiral bundle but was also heavy at the base of the outer hair cell and at the outer spiral bundle. Using similar techniques, but with the added power of the electron microscope, Smith and Rasmussen (1963) traced efferent fibers from the habenula perforata to the hair cells.

Moscovitch and Gannon (1965) reported that perfusion of the scala tympani (in guinea pigs) with a calcium-rich solution mimics the inhibitory effects of electrical stimulation of the olivo-cochlear, or Rasmussen's bundle.* These olivo-cochlear inhibitory effects reduce the magnitude of the whole-nerve response (Galambos, 1956) by an equivalent of a 15 to 20 dB reduction in the strength of the acoustic click (Desmedt, 1962). Along with the reduction in the neural response, the cochlear microphonic is enhanced by five to ten percent (Desmedt, 1962; Fex, 1962). Olivo-cochlear inhibition has also been elicited in first-order single units of the auditory nerve by a strong acoustic stimulation of the contralateral ear (Fex, 1962).

Tanaka and Katsuki (1966) added other pharmacological information on cochlear function by showing that acetylcholine, iontophoretically injected into the scala media strongly *reduces* the cochlear microphonic response. Other substances — sodium, potassium, chlorine, and calcium — similarly injected, have no effect. Along with the reduction in cochlear microphonic response, unit activity in first-order neurons is also reduced. The effect of acetylcholine is blocked by d-tubocurarine. The endolymphatic potential, also reduced by acetylcholine, is unaffected by the d-tubocurarine. These agents have no effect on olivo-cochlear inhibition elicited by electrical stimulation in the floor of the fourth ventricle where the inhibitory fibers originate.

B. Nutrition

All studies confirm that the cochlea does not store a large surplus of energy. Anoxia in various forms reduces the electrical output of the cochlea severely and quickly (Tonndorf et al., 1955). Vosteen's (1963) review is a helpful overview of the biochemical techniques used to investigate these processes in the cochlea.

Electrical Signs. The chemistry of the fluid in the spaces within the organ of Corti and the details of the electrical properties of the fluid are difficult matters. They are important because the fluid bathes and may provide nutrition for the hair cells and nerve fibers. Engström and Wersäll (1953) suggested that the fluid in these spaces is neither endolymph nor perilymph, but "cortilymph" of unknown composition. They reported that there is never any communication between the spaces within the organ of Corti and the other scalae throughout development. Lawrence and Clapper (1961), on the basis of a stain selective for endolymph, concluded that the basilar membrane is a clear barrier to the perilymph of scala tympani. The basilar membrane is permeable to KCl introduced into scala tympani.

---

*However, other hypertonic solutions may produce similar effects.

Investigators do agree that outside the organ of Corti region, but within scala media, the endolymph shows about 60 to 80 mV positive potential relative to perilymph, and that the fluid is similar in chemical composition to the interior of cells. The source of this endolymphatic potential (EP) appears to be stria vascularis. Removal of hair cells does not affect the potential (Konishi et al., 1961), nor does perfusing scala tympani with a potassium-rich medium (Tasaki et al., 1954). The latter operation does reduce the electrical responses to acoustic stimuli, however. The EP is greater close to the stria vascularis (Tasaki et al., 1954), is present in waltzing guinea pigs without hair cells, and also is reduced by interruption of the blood supply (Konishi et al., 1961).

Misrahy et al. (1957) showed that the EP drops in local regions of the cochlear partition when oxygen is rapidly depleted. Butler et al. (1962) reported that the decline of EP under anoxia is retarded when scala vestibuli is perfused with Ringer's solution, even though the solution is previously bubbled with nitrogen. The implication is that waste products were removed by the perfusion, since increases in perfusion rate aided in maintaining EP. Therefore, the pattern of steady potentials through different regions within the cochlea may be indicative of nutritional processes.

Within the organ of Corti region, Tasaki et al. (1954) reported that the *intra*cellular potentials are of the order of −60 to −70 mV. However, Tasaki and Spyropoulos (1959) and also Butler (1964) reported that microelectrodes too large to penetrate cells (25μ) also record a large negative steady potential when they are inserted into the organ of Corti region. These observations suggest that the organ of Corti region is iso-potential — that the inside and outside of cells in that region are not electrically different. This proposition is difficult to reconcile with the potential difference required for the excitation of nerve, i.e., in order for depolarization to occur, there must first be a polarization.[*]

There is also some evidence that the hair cells and nerve fibers receive nutrition from different sources, (although there may be alternative routes). Vosteen (1963) concluded that although the hair cells seem to derive their oxygen supply from the stria vascularis, the oxygen supply to the nerve fibers comes from accompanying blood vessels. He suggested that the high positive polarization has no functional significance and that endolymph is a nutritive source for the

---

[*]Dallos (1969) suggests that the negative potential is produced by the large electrode rupturing cells.

hair cells. That is, the EP may be only a by-product of the nutritional system, and may not contribute directly to excitability.

Davis (1961a) suggested that the EP is a battery in series with an *intra*cellular potential. Biological amplification is said to occur as the hair cells modulate the flow of current in the circuit. However, Tasaki *et al.* (1954) were unable to find the flow pattern demanded by the theory. The theory is still useful, of course (Davis, 1959).

Butler's (1964) observations of the cochlear microphonic (CM) in relation to the EP and to the negative organ-of-Corti potential show that the changes in CM magnitude vary with the *gradient* of potential and that under anoxia the positive EP, the negative organ of Corti potential, and the CM all fall to zero. Butler concluded that the decline of the CM follows the *algebraic difference* between the EP and the organ of Corti potentials more closely than it follows the decline of the EP alone. This relation suggests that the CM is a modulation of the sum of the two potentials, i.e., of the 150–160 mV across the reticular lamina. However, this formulation by itself says nothing regarding the excitability of the nerve fibers, also in the organ of Corti region.

Across the reticular lamina there is about 160 mV potential difference. There are conflicting and puzzling data regarding the negative half of the total potential. On one hand, the negative potential is intracellular; on the other, the negative potential is found throughout the organ of Corti region, thus suggesting that the region is iso-potential. Although puzzling, this conclusion does serve to emphasize the problems of the relations between electrochemical properties of the endolymph and the organ of Corti region.

Circulation. Figure 5 illustrates the blood supply within the cochlea according to Perlman and Kimura (1955b). The movement of clusters of corpuscles in the stria vascularis has been studied by at least two groups of investigators (Perlman and Kimura, 1955a; Weille, 1955). There is a complex system of arcades that permit much shunting and alternative routing of the blood supply. Only a thin wall between the corpuscles and the endolymph obstructs filtration through the stria vascularis (Vosteen, 1963).

Consideration of nutritional routes must also include consideration of resorption routes. There appears to be some ambiguity. One report (Saxén, 1951) suggested that resorption takes place throughout the cochlear partition. Another investigation (Butler *et al.*, 1962) suggested that, following venous obstruction, most of the resulting debris remains in the scalae and that resorption is slow, indicating that electrophysiologic experiments following sectioning of the audi-

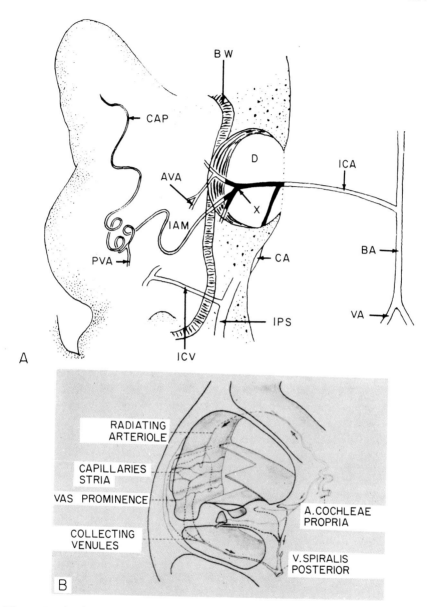

Figure 5 Blood supply routes of the cochlea. (A) For surgical interruption of blood supply. VA, vertebral artery; BA, basilar artery; ICA, anterior inferior cerebellar artery; AVA, anterior vestibular artery; PVA, posterior vestibular artery; CAP, cochlear artery; ICV, inferior cochlear vein; IPS, inferior petrosal sinus; CA, cochlear aqueduct; BW, bullar wall; D, surgical defect; IAM, internal auditory meatus; and X, point of arterial obstruction. (Kimura and Perlman, 1958.) (B) Cross sectional detail of scala media blood supply routes. (Perlman and Kimura, 1955b.)

tory nerve but leaving the blood supply intact should be interpreted with caution (Kiang and Peake, 1960; Peake and Kiang, 1962).

These biochemical problems of nutrition and resorption require the use of both biochemical and electron microscopic techniques. Generally, these are not familiar techniques to physiological or psychological acousticians. The merging of the techniques with the experimental interests of bioacoustics could be a fruitful, if exacting, area of research.

III. ELECTROPHYSIOLOGICAL PRINCIPLES

The cat and the guinea pig rival each other in popularity for physiological experiments on cochlear function. Each animal presents the investigator with a different set of limitations and advantages.

A. Guinea Pig

The cochlea in the guinea pig (gp) contains approximately three and three-quarter turns. The full length of the bony cochlea can be exposed by opening the bulla ventrally. The thin portions of the cochlear wall show the stria vascularis clearly and its spiral course can be followed. These visual markings provide guides for drilling small holes into the scalae. Fine wire electrodes can be safely inserted into the scala tympani and scala vestibuli. For the scala media, still finer, nonpolarizable electrodes must be used.

If pairs of wire electrodes, placed equidistant from the cochlear partition and oriented normal to its slope, are inserted into the scala tympani and scala vestibuli, and if their outputs are led to a differential amplifier, only the voltage generated within an estimated radius of 1.5 to 2.0 mm is recorded (Tasaki *et al.*, 1952). Since the ventral aspect of the three and three-quarter turns is accessible in the guinea pig, the locally generated potential can be sampled at four or five positions along the cochlear partition (Teas *et al.*, 1962). One can thus investigate the cochlear microphonic response, an important locally generated potential, in some detail as a function of position along the cochlear partition. Note that these electrodes are in the scala vestibuli and scala tympani and are, therefore, some distance from the generators of the potentials.

The cochlear microphonic is a graded response generated by movement of the cochlear partition, and is closely associated with the movements of the hair cells. First, let me discuss three factors: *(a)* the generator of the cochlear microphonic, *(b)* the two scalae, vestibuli and tympani, and *(c)* the electrode positions.

Local Potentials. If an electrode is advanced through the scala tympani toward the basilar membrane, the polarity of the CM response (referred to the neck) is first in one direction. As the electrode is further advanced, it penetrates the basilar membrane, passes through the organ of Corti, the reticular lamina, and finally emerges into the scala media. At the instant the microelectrode shows the high positive steady potential characteristic of scala media, the CM reverses its phase. Thus, the CM appears to be localized at the border between hair cells and scala media (Tasaki *et al.*, 1954; Konishi and Yasuno, 1963).

An electrode in the scala tympani sees the CM response from nearby hair cells with one polarity, while an electrode directly opposite in scala vestibuli sees the CM response from the same hair cells with the opposite polarity. However, both electrodes record the same polarity from remotely located generators. A differential amplifier discriminates against the signals that are in-phase at the two electrodes. With properly placed intracochlear electrodes, the relation between the voltage source (hair cells) and anatomy (the two scalae) allows one to differentiate between locally generated CM and the electric responses from generators remote to the electrode site.

With two pairs of intracochlear electrodes, one can show the rejection of voltage originating from remote generators for each pair. Local destruction of hair cells can cause loss of CM at one pair but not at the other (Tasaki and Fernández, 1952). Frequencies may appear at one recording site and not at the other (Tasaki *et al.*, 1952).

The local recording also provides a basis for determining the adequacy of the preparation. If, for example, the hair cells between one pair of electrodes are destroyed, the phase relation between two recording sites along the partition will be altered. The relations between input-output functions from two sites provide checks of the adequacy of preparation. Finally, the output from each electrode can be displayed alone as a test of equality. For the basal turn, the electrical configuration for this single cochlear electrode is similar to that for a round window electrode.

Remote Potentials. If the electrical outputs from the two intracochlear leads are added, the CM voltage, in phase-opposition, is cancelled and any voltage in phase agreement can be amplified. One large in-phase voltage comes from the group of auditory-nerve fibers that is excited by the acoustic signal. This whole-nerve action potential (AP) can be displayed alone on one beam of an oscilloscope and the locally-generated CM can be displayed on another beam, provided that the outputs of the two electrodes are equal in magnitude and the CM is opposite in phase at each one. In practice, one uses a resistance network to balance the outputs, and correct placement of the electrodes to achieve the proper phase relation (Tasaki *et al.*, 1952). Note, however, that although the recording procedure permits a direct analysis of CM source, the voltage sum of *all* auditory fibers activated by the particular acoustic signal is recorded at once (Teas *et al.*, 1962).

Applications. Informative experiments have been carried out by altering the blood supply to the cochlea (Kimura and Perlman, 1956; Davis *et al.*, 1958a; Kimura and Perlman, 1958; Perlman *et al.*, 1959). The visibility of the stria vascularis through the thin wall of the bony cochlea is also important for the general study of circulation in small blood vessels (Perlman and Kimura, 1955b; Weille, 1955). With little more surgery, the arterial blood supply to the cochlea can be seen at a point where the cochlear artery branches from the anterior inferior cerebellar artery (Konishi *et al.*, 1961). Occlusion at this point produces obstruction of the arterial supply to the cochlea.

Finally, the ventral approach to the cochlea has also been used in the study of single units of the auditory nerve (Tasaki, 1954). An advantage to this approach is the option one has of comparing locally-generated CM responses to single unit activity. A disadvantage is the lack of good visual control for the entry into the auditory nerve. For access, one must drill through the cochlear wall below turn I at an angle normal to the course of the internal auditory meatus. Visibility is limited. But with a slight change in angle, one also has access to the cochlear nucleus (Tasaki and Davis, 1955).

Complications. Any animal is difficult to hold at a constant level of anesthesia. The guinea pig is particularly difficult to keep at a sufficiently deep level to prevent movement, even with a long-lasting anesthetic. There seems to be a very critical level: below it the guinea pig dies, and above it movement artifacts may be severe. However, usual surgical anesthesia followed with a muscle-paralyzing drug produces a good preparation, even for microelectrode work.

In contrast, a cat can be made quiet much more safely. Supposedly size is a factor. However, the chinchilla and young guinea pigs are similar in size, but the chinchilla takes anesthetic more satisfactorily than the guinea pig. The chinchilla too has an accessible, thin-walled cochlea. In this respect, as well as others, it is a compromise experimental animal for research on the auditory system.

All physiological techniques can be buttressed by following them with histology. The processes of perfusion, decalcification, sectioning, and staining of the cochlea require several months for completion. The effects of exposure to noise have been studied with intracochlear electrodes, sampling the CM before and after the exposure, and following the electrical measurements with histological specification of damage to the organ of Corti (Eldredge and Covell, 1958). Such studies, using the electron microscope to detect small changes due to moderate intensities of acoustic stimulation, should provide information for localizing minor, perhaps reversible, changes along the organ of Corti (Spoendlin, 1962).

B. Cat

In contrast to the easy access of the entire ventral aspect of the cochlea once within the bullar cavity of the guinea pig, the cat's bulla is partitioned, and the base is separated from the apex. The bony cochlea in the cat is also thicker than in the guinea pig. Thus, intracochlear electrodes have not been used as generally as they have with the guinea pig, although some experiments have been reported (Tonndorf and Tabor, 1962; Simmons, 1964).

The cat has been used principally with an electrode on the round window (RW) membrane (Wever and Bray, 1930a; 1930b); with a postero-ventral approach one can observe the RW directly for placement of the electrode. When the RW electrode is referred to a remote point, one records a mixture of the CM and AP responses. Since the CM response has no latency but the AP does, the two potentials can be separated for some brief acoustic signals at some intensities (Rosenblith, 1954).

Relations Among Electrical Signs. The whole-nerve AP response exhibits fundamentally the same electrical configuration with both RW and intracochlear electrodes. Although there may be slight differences in waveforms due to minor electrical differences, it is mainly in the resolution of the locus of CM voltage that the RW configuration is deficient. If one's interest is in the whole-nerve AP response, then the problem is to remove the contaminating CM. One way CM has been eliminated from the complex recording is by electronically averaging many responses to a short burst of noise (Peake *et al.*,

1962). The distribution of instantaneous noise amplitudes is random and averages zero, leaving the time-locked AP response free from CM. Another procedure is to average equal numbers of responses to stimuli that are opposite in polarity. In denervated preparations this procedure leaves a slight, but systematic, shift of the baseline, referred to as the slow potential (Kiang and Peake, 1960; Peake and Kiang, 1962). Reports have also described certain electrode locations in the cat's bulla that yield microphonic-free recordings (Rosenblith, 1954). Since round-window electrode records cochlear-microphonic activity principally in the first turn (Simmons and Beatty, 1962; Tasaki and Fernandez, 1952), one cannot investigate the variation of the CM response as a function of distance along the cochlea. One does, of course, observe the presence or absence of the CM and changes in its magnitude.

Conventional recording (an active lead and a remote reference) from two different places along the cochlea will show smaller differences between the two leads than will comparisons from similar locations for pairs of intracochlear electrodes. Békésy's (1960, pp. 684–703) data show how voltage from a source in the basal turn spreads along a scala, and also how a source in the scala media spreads across the basilar membrane and Reissner's membrane. When the electrode source is located within the scala media, spread along scala media falls off fairly quickly with distance. For the scala tympani and scala vestibuli, the coupling is capacitative across the separating membranes. The potential in these adjacent regions is less steeply differentiated spatially, i.e., it is spread over a greater distance and is reduced in magnitude.

There are techniques for studying the reduction of cochlear responses. Let me point out only two: (a) the middle-ear muscles are available for recording electromyograms, and a RW electrode permits one to study the reduction in electrical response from the cochlea due to the contractions of middle-ear muscles; and (b) inhibitory efferent processes may also be studied.

Unitary Electrical Signs. An appropriate use of the anatomy of the cat is made in experiments on single units of the auditory nerve or on the central nervous system. By approaching the internal auditory meatus of the cat from an opening over the cerebullum, tissue can be removed by suction: the remaining part can be retracted and the proximal side of the internal auditory meatus seen. Thus, the distal portion of the auditory nerve may be reached through the meatus, and on the proximal side the cochlear nucleus is also relatively easy to expose. The position of microelectrodes can be adjusted under visual control so that the part of the auditory nerve thought to be peripheral (distal) to the glial margin can be penetrated. One is then fairly sure that the units sampled are first-order units. We note here that stimulus coding in first-order fibers will include transmission across at least one synapse-like relation between nerve ending and hair cell (Smith and Sjöstrand, 1961). With visual control and careful preparation of micro-electrodes, investigators can remain close to a cell, maintaining contact long enough to carry out parametric experiments to investigate its statistical properties. Note that the single unit may be an ultimate level for studying the spatial correlate of cochlear responses.

When a microelectrode penetrates the auditory nerve, fibers with high best frequencies are encountered first. As the electrode advances to the core of the nerve, fibers with lower best frequencies are en-countered (Kiang et al., 1962). This pattern reflects the organization of the nerve trunk, i.e., fibers from the apex are located in the center of the twisted nerve trunk while fibers arising from basal regions lie toward the outside. The twisting of the trunk proceeds as the ear and the auditory nerve develop.

The pattern of best frequencies encountered is an important ana-tomical 'safeguard in interpreting the data. A second check on whether units are first-order is to verify the position of the microelectrode to be peripheral to the glial margin. The latency of the unit response with respect to the CM from turn I (CM_I) or the CM from the round window (CM_{RW}) correlates highly with this anatomical locus. From the latency alone, however, some apical first-order units could be confused with early-firing cochlear nucleus units. Thus, one might exclude fibers that are truly first-order.

A contralateral anatomical approach has been used by some in-vestigators (Rupert et al., 1963). With the proper stereotaxic coordi-nates, a microelectrode can be directed from above one ear to enter the internal auditory meatus of the opposite side. Note that in this contralateral approach, one progresses through much neural tissue before entering the auditory nerve and passing through the glial margin.

If the final position of the electrode tip is specified in an unambigu-ous manner, then the electrode track can be reconstructed. One then regards as primary those units recorded from when the electrode tip is estimated to be beyond the glial margin. An important difference between the two anatomical approaches, contralateral and ipsilateral, is the difference in visual control.

IV. COCHLEAR MICROPHONIC AND MOVEMENT OF THE COCHLEAR PARTITION

A. Background

The movement of the cochlear partition in response to acoustic signals and the principles underlying it are largely the work of G. von Békésy. His book, *Experiments in Hearing* (1960) is an eloquent statement of his work.[*]

Probably the most significant contributions made by Békésy are those that show that the various theories of wave motion in the cochlea belong to one great family (Békésy, 1962). By varying only the elasticity of a rubber membrane, a substitute for the basilar membrane in dimensional models of the cochlea, Békésy produced wave motions demanded by resonance theory, telephone theory, standing-wave theory, and traveling-wave theory. The gradation of elasticity along the membrane and the coupling between its segments, in addition to its overall elasticity, were significant variables that determined its pattern of vibration (Békésy, 1960, pp. 437–440 and pp. 514–534).

In the simple resonance theory, the basic problem of frequency resolution along the cochlea was solved in principle by postulating that the basilar membrane is under radial tension (Helmholtz, 1912). The tension was said to vary in strength along the basilar membrane, inversely to its width: short with greater tension at the base, long with less tension at the apex. The coupling between segments was assumed to be negligible. Békésy (1960, pp. 469–480) directly investigated this assumption of radial tension. He pressed upon the basilar membrane with a fine glass thread; the depression produced by the thread was round. He cut longitudinal slits in the basilar membrane; the cut edges did not pull apart. Thus, radial tension in the basilar membrane was shown not to exist.

The coupling between adjacent segments of the cochlear partition is not negligible, but varies with the elasticity. The elasticity of the membrane is graded from stiff near the stapes, to flexible near the apex. Békésy, applying a constant force, found that the displacement

---

[*]Two other sources serve as bases for material in this chapter. One is the 1962 Békésy Commemorative Issue of the *Journal of the Acoustical Society of America* (in honor of his receiving the Nobel Prize for Physiology in 1961). The other source is Davis's 1957 review paper in *Physiological Review*. These sources, with their bibliographies, provide extensive coverage of cochlear physiology.

was small at the base, but a hundred times larger at the apex. The gradient of stiffness is determined almost entirely by the basilar membrane itself.

The problem of frequency resolution along the basilar membrane remains, but Békésy's direct observations altered the nature of questions appropriate to the problem. For example, in the guinea pig, the whole cochlear partition moves as a unit in response to a 300 Hz tone (Békésy, 1960, pp. 460–469). As frequency increases, an amplitude maximum occurs along the membrane at a position congruent with its elasticity. The displacement amplitude maximum moves toward the base of the cochlea as the driving frequency is increased. Thus, in order to understand frequency resolution in the cochlea, we must first understand the movement of the cochlear partition as a function of frequency.

B. Traveling Wave

The displacement of the cochlear partition travels in a fixed direction (Békésy, 1960, pp. 510–524). The graded stiffness of the partition, along with the fast compression wave consequent to an acoustic signal, provide for a constant direction of travel of the ensuing displacement wave, regardless of the position in the cochlea at which the driving force is administered. The stiffer parts of the membrane drive the more flexible parts when the driving force is applied to a large segment of the membrane, which condition is provided by the fast compression front (Békésy, 1960, pp. 520–524). Thus, the traveling wave of displacement invariably travels from the stapes end of the cochlear partition toward the apical end.

As the traveling wave progresses along the cochlear partition, the displacement amplitude gradually increases, reaching a maximum in the region where the partition is tuned, due to its elasticity, to the driving frequency. Only in this sense is the term *resonance* properly used to describe the response of the cochlea. Apical to the maximum, the displacement becomes small rather abruptly. A plot of maximal amplitudes as a function of distance from the stapes, the envelope, shows two slopes: basal to the maximum, the slope is more gradual than it is apical to the maximum. According to Greenwood (1962), the amplitude at a point 8 mm basal to the maximum has an amplitude of 20% of the maximum in man. The corresponding figure for the guinea pig is about 2.5 mm. He calculated (from Békésy's data) that, apical to the maximum, no displacement (0%) occurs at 2 mm for the guinea pig and at 4.4 mm for man.

For sinusoidal stimuli, Békésy (1960, pp. 37–40) used the phase relation between stapes movement and the movement of a point along the cochlear partition as a descriptive measure. Phase lag differentiates between a simple resonance vibration and a traveling-wave phenomenon. The phase difference continues to increase as a function of distance along the cochlear partition and the driving frequency. At the point of maximum amplitude, the phase angle was π and it continued to increase beyond that point to 3π. In a simple resonant system, the phase lag is zero at the point of maximum amplitude. Thus, the test differentiates the wave motion in the ear from that due to a simple resonant system.

Compared to psychophysical measures of frequency discrimination, frequency resolution in the movement of the cochlear partition is broad. One mm along the cochlear partition probably includes between 700 and 1200 hair cells. Suppose that a low intensity, 1–kHz signal does indeed lead to a maximum displacement amplitude about 1 mm in extent and that movement of the hair cells located there leads to excitation of the nerve fibers ending at their bases. If we change the frequency of the signal, how many different hair cells must we move in order to differentiate the second signal from the first? The answer must certainly lie in the ratio between the hair cells common to the two signals and the hair cells unique to each sample, modified by the noise inherent in the system. Although the effective noise in the system may vary with frequency, the statistical principle should not. We must, therefore, look farther than the overall movements of the cochlear partition to the movements of hair cells themselves or to the nerve fibers innervating them to understand frequency resolution.

C. Relations Between Movement of the Cochlear Partition and Electrical Potentials

Békésy has also provided important information relating movement of the structures of the cochlear partition to the cochlear microphonic potentials. With a vibrating electrode, small bits of tissue could be moved, and the resulting microphonics recorded (Békésy, 1960, pp. 672–684). He impressed a trapezoidal waveform upon the vibrating element. The CM responses to *displacement* of the membrane would duplicate the trapezoid; responses to *velocity* of the displacement would show a pulse whenever the displacement was changing.

When the vibrating electrode was placed on the basilar membrane, a displacement response was recorded. When the vibrator was placed on Reissner's membrane, the responses included a small velocity component. There is then a direct relation between the CM and the displacement of the cochlear partition.

With a vibrating needle, Békésy applied lateral vibratory motion to the tectorial membrane. An active electrode placed nearby recorded the microphonics produced by the applied vibration. The lateral vibration primarily produced shearing forces (Békésy, 1960, pp. 703–710). When the outer edge of the tectorial membrane was moved at a frequency of 300 Hz, the greatest amplitude of the microphonic was produced by lateral vibration in a radial direction. At the inner (modiolar) edge of the tectorial membrane, the greatest amplitude for the microphonics was produced by lateral vibration in a longitudinal direction. Whether the lateral movement was toward or away from the generator cells made no difference in magnitude of the response, so Békésy concluded that the shearing forces are indeed the critical forces in producing the microphonics.

The large microphonic when the tectorial membrane is vibrated in a radial direction is consistent not only with the relation between the stiff reticular lamina and the soft mass of the organ of Corti, but also with the relation between the modiolar attachments of the tectorial membrane and the basilar membrane. The relative positions of the modiolar attachments, acting like hinges, are such that the tectorial membrane and reticular lamina can slide with respect to each other. If the tops of the hairs are imbedded in the tectorial membrane, there is adequate anatomical substrate for effective shearing action. If the tops of hairs are not imbedded, then perhaps some other critical event occurs. Or perhaps the important difference is the one between the reticular lamina and the organ of Corti.

Békésy (1960, pp. 485–500) also observed movement of hair cells during acoustic stimulation. The movements of hair cells that are located at the position of maximum displacement are longitudinal. Basal to the amplitude maximum, movements of the hair cells are up and down. Still more basal, their movements are radial, in the same direction as the fibers of the tectorial membrane. Apical to the amplitude maximum, hair-cell movement decreases markedly. An increase in frequency of the stimulus moves the entire pattern toward the stapes.

At a position just basal to the region of maximum amplitude, the radial shear motion is the greatest, suggesting that the maximum cochlear microphonic output arises somewhat basal to the region where the displacement is greatest. Also recall that between the region of maximum amplitude of the displacement and the region of maximum radial movement of hair cells, the movements are up and down, like pistons.

D. Cochlear Microphonic Response

The CM is an electrical response that may be recorded from an electrode placed in various positions close to the cochlea. Its existence has been known for many years; its role is still not specified. Today, the source of the microphonic is specified and techniques are available to permit sampling from restricted regions along the cochlear partition. With the use of generally improved techniques, the CM is no longer the only candidate for a role in stimulating nerve fibers. A dishearteningly large number of potentials can be sampled from the inner ear. The roles these potentials portray in the excitation of nerve fibers and in indicating nutritive processes are still to be completely specified. Let me first treat the CM.

Békésy (1960, pp. 684–703) found that the basilar membrane and Reissner's membrane are good insulators. Within the scala media, he found a high, positive, steady (DC) potential, the endocochlear or endolymphatic potential. For this positive potential to be effective in some way for excitation, it must be contained. Reissner's membrane and the basilar membrane, as good insulators, do contain the DC.

Tasaki and Fernández (1952) showed that pairs of electrodes (differential or intracochlear electrodes) oriented perpendicularly to the cochlear partition record electrical activity from restricted regions along the cochlea. Thus, they were able to sample the CM at various positions. Although the apical end of the cochlea, turn III and the apex, responds only to low frequencies, the basal turn, turn I, responds to all frequencies. The response from a round window electrode compared with the response from a pair of electrodes in turn I showed that the source of both potentials is the basal turn.

Since the cochlear partition is insulated from the perilymph on either side, sampling the CM with electrodes in the scala vestibuli and scala tympani yields an attenuated signal. With modern methods of amplification such attenuation presents little difficulty. But there are questions of validity. For example, can capacitative coupling across the insulating membranes distort the electrical recording? Such capacitance could alter the time course of the CM recorded from perilymph as compared to the CM within scala media. Békésy's

(1960, pp. 684–703) studies of cochlear electrophysiology imply that the capacitance is sufficient to cause differences in the time course between a local CM recorded from the scala media and one recorded from the perilymph with pairs of intracochlear electrodes. These conclusions are based on the electrical synthesis of patterns similar to those measured in the cochlea.

Alternative to synthesizing similar conditions, one can correlate electrophysiological responses and histological evidence, in order to show causal relation. Davis *et al.* (1953) compared histological with electrophysiological evidence to determine whether the maximum CM, recorded with electrodes, corresponds to sites where the greatest destruction is produced by tones appropriate to that location along the basilar membrane. They stimulated the ear with tones that were estimated (from the CM) to produce maximal amplitude at the electrode site. The region of greatest damage corresponded with the CM maximum. Such comparisons grossly estimate that the CM response recorded with intracochlear electrodes in perilymph is a valid indicator of movement of the cochlear partition.

A precise indication of longitudinal movement is the phase relation between pairs of points. Tasaki *et al.* (1952) constructed Lissajous patterns by placing the output of one pair of intracochlear electrodes on the vertical plates of an oscilloscope and the output of another pair on the horizontal plates. Such patterns are used to measure the phase relation between two signals. Converted to time differences, these phase differences show a delay similar to that of the traveling wave. Tasaki *et al.* (1952) concluded that intracochlear electrodes sample the CM within a 1–2 mm range.

With a transient stimulus, measuring phase relations becomes inappropriate; the delay itself must be measured instead. Teas *et al.* (1962) measured this travel time for the CM response sampled at five places in the guinea-pig cochlea. The CM travels quite rapidly in the basal turn, gradually slowing as it reaches the position at which the voltage is greatest. This pattern of travel is consistent with the variation in stiffness along the cochlear partition.

Measurements of the velocity of the traveling wave in response to different frequencies of acoustic signal should reflect any capacitative pick-up across the membranes. Sufficiently precise measurements have not yet been made to allow this determination. Sufficient precision is available, however, to determine several relations. The acoustic pressure leads to displacement of the stapes. The CM response in turn I follows the velocity of stapes movement (Teas *et al.*, 1962; Tonndorf, 1962; and Eldredge, personal communication, 1960).

Since the CM is proportional to the displacement of the cochlear partition (Békésy, 1960), it follows that displacement of the partition also follows the derivative of stapes movement. Note that this relation implies that the phase lag progresses along the cochlear partition from 90°, not from zero. Note also that the cochlear partition itself can still move as a unit, i.e., in phase, to low frequency signals, but lag 90° behind stapes displacement.

Input-Output Relations. Since pairs of intracochlear electrodes do record CM from restricted regions of the cochlear partition, one can measure input-output functions for different electrode locations. Input-output functions were reported by Tasaki *et al.* (1952) for tone bursts and by Teas *et al.* (1962) for low-pass transients. The simplest measure is afforded by relatively narrow-band stimuli. For the frequencies of 4 kHz and above, Davis (1961b) and his co-workers used a gated sinusoid with a rise time of 1 msec, a duration of 3–4 msec, and fall time of 1 msec. For lower frequencies, they used tone pips, rising to a maximum in 2–3 cycles, staying at maximum for 2 cycles, and then decreasing again in 2–3 cycles. Such stimuli, tone pulses or tone pips, are compromises between brief clicks with their wide-band characteristics and long-duration tones with their narrow bands. It is difficult to study long segments of time in detail, and wide-band stimuli such as clicks do not permit stimulation of restricted regions of the cochlear partition.

Input-output functions for the CM show a range of linear growth; then they begin to bend. The maximum output before bending over depends upon frequency and the position of the electrodes. For a 500 Hz tone pip, the maximum linear growth in turn III is reached at about 100–200 μV, whereas for turn I the maximum linear growth approaches 3–4 mV. For a 7 kHz tone burst, there is no output from turn III. At turn I, the maximum linear growth may reach 1 mV, but is definitely less than it is for the low-frequency tone pip. Similar frequency and intensity relations between the input and output hold for turn II recordings.

Since parts of the input-output curves are linear, a measure of the filtering between turn I and turn III can be derived from them. For equivalent output from turn III and turn I for a 500 Hz tone pip, there is about a 15 dB difference in signal strength. Thus, with intracochlear electrodes, the slope of the filtering between turn III and turn I for 500 Hz is about 2 dB/mm. This figure reflects the increased amplitude of the mechanical movement at the basal location.

CM Envelope. The linear growth of the input-output curves also permits the construction of an envelope for the traveling wave. The baseline-peak (positive and negative) voltages at each location can be plotted on the abscissa at points corresponding to the positions of the electrodes along the cochlear partition. A smooth curve fitted to the points represents the maximum amplitudes of voltage along the membrane.

With the curves describing the velocity of the traveling wave, the voltage envelope permits a construction of successive instantaneous values of CM voltage as a function of position along the cochlear partition. Figure 6 shows a succession of such curves for a low-pass acoustic transient.

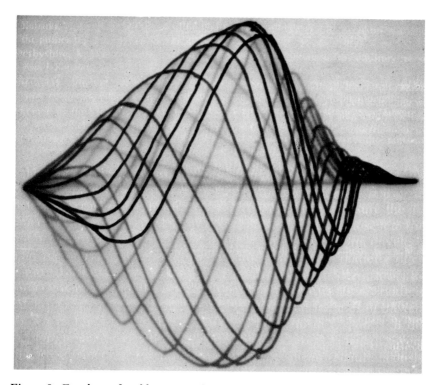

Figure 6 Envelope of cochlear microphonic response to a low-pass acoustic transient constructed by superimposing successive single voltage curves along the cochlea at instants in time after the delivery of the acoustic signal. Time between successive curves is 0.05 msec. Darkest curves are most recent in time. (Teas *et al.*, 1962. By permission from *Journal of the Acoustical Society of America*.)

The observation that the input-output curves for the CM bend at strong signal levels and even give decreasing outputs with further increases in signal strength does not coincide with Békésy's (1960, pp. 480–484) observations of the amplitude of movement of the cochlear partition. He used signal strengths approaching the threshold of feeling and never reported any decrease in the amplitude of movement. But remember that Békésy recorded the microphonics produced by lateral vibration of the tectorial membrane and lateral vibration imparts shearing forces to the hair cells. Thus, although the amplitude of movement of the organ of Corti appears to increase, the microphonics, if due to shearing forces, could reach a maximum and fail to grow further.

The frequencies contained in *wide-band* acoustic signals are sorted out as a function of distance from the stapes. The response to a click will be a faithful reproduction of stapes movement only when recorded from the basal turn. The response from turn III, on the other hand, will be similar to the electric response from a filter set to pass frequencies from 500 Hz on down to 0. That is, each region of the cochlear partition can be made to respond only as fast as its properties of elasticity will permit. If a stimulating earphone rings at 3 kHz, the oscillations will be evident at locations along the partition appropriate to 3 kHz, and also in regions basal to that if their strength is great enough. They will *not* appear in regions apical to the region of maximum response for 3 kHz, provided the operating level is within the linear range of the input-output functions.

E. Summating Potential

Davis, *et al.* (1958b) described another potential, the source of which is also the hair cells. The summating potential (SP) appears as a shift in the baseline on which the CM occurs. The SP may be either positive or negative, a fact that can obscure its growth and behavior under various experimental conditions. The SP is most clearly seen in response to high-frequency signals from turn I electrodes.

When the CM response to a 7 kHz tone burst begins to grow nonlinearly, and then to decrease, the negative SP continues to increase. However, at SPLs of 100 dB and greater, there is a transient response to the 1 msec onset and fall of the tone burst. This transient is propagated toward the apex of the cochlea. At turn III, after a delay appropriate to the traveling wave, a CM is recorded that corresponds to the onset and fall time of the tone burst. The turn III response is not the

SP; only the baseline shift at turn I during the signal presentation is to be regarded as SP (Davis *et al.*, 1958b).

Békésy (1960, pp. 636–646) found a steady positive potential in the scala media throughout the endolymph. He also recorded both the cochlear microphonic responses and the changes in the steady potential during stimulation with acoustic signals. The DC becomes less positive during stimulation by sound. Upon cessation of the acoustic signal, the steady potential recovers to its initial value. The question arises whether the SP recorded by intracochlear electrodes is a manifestation of the shift in the endocochlear potential reported by Békésy.

At least one paper has stated this proposition explicitly. Konishi and Yasuno (1963) said that the SP and the shift of the endocochlear potential are different manifestations of the same underlying events. They inserted microelectrodes into the scala media at each turn of the guinea pig's cochlea. The SP was measured for a range of frequencies and intensities. Their stimuli were of long duration with slow rise and fall times. Generally speaking, the SP measured in turn I is positive for low frequencies and negative for high frequencies. The authors stressed that the polarity and magnitude of the SP to long tones depend strongly on the position of the recording electrode.

Konishi and Yasuno also recorded the SP under electrical polarization of the endolymph. When the scala vestibuli was made positive, the SP became more negative, and the CM became larger. With the scala vestibuli negative, the CM was reduced, and the SP became only slightly positive.

Tasaki *et al.* (1954) reported more extensive manipulation of DC pressure changes as well as of electrical polarization. These earlier data on electrical polarization and the new data by Konishi and Yasuno are consistent with each other. An important additional feature of the earlier data is the similarity between increasing pressure in scala tympani and increasing polarization in scala vestibuli. The effect on the SP is the same, an increase in the negative SP.

The important information added by Konishi and Yasuno (1963) is that the SP as well as the CM reverses its polarity upon penetration of the reticular lamina. Its source is thereby located at the hair cell. However, positive endolymphatic potentials have been found in waltzing guinea pigs with no hair cells, but with the stria vascularis intact. On this basis, the source of the endolymphatic potential was thought to be an active process of the stria vascularis and *not* due to the hair cells. Thus, equating the SP with a transient decrease in the endolymphatic potential while demonstrating that the hair cell is the generator for the SP raises critical questions.

Butler (1964) clarified some aspects of the problem. His data suggest that the organ of Corti region is isopotential and negative in sign. The scala media is positive. If hair cells modulate the DC, they modulate the difference or gradient between the electrically positive and electrically negative sources.

Tasaki's (1960) suggested interpretation of microphonic responses is consistent with the Butler data. A nerve fiber immersed in a potassium-rich medium does not respond to electrical stimulation. However, if that nerve fiber is subjected to anodal (positive) polarization, it becomes highly sensitive to mechanical deformation. The membrane potential fluctuates between a high positive value and a low negative value. Thus, its response depends upon its state. Tasaki's suggestion is that the CM is the response, in concert, of a great many hair cells changing their state together. The gradations in magnitude of the CM represent gradations in the number of cells responding in concert. Konishi and Yasuno (1963) suggested that the vagaries of their SP recordings, under the conditions of their experiments, is compatible with Tasaki's suggestion.[*]

Although these data and their interpretation may account for generator potentials, they do not clarify the problem of how unmyelinated nerve fibers are excited to produce the action potential propagated to the cochlear nucleus. If the organ of Corti region is isopotential, with the inside and the outside of nerve fibers identical electrically, it is difficult to understand the triggering mechanism. Békésy (1960, pp. 485–500) reported a variety of movements of hair cells under acoustic stimulation, so there is some basis for supposing that the CM and SP are due to different kinds of movements. Engström et al. (1962) suggested that inner hair cells are structurally suitable for sensitivity to radial shear, but that outer hair cells are structurally suitable for sensitivity to a *variety* of shear movements. From a correlation of histological and electrophysiological evidence, Davis et al. (1958a) found that the SP is present when only inner hair cells remain intact, suggesting that the outer hair cells are responsible for the CM. Békésy's data showing that the inner hair cells are most sensitive to longitudinal shear also fit with Davis's hypothesis.

Because of the variety of motions possible along the cochlear

---

[*]Harris et al. (1970) report that the microphonic response from a single hair cell in the tail of the mudpuppy is graded.

partition and because of the variety of electrical potentials that are present, it is useful to consider simpler systems. Flock (1965) investigated the ultrastructure and the physiology of the lateral-line organ. In contrast to the ordered arrangement of hairs on the outer hair cells in the cochlea, the lateral line organ (and the vestibular apparatus) has the hairs in two clusters, each on one side of a kinocilium. Flock found further that displacement of the cupula toward the kinocilium leads to depolarization but that displacement away from the kinocilium leads to hyperpolarization. Therefore, in the lateral-line organ, the "double-frequency" of its microphonic is traced to the dual clusters of hairs.

We should, therefore, be aware of possibilities for both depolarization and hyperpolarization in the more complicated system of the mammallian cochlea. If, for example, the suggestion of Engström *et al.* (1962) is correct that the morphological relations of the outer hair cells are suitable for a variety of shear movements, then details of the movement of hair cells may be important in the encoding of mechanical activity into neural excitation.

V. ACTION POTENTIAL

The CM and the SP are graded responses, and they are local, confined to the sense organ itself. They are easily measured and undoubtedly are highly correlated with the immediate stimulus to the nerve fibers. However, the point of departure for conceptualizing the excitatory events leading to neural activity is the traveling wave of displacement of the cochlear partition.

The study of auditory nerve fiber responses should give information that can be related to the mechanical movement, and, therefore, to the CM and SP. One everpresent problem in working with neural responses at the ear is the difficulty of being certain of the sources from which one is recording. Not only is there a problem of differentiating the AP from the receptor potentials, the CM and SP, but there is also a problem of differentiating between the relatively synchronous population responses of the cochlear nucleus and the responses from first-order neurons.

The electrical sign of population responses varies depending upon the geometry of the active and reference electrode, and the source of the response. In the case of a large electrode on or in the cochlea with a remote reference electrode, the situation is complicated because activity across the whole nerve is recorded. In the case of a microelectrode, the response is unitary.

A. Whole-Nerve Response

Teas *et al.* (1962) found that the response waveform of a highly synchronous group of nerve impulses from the basal turn was diphasic: first negative, then positive. They developed a graphic model of the electrical response of a neural element as it would appear between an active electrode in the cochlea and a remote reference. With this diphasic model, they showed that late-occurring, initially negative nerve impulses are obscured by the positive voltage from early nerve impulses. Therefore, only the most synchronous part of the whole-nerve response is seen unless special procedures are applied.

If the CM and the AP responses are separated from each other and viewed on the same time base, the time relations between them can be estimated. For a low-frequency signal, the AP response appears during a fixed segment of the CM_I waveform. With intracochlear electrodes, the segment is one during which the scala vestibuli changes from positive to negative re scala tympani (Deatherage *et al.*, 1959). The change occurs during a half-cycle of the period of the stimulus. The time required for this half-cycle to travel from the base of the cochlea to the point of maximum amplitude along the cochlear partition varies with the frequency of the acoustic signal. The duration over which nerve impulses are produced also varies, as does the length of the partition over which the traveling wave is effective.

To explain the diphasic character of the whole-nerve AP response, it is necessary to recall the nature of the traveling wave. The direction of travel from base to apex of the cochlea, i.e., from a region most sensitive to high frequencies to a region most sensitive to low frequencies, from stiff to flexible, is invariant and leads to certain consistent features for the volleys of neural impulses consequent to a brief acoustic signal.

Sensitivity and Synchrony. The lowest signal strengths that elicit detectable AP responses on the oscilloscope belong to high-frequency tone bursts or tone pips with rapid rise times. These stimuli are maximally effective in the basal turn, which comprises about one-half the longitudinal extent of the cochlea in the guinea pig. In cat and man, the basal turn includes somewhat more than half of the cochlea.

For low-frequency tone pips or low-pass transients, the CM responses from turn III can be detected at lower signal strengths than can the AP response. It is unlikely that no neural impulses are excited by these signals at these levels, however. The oscilloscope trace may show only an upper portion of the intensity function for the whole-nerve AP in response to these low-frequency signals. The detectability of the whole-nerve response on the oscilloscope depends in part upon the synchrony of the nerve impulses, the less synchronous impulses not being seen. Even though 5–kHz tone bursts are used for stimuli, if their rise times are greater than 4 msec, the whole-nerve response is not detectable (Goldstein and Kiang, 1958). However, there is a detectable evoked response at the cortex. Thus, synchrony and AP detectability vary together, but they are not necessarily measures of physiological effectiveness.

An earphone transduces a square wave so that both low and high frequencies are present. They are also present in the CM. However, the nerve impulses from the basal turn, excited relatively synchronously by the high frequencies since this part of the partition moves nearly as a unit, occur first in time, are more easily detected, and grow faster to a greater magnitude and contribute more to the voltage sum than do nerve impulses from the apical locations. Nevertheless, the less synchronous nerve impulses from apical locations in response to these broad-band signals, although difficult to detect, are present and may be studied with appropriate analytical procedures.

The term synchrony is a useful one, although difficult to apply experimentally. Broadly speaking, the greater the synchrony, the larger the number of nerve fibers per millisecond that are excited. A whole-nerve response can become larger because of an increase in synchrony or because of an increase in the number of nerve impulses. For illustrative purposes, consider a segment of the cochlear partition with a maximum CM response to 500 Hz. Nerve impulses are excited between 90° and 270° in each cycle of the sinusoid, i.e., over a 1 msec duration. If there are 1000 excitable nerve fibers within the segment, then at maximum signal strength, synchrony within the segment is 1000 fibers per msec. Unfortunately, the simplicity is only theoretical. Probably the thresholds of the 1000 fibers are distributed in sensitivity and the sensitivities probably vary with time. At signal strengths below the maximum, fewer than 1000 fibers will be excited, but, at the maximum, the signal strength will be strong enough to exceed the thresholds of some nerve fibers located in more basal regions. Consequently, the velocity of the traveling wave must also be considered. Since the traveling wave moves more rapidly in the basal regions, more nerve fibers per unit time are excited and response magnitudes grow more rapidly than at the lower signal strengths.

Magnitude. The complexity of the whole-nerve AP (owing to the diphasic waveform of the neural element and the asynchronous excitation of nerve fibers) leaves measurements open to question. The response element derived by Teas *et al.* (1962) is a useful basis for evaluating measures of the whole-nerve response.

The initial phase of the response element is negative; its duration is about 0.25 msec. Therefore, a measure of the magnitude of neural activity may be made within 0.25 msec of the beginning of the whole-nerve response. At greater times, the positive phase from previous nerve impulses begins to interfere with the negative phase of new neural activity and the measure from the baseline or any other point becomes complicated.

For estimates of magnitude of neural activity after the initial negative phase, detailed comparisons of waveforms must be made. Generally speaking, one compares the response to the signal in question with the response to the same signal plus noise. If all other experimental conditions have been held constant, then the difference between the two response waveforms reflects the neural activity. Computer processing aids greatly in these experimental comparisons.

Latency. Most properly, the latency of the whole-nerve response should be measured from the CM arising in the same region of the cochlear partition from which the nerve impulses arise. The figure would then reflect the temporal properties of the excitation of those nerve impulses at that position. In practice, latency may be measured from the occurrence of the electrical signal, from the movement of the stapes, or from the CM from turn I or the round window. For low-frequency stimuli, the positive peak of the CM, as one traveling wave proceeds along the cochlea, should give the reference time for the respective location.

The peak of the small whole-nerve AP that is just detectable on the oscilloscope in response to a low-pass signal occurs slightly less than 1 msec after the positive peak of CM_{III}. When the positive peak of CM_I is the reference, the latency to the low intensity signal is slightly more than 2 msec. At strong signal strengths, the latency measured from CM_I is about 1.2 msec to such a signal, earlier than the positive peak in CM_{III}.

Pestalozza and Davis (1956) measured the latency to high frequency tone pips from 8 kHz to 38.5 kHz. They found a systematic effect for both frequency and intensity. Their highest frequency, 38.5 kHz, showed a decrease of latency with increasing intensity of only about 0.30 msec, whereas for the 8 kHz pip, the latency range from near detectability to 75 dB SPL was about 1.1 msec. These tone pips had rise times of 1 msec. As intensity increased, nerve impulses occurred earlier. Presumably these time differences indicate spatial differences due to different frequencies being most effective at different locations along the cochlear partition. (These latencies also include time for conduction to the effective recording site in the internal auditory meatus as well as possible differences in excitation time.)

Comparisons of the effects of various narrow bands of noise in removing some of the nerve impulses from the synchronous response to a low-pass signal show that the higher the signal strength, the higher the frequency of the noise band that most effectively removes nerve impulses. The latency of the nerve impulses removed by a given band of noise is invariant with signal strength; the magnitude is not. With signal strength constant, the latency of the nerve impulses removed by bands of noise successively higher in frequency decreases. Therefore, as signal strength increases, nerve fibers from successively more basal locations are excited. Latency correlates well with frequency and therefore with location along the cochlear partition. This decrease in latency for the whole-nerve AP response represents a *basal extension* of excitation from the more flexible to the stiffer parts of the cochlear partition as signal strength increases. This principle accounts for the finding that the lower the frequency of the signal, the greater the range of latency shift that can be expected.

A click signal adds other complicating features. The cochlear partition in turn III cannot respond faster than about 0.5 kHz, but turn I responds readily to higher frequencies. Below 4 kHz, the rate of change of the CM appears to be critical for neural excitation. Therefore, for a broad-band transient signal, nerve fibers at turn I respond first and faster than those at turn III because the stimulus is there first. Later neural activity originating apically is obscured. Latency of the peak of the whole-nerve AP, measured from CM_I, includes the traveling wave delay, the difference between excitation processes occurring at all positions along the cochlea, and represents only the most synchronous group of nerve impulses. Because of the asymmetric response pattern seen both in the CM and in the whole-nerve AP, the latency problem is also complicated by excitation of nerve fibers basal to the region of maximal amplitude for the traveling wave.

Overlaying these factors is the diphasic waveform for the neural element in the whole-nerve AP. Experiments calculated to inactivate basal regions should permit examination of the synchrony of excitation for apical nerve impulses. Further analysis of latency and synchrony of nerve impulses, recorded as population responses but broken down into small groups, may tell us more about the excitation processes along the cochlear partition.

B. Computer Processing

Several developments in research on the cochlea and its nerve fibers lend significance to the analysis of responses to low-level signals. A problem arises in the analysis of small responses because of the noise inherent in physiological recording. This problem is a general one which extends across recording methods and across particular experiments, from population responses to single-unit responses. For low-frequency acoustic signals, strength of stimulation is related to that position along the cochlear partition from which the nerve impulses arise. Thus, if our detection level depends on synchrony, there is an inherent artifact in our data: the lower end of the input-output function is not retrievable except with special analytical techniques, and perhaps not retrievable at all except with the improvement in the signal-to-noise ratio (S/N) afforded by computer techniques. The use of computers to extend downward the signal strengths that elicit reliable responses is, therefore, important for our understanding of the precision of tuning in the cochlea. By now enough information is available to indicate that, at the cochlear level, tuning becomes broader as intensity is increased.

With respect to single-unit data, the problem of the S/N is also critical, but it is manifested in a different way. The effect of an acoustic signal is detected in the response of a single primary auditory unit as a change in the rate of spontaneous activity, e.g., as a change in the rate of pulses heard over a loudspeaker monitoring the output of the electrode. With no acoustic signal delivered there is always a base rate of "spontaneous" activity in first-order auditory neurons. An increase in rate of firing is defined as an excitatory effect; a decrease in rate of firing is an inhibitory effect. Objective, sensitive, and highly reliable means of detecting changes in the recurrent activity of a unit would help to get consistent and lawful data. Criteria based on electronic counters or other objective devices are more desirable than is reliance on human judgment.

Computers also increase the number of data that can be processed. This facility allows more detailed study of physiological responses to signals varied parametrically. Without computer techniques, one is faced either with a forbidding task of analysis (with questionable validity) or with no analysis at all (Rosenblith and Vidale, 1962).

With the computer, there can also be immediate feedback of processed data so that a consistency judgment can be made. One can evolve a considerable degree of sophistication with regard to the data and physiological experiments can be made quite precise (Kiang, 1961).

C. Single Units

The responses of single units of the auditory nerve are not as complex as is the whole-nerve response. The single-unit responses recorded extracellularly are all-or-none and, therefore, the complicated voltage summations that can arise in recording from populations are not present. Magnitude of response is irrelevant for understanding the role of the fiber in transmitting information about the acoustic stimulus. The only relevant information is the timing of the unitary response. The single-unit response also lends itself well to processing by electronic equipment, since it is essentially a pulse, and can be shaped in any way that will make analysis easy. The only property one must preserve is the time of occurrence.

With the appropriate synchronization, then, computers can total the number of impulses, count the number of impulses within a time interval, or specify the time interval between impulses. The sample of responses over which the computation is made can be as large as necessary. These automatic counting procedures lead to histograms showing the number of responses appearing at different latencies and the number of intervals occurring for different durations between pulses. The form of the distribution of intervals for a sample of spontaneous activity can be ascertained (Gerstein 1960; Gerstein and Kiang, 1960) and, in some cases, summary statistics such as the mean and variance can be calculated. Generally speaking, at this stage of our experimental sophistication, we must accept (or at least test for) the statistical properties of single units anywhere in the nervous system.

Statistical descriptions of response properties are still relatively new and their fruitfulness is perhaps yet to be fully realized. But classical concepts of response measures remain quite valuable, e.g., the concept of the response area (Galambos and Davis, 1943).

Excitation. A response area includes all combinations of frequency and intensity of tonal stimuli for which a unit's firing rate is increased over the level of spontaneous activity. At some frequency, defined as the unit's best or characteristic frequency, the unit will be excited by a minimal intensity. Response areas may have holes in them, subareas describing combinations of frequency and intensity for which the spontaneous firing rate is reduced. Such gaps in the response area or perturbations of its outline are interpreted to represent inhibition.

It is in the determination of best frequencies that the question of S/N becomes important. The experimenter's judgment can determine the minimum detectable change in rate from the spontaneous activity due to the acoustic signal. Katsuki et al. (1958, 1959) described the difficulties in determining best frequencies for tone pulses as contrasted with continuous tones, an example of determinations made by the same group of investigators using two different stimuli that yield responses differing in the S/N. The response areas for continuous tones extended to lower intensities for the best frequencies and were sharper. At higher intensities, the response areas became broader, often showing two slopes, a steep one for about 20 dB, then a less steep one at higher intensities.

Katsuki et al. further commented that the 2 kHz threshold for the human ear is about 100 dB below their reference level. Man's threshold is 10 to 15 dB higher than the cat's at 2 kHz (Miller et al., 1963). Thus, the minimal intensities for best frequencies in the Katsuki et al. data are probably high if one accepts the audibility curve for the experimental animal as a criterion. Sensitivity near the behavioral criterion is likely to be necessary in order to establish valid bases for interpretations concerning relations between physiological measures and psychoacoustic judgments.

There are still questions regarding the narrowness of the response areas for high frequency single units, the tuning curves for the CM along the cochlear partition, and interpretations of the whole-nerve response. Response areas determined by Tasaki and Davis (1955) are broad and qualitatively consistent with the slope of -12 dB per octave demanded by a chronaxie hypothesis of stimulation of nerve fibers by the CM. Data by Kiang et al. (1962) show sharper response areas than can be accounted for on the basis of previous conceptualizations. The data from Kiang et al. and Katsuki et al. are on the cat, whereas previous data are on the guinea pig. However, the species differences are probably not as great as the differences between the two sets of single-unit data. Differences due to sensitivity of recording are in the proper direction.

On the basis of the CM responses and the whole-nerve AP responses, we would expect that single nerve fibers in the basal turn should show broad response areas. That is, the nerve fiber should cut off fairly abruptly at frequencies above its characteristic frequency, but be capable of excitation by a lower frequency, depending on signal strength. Thus, the higher a fiber's characteristic frequency, the more basal its termination along the cochlear partition and the broader its response area should be toward the low-frequency side. characteristic frequency.

The response areas reported by Kiang et al. are generally asymmetric, but units with high characteristic frequencies do not show the expected broad response areas. The response area appears broader as characteristic frequency decreases, that is, for apical fibers.*

The relation between the bandwidth of the unit and its characteristic frequency can be studied with post-stimulus-time histograms for uniform clicks (Kiang et al., 1962) taken from units with different characteristic frequencies. Units with characteristic frequencies below 4 kHz show histogram peaks separated by the reciprocal of their characteristic frequency.

The periodicities in the single-unit responses refer to the successive stimulations of that fiber at its position along the cochlear partition and hence to critical events in the movement of the basilar membrane. A plot of these intervals-between-firings-of-single-units vs. the periods of their characteristic frequencies gives a distribution with a slope of 1.0. This relation is strong evidence for an orderly and straightforward organization of the nerve fibers and the processes leading to their excitation along the cochlear partition.

Above 4 kHz, the intervals between peaks cannot be discriminated. These high-frequency units show only a single peak of activity in response to a click. If the nerve has a time constant of excitation, then at some frequency the period of the signal will be less than that time constant. At that frequency, some summative effect might occur. In a computer simulation of the Kiang et al. single-unit data on the auditory nerve, Weiss (1964) considered some of these properties. One of his conclusions was that the excitability of auditory nerve fibers increases with frequency independently of acoustic resonances.

Both Tasaki (1954) and Katsuki et al. (1958, 1959) gave the dynamic

---

*For a complete description of characteristics of primary auditory nerve fibers, see Kiang (1965).

range of a single fiber. Katsuki *et al.* showed a sigmoidal curve for the frequency of nerve impulses vs intensity, ranging over about 20 dB. Tasaki's curve, may be only the top half of the sigmoid. Kiang *et al.* (1962) reported a very low frequency of repetitive responses in single units; Tasaki reported a higher percentage. This finding also suggests greater sensitivity in the more recent data.

In the Kiang *et al.* data, the latency of the unit responses changed only slightly as a function of signal strength. With increasing signal strength, new and earlier peaks developed in the histograms, but those peaks were still separated from the later ones by the period of that unit's characteristic frequency. The dynamic range of any single nerve fiber is probably not greater than 15–20 dB.

Inhibition. The response areas from the three studies, Tasaki (1954), Katsuki *et al.* (1958, 1959) and Kiang *et al.* (1962), are straightforward reflections of properties of the excitation along the cochlear partition. Reduction in rate of firing with the simultaneous presentation of two acoustic signals was reported by Kiang (1963), and more extensively by Nomoto *et al.* (1964).* Note that the requirements of two acoustic signals leaves open the possibility that the inhibitory-like effect depends upon mechanical events in the cochlea preceding the neural events.

A fourth group of investigators, Rupert *et al.* (1963), reported both an immediate reduction in the *spontaneous* rate of response upon acoustic stimulation and also a reduction with a long time-course of onset and recovery. Such reductions in spontaneous response rate constitute an empirical definition of inhibition.

Rupert *et al.* (1963) noted a single unit with a high spontaneous rate. Upon stimulation with a 1 kHz continuous tone, there was a sharp reduction in its spontaneous rate of response. Other frequencies at other intensities also reduced the spontaneous rate, i.e., the inhibitory effect was not limited to one frequency. No detailed parametric study of the unit was presented.

A second type of change in rate of firing developed more slowly. First, there was a brief increment in the response rate upon stimulation by a tone, followed by a gradual reduction to levels below the prestimulation level. Upon cessation of the tone, the spontaneous rate

---

*For a more recent and quantitative study of two-tone inhibition, see Sachs and Kiang (1968).

slowly returned to the prestimulation level, requiring about one minute for recovery.

From a study of single units in the frog, Frishkopf and Goldstein (1963) reported two categories of unit activity, termed by them *simple* and *complex*. Units in the simple category respond to acoustic signals above 1 kHz, and show spontaneous activity. These units can not be inhibited. Units in the complex category may be activated by acoustic signals between 200 and 700 Hz, or by vibration or by both modes of stimulation; they may or may not show spontaneous activity. Units in this category can be inhibited by an acoustic signal.

The inhibitory effects these authors described are stimulus-dependent. They observed one spontaneously active complex unit with an inhibitory *tuning curve*. As with the response area, this curve defines combinations of frequency and intensity that, in this case, shut off the spontaneous activity. For units excited by acoustic signals, they reported that the second acoustic signal (inhibitory) must be 6 dB larger to inhibit totally. It is important to remember the stimulus dependency of the inhibitory effects.

Nomoto *et al.* (1964) also reported stimulus dependencies for short-latency inhibitory effects in the monkey. Figure 7 shows the inhibitory effects occurring on the skirts of the response area. The procedure is to stimulate with a continuous tone, inserting a tone burst of appropriate frequency and intensity from another source at different times. With the background and inhibitory frequencies appropriately chosen, they found inhibitory effects only for high-frequency units and failed to detect any such effects for units with characteristic frequencies of 1 kHz or less. Strong signals are required.

The fact that neural responses, both whole-nerve and single-unit, occur in periodic relation to low-frequency acoustic signals is well known. Tasaki (1954) showed that the unit response is correlated with the phase of the cochlear microphonic, not with the signal. The traveling-wave delay between turn I and turn III in the guinea pig's cochlea is about 1 msec. If one uses the CM_{RW} or the electrical waveforms as his reference, the unit responses from different neurons can indicate firing throughout a complete cycle of a 500 Hz signal, when actually there is a traveling-wave delay and the excitation of neural impulses occurs for comparable phase at the different locations along the cochlear partition. Thus, periodicity may be present but obscured when one inspects different single units. This temporal spread of the neural activity is evident in the whole-nerve response. Gold-

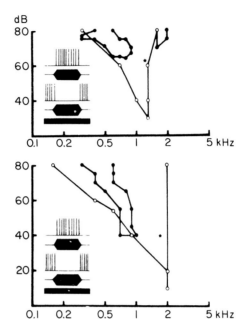

Figure 7 Response areas and inhibitory areas from two neurons in the VIIIth nerve of the monkey. Open circles, response area; closed circles, inhibitory area; °, background tone. Frequency and intensity of tone bursts which decreased unit responses occurring to background tone can be read from the abscissa and ordinate, respectively. (Nomoto *et al.*, 1964. By permission from *Journal of Neurophysiology*.)

stein and Kiang (1958) showed that the overlap of waveforms from successive stimuli can distort the electrical sign of neural activity, thus placing a limit on the usefulness of this sign for determining the upper limit for periodicity.

Rupert *et al.* (1963) reported unit responses that, although periodic, show a variety of relations with the signal. Some units respond with interspike intervals approximating the frequency of the stimulus. Others hold fast to preferred interspike intervals and still others vary their intervals with the intensity of the tone. Such variations in response properties might be understood in terms of the signal and the ensuing traveling wave along the cochlear partition. But to attempt such an interpretation requires more detailed information than we have concerning the response areas for those units. The temporal pattern of response to impulsive broad-band signals might also help in understanding these phenomena.

VI. OVERVIEW

The physiological questions for which we can expect reasonable answers are changing. Microtechniques such as electronmicroscopy and histochemistry are being applied to the study of the ear and we are learning about its biochemical substrate. The appearance of this research interest is significant both for our understanding of the mechanism of neural excitation and for medical diagnosis and treatment.

For electrophysiology in particular, there is another dimension of change in research questions. The capacity for processing large amounts of electrophysiological data leads to treating more complex problems. This ability, accompanied by a sophistication in experimental techniques, brings within reach the investigation of relations among several separate events. The processing of representative samples of simultaneously recorded, separate electrical events in the auditory system can give important data on the physiological processing of acoustic events at the ear as well as at more central sites.

Single unit activity in primary auditory nerve fibers represents an important stage in neural processing, between the mechanical movement of the cochlear partition and the neural encoding of that movement. In the anesthetized animal, there appears to be a straightforward relation between the anatomical location at which the nerve terminates in the cochlea and its response to acoustic signals.

Although we understand many properties of single-unit responses, other problems remain to be worked out. One of these centers around the question of an inhibition in primary fibers in anesthetized preparations. It would help to know the pattern of mechanical movement of the cochlear partition for those single units showing inhibition. Studies relating the cochlear microphonic to single-unit activity are difficult and require special experimental design. Such studies should show how well the electrical signs of mechanical movement and neural activity correlate with each other. For example, is the physiological mechanism that reduces spontaneous activity following stimulation by a tone different from the one that reduces firing rate during the simultaneous presentation of two signals? Specification of stimulus-response relations for single-units and also of the relations between mechanical movement and single-unit activity could resolve this question.

Single-unit activity should be related not only to its antecedents such as the cochlear microphonic, but to contemporaneous events such as population responses, and also to subsequent behavioral events. Probably the population responses will be important in the study of physiological correlates of psychoacoustic judgments, since such judgments are probably based on the activity of many rather than few neurons. The small dynamic range of single units suggests that loudness may be mediated by large numbers of nerve impulses.

Actually, there are relatively few studies of physiological correlates, that is, studies in which measurements of electrical activity of the auditory system are reported. Frishkopf and Goldstein (1963) reported relations between excitatory and inhibitory properties of single units in the frog together with the spectrum of the frog's croak. For the auditory system of the frog, parallels between the spectrum of emitted sound and receptive capacity are useful and informative.

For animals with broader frequency response and wider auditory repertoire, the parallels between single-unit responses and spectra of emitted sound may be less fruitful. However, comparisons of the audibility curve of the experimental animal with response areas of single units would be useful.

There has been a progressive improvement in the sensitivity of measures of single-unit activity. Much improvement is due to recording procedures and techniques, but probably more could be expected if automatically applied statistical criteria were used to discriminate between the spontaneous background activity and activity related to the acoustic signal. Weiss's simulation study of single-unit responses in the cat indicates that such an improvement in sensitivity could be achieved.

Another improvement in physiological data afforded by computer processing lies in the representativeness of the response indicators. The averaging process alone extends the generality of physiological data in two important ways. One illustration is the basal extension of excitation for low-frequency signals: the nerve fibers at progressively more basal sites are stimulated as signal strength is increased. This observation may be the analogue for population responses to the problem of response area and sensitivity for single units. Improvement in response resolution can, therefore, lead to the study of population responses from a restricted set of nerve fibers that arise from the apical locations. These groups of nerve fibers carry information not available from the separate study of their single units since the space-time pattern of activity among the nerve impulses is not recorded in the latter case. The space-time pattern of nerve impulses does contribute information that is used by the central nervous system, for example, in lateralization.

In studies of whole-nerve activity in response to transient acoustic signals, response strength and anatomical origin of nerve impulses along the cochlear partition are not independent. Since neural activity is best seen as a transient response against a steady-state noise background, there is reason to use acoustic signals in which the theoretically simple or pure dimensions of frequency and intensity are deliberately confounded. Study of the discrimination of tailored transient signals and of the electrical signs of the neural activity evoked by them should be fruitful in specifying physiological correlates for their pitch, loudness, and localization.

A second improvement in physiological data resulting from on-line computer processing is that statistical-physiological responses no longer must represent the speciously typical example. Enough data can be processed to arrive at statistically representative estimates of the electrical signs of neural activity. One can include similar numbers of events for both psychoacoustic judgments and the electrical signs of the neural activity underlying them. Quantification is possible because large numbers of events are assessed. Although the experimental procedures themselves may present problems, it becomes reasonable to record both behavioral and physiological data simultaneously. In this context, it is clear that we know a good deal about designing experiments to show either behavioral or physiological effects, but much less about designing informative experiments to recover both types of data. However, simultaneous recording of the two aspects of the same overall events is an important principle to retain.

ACKNOWLEDGMENT

The preparation of this chapter was supported by Career Research Development Award NBK3–8600, by Research Grant NB–04740, both from the National Institutes of Health, and in part by The Edwards-Lazear Foundation for Auditory Research. Special acknowledgment is made for the assistance of Mrs. Betty Schacter in handling details extending beyond usual secretarial tasks.

REFERENCES

von Békésy, G. (1960). *Experiments in hearing*. McGraw-Hill, New York.
von Békésy, G. (1962). Concerning the pleasures of observing, and the mechanics of the inner ear. *Prix Nobel, 1961*. Norstedt Söner, Stockholm.
Butler, R. A. (1964). Experimental observations on a negative d.c. resting potential in the cochlea. *J. Acoust. Soc. Am.*, **36**, 1016 (A).

Butler, R. A., Honrubia, V., Johnstone, B. M., and Fernández, C. (1962). Cochlear function under metabolic impairment. *Ann. Otol. Rhinol. Lar.*, **71**, 648–656.

Churchill, J. A. and Schuknecht, H. F. (1956). Acetylcholinesterase activity in the cochlea. *Laryngoscope*, **66**, 1–15.

Dallos, P. J. (1968). On the negative potential within the organ of Corti. *J. Acoust. Soc. Am.*, **44**, 818.

Davis, H. (1957). Biophysics and physiology of the inner ear. *Physiol. Rev.*, **37**, 1–49.

Davis, H. (1959). Excitation of auditory receptors. In J. Field (Ed.) *Handbook of physiology.* Vol. 1, pp. 565–584. American Physiological Society, Washington.

Davis, H. (1961a). Peripheral coding of auditory information. In W. A. Rosenblith (Ed.) *Sensory communication.* pp. 119–141. M.I.T. Press *and* Wiley, New York.

Davis, H. (1961b). Some principles of sensory receptor action. *Physiol. Rev.*, **41**, 391–416.

Davis, H. and Associates (Benson, R. W., Covell, W. P., Fernández, C., Goldstein, R., Katsuki, Y., Legouix, J.-P., McAuliffe, D. R., and Tasaki, I.) (1953). Acoustic trauma in the guinea pig. *J. Acoust. Soc. Am.*, **25**, 1180–1189.

Davis, H., Deatherage, B. H., Rosenblut, B., Fernández, C., Kimura, R. S., and Smith, C. A. (1958a). Modification of cochlear potentials produced by streptomycin poisoning and by extensive venous obstruction. *Laryngoscope*, **68**, 596–627.

Davis, H., Deatherage, B. H., Eldredge, D. H., and Smith, C. A. (1958b). Summating potentials of the cochlea. *Am. J. Physiol.*, **195**, 251–261.

Deatherage, B. H., Eldredge, D. H., and Davis, H. (1959). Latency of action potentials in the cochlea of the guinea pig. *J. Acoust. Soc. Am.*, **31**, 479–486.

Desmedt, J. E. (1962). Auditory-evoked potentials from cochlea to cortex as influenced by activation of the efferent olivo-cochlear bundle. *J. Acoust. Soc. Am.*, **34**, 1478–1496.

Eldredge, D. H. and Covell, W. P. (1958). A laboratory method for the study of acoustic trauma. *Laryngoscope*, **68**, 465–477.

Engström, H. and Wersäll, J. (1953). Is there a special nutritive cellular system around the hair cells in the organ of Corti? *Ann. Otol. Rhinol. Lar.*, **62**, 507–512.

Engström, H., Ades, H. W., and Hawkins, J. E., Jr. (1962). Structure and functions of the sensory hairs of the inner ear. *J. Acoust. Soc. Am.*, **34**, 1356–1363.

Fernández, C. (1951). The innervation of the cochlea (guinea pig). *Laryngoscope*, **61**, 1152–1172.

Fex, J. (1962). Auditory activity in centrifugal and centripetal cochlear fibres in cat: a study of a feedback system. *Acta Physiol. Scand.*, **55**, *Suppl. 189*, 1–68.

Flock, Å. (1965). Electron microscopic and electrophysiological studies on the lateral line canal organ. *Acta Oto-Lar.*, *Suppl.* **199**, 1–90.

Frishkopf, L. S. and Goldstein, M. H., Jr. (1963). Responses to acoustic stimuli from single units in the eighth nerve of the bullfrog. *J. Acoust Soc. Am.*, **35**, 1219–1228.

Galambos, R. (1956). Suppression of auditory nerve activity by stimulation of efferent fibers to cochlea. *J. Neurophysiol.*, **19**, 424–437.

Galambos, R. and Davis, H. (1943). The response of single auditory-nerve fibers to acoustic stimulation. *J. Neurophysiol.*, **6**, 39–57.

Gerstein, G. L. (1960). Analysis of firing patterns in single neurons. *Science*, **131**, 1811–1812.

Gerstein, G. L. and Kiang, N. Y-s. (1960). An approach to the quantitative analysis of electrophysiological data from single neurons. *Biophys. J.*, **1**, 15–28.

Goldstein, M. H., Jr. and Kiang, N. Y-s. (1958). Synchrony of neural activity in electric responses evoked by transient acoustic stimuli. *J. Acoust. Soc. Am.*, **30**, 107–114.

Greenwood, D. D. (1962). Approximate calculation of the dimensions of traveling-wave envelopes in four species. *J. Acoust. Soc. Am.*, **34**, 1364–1369.

Guggenheim, L. (1948). *Phylogenesis of the ear*. Murray and Gee, Culver City, California.

Harris, G. G., Frishkopf, L., and Flock, A. (1970). Receptor potentials from hair cells of the lateral line. *Science*, **167**, 76.

von Helmholtz, H. (1912). *On the sensations of tone*. (Fourth English ed. of the fourth German ed. of 1877). Longmans, Green, London *and* New York.

Katsuki, Y., Sumi, T., Uchiyama, H., and Watanabe, T. (1958). Electric responses of auditory neurons in cat to sound stimulation. *J. Neurophysiol.*, **21**, 569–588.

Katsuki, Y., Watanabe, T., and Suga, N. (1959). Interaction of auditory neurons in response to two sound stimuli in cat. *J. Neurophysiol.*, **22**, 603–623.

Kiang, N. Y-s. (1961). The use of computers in studies of auditory neurophysiology. *Trans. Am. Acad. Ophthal. Oto-Lar.*, **65**, 735–747.

Kiang, N. Y-s. (1963). Spontaneous activity of single auditory nerve fibers in cats. *J. Acoust. Soc. Am.*, **35**, 793 (A).

Kiang, N. Y-s. and Peake, W. T. (1960). Components of electrical responses recorded from the cochlea. *Ann. Otol. Rhinol. Lar.*, **69**, 448–458.

Kiang, N. Y-s., Watanabe, T., Thomas, E. C., and Clark, L. F. (1962). Stimulus coding in the cat's auditory nerve. *Ann. Otol. Rhinol. Lar.*, **71**, 1009–1026.

Kiang, N. Y-s. (1965). Discharge patterns of single fibers in the cat's auditory nerve. M.I.T. Research Monograph No. 35, M.I.T. Press, Cambridge, Mass.

Kimura, R. S. and Perlman, H. B. (1956). Extensive venous obstruction of the labyrinth. *Ann. Otol. Rhinol. Lar.*, **65**, 332–350.

Kimura, R. S. and Perlman, H. B. (1958). Arterial obstruction of the labyrinth. *Ann. Otol. Rhinol. Lar.*, **67**, 5–40.

Konishi, T. and Yasuno, T. (1963). Summating potential of the cochlea in the guinea pig. *J. Acoust. Soc. Am.*, **35**, 1448–1452.

Konishi, T., Butler, R. A., and Fernández, C. (1961). Effect of anoxia on cochlear potentials. *J. Acoust. Soc. Am.*, **33**, 349–356.

Lawrence, M. and Clapper, M. (1961). Differential staining of inner ear fluids by Protargol. *Stain Technol.*, **36**, 305–308.

Miller, J. D., Watson, C. S., and Covell, W. P. (1963). Deafening effects of noise on the cat. *Acta Oto-Lar.*, *Suppl.* **176**.

Misrahy, G. A., Shinabarger, E. W., Hildreth, K. M., and Gannon, W. J. (1957). Bioelectric studies of the cochlea. *Fedn Proc. Fedn Am. Socs Exp. Biol.*, **16**, 88 (A).

Moscovitch, D. H. and Gannon, R. P. (1965). Effects of calcium on sound-evoked cochlear potentials. *J. Acoust. Soc. Am.*, **37**, 1201 (A).

Nomoto, M., Suga, N., and Katsuki, Y. (1964). Discharge pattern and inhibition of primary auditory nerve fibers in the monkey. *J. Neurophysiol.*, **27**, 768–787.

Peake, W. T. and Kiang, N. Y-s. (1962). Cochlear responses to condensation and rarefaction clicks. *Biophys. J.*, **2**, 23–34.

Peake, W. T., Goldstein, M. H., Jr., and Kiang, N. Y-s. (1962). Responses of the auditory nerve to repetitive acoustic stimuli. *J. Acoust. Soc. Am.*, **34**, 562–570.

Perlman, H. B. and Kimura, R. S. (1955a). Observations of the living blood vessels of the cochlea. *Ann. Otol. Rhinol. Lar.*, **64**, 1176–1192.

Perlman, H. B. and Kimura, R. S. (1955b). Physiology of the cochlear blood vessels. *Angiology*, **6**, 383–393.

Perlman, H. B., Kimura, R. S., and Fernández, C. (1959). Experiments on temporary obstruction of the internal auditory artery. *Laryngoscope*, **69**, 591–613.

Pestalozza, G. and Davis, H. (1956). Electric responses of the guinea pig ear to high audio frequencies. *Am. J. Physiol.*, **185**, 595–600.

Rosenblith, W. A. (1954). Electrical responses from the auditory nervous system. *Ann. Otol. Rhinol. Lar.*, **63**, 839–860.

Rosenblith, W. A. and Vidale, E. B. (1962). A quantitative view of neuroelectric events in relation to sensory communication. In S. Koch (Ed.) *Psychology: a study of a science*. Vol. 4, pp. 334–379. McGraw-Hill, New York.

Rupert, A. L., Moushegian, G., and Galambos, R. (1963). Unit responses to sound from auditory nerve of the cat. *J. Neurophysiol.*, **26**, 449–465.

Sachs, M. B. and Kiang, N. Y-s. (1968). Two-tone inhibition in auditory nerve fibers. *J. Acoust. Soc. Am.*, **43**, 1120.

Saxén, A. (1951). Histological studies of endolymph secretion and resorption in the inner ear. *Acta Oto-Lar.*, **40**, 23–31.

Schuknecht, H. F., Churchill, J. A., and Doran, R. (1959). The localization of acetyl-cholinesterase in the cochlea. *Archs Otolar.*, **69**, 549–559.

Simmons, F. B. (1964). Electrodes permanently placed within cochlea. *Fedn. Proc. Fedn. Am. Socs. Exp. Biol.*, **23**, 414 (A).

Simmons, F. B. and Beatty, D. L. (1962). The significance of round-window-recorded cochlear potentials in hearing. *Ann. Otol. Rhinol. Lar.*, **71**, 767–800.

Smith, C. A. and Rasmussen, G. L. (1963). Recent observations on the olivo-cochlear bundle. *Ann. Otol. Rhinol. Lar.*, **72**, 489–506.

Smith, C. A. and Sjöstrand, F. S. (1961). Structure of the nerve endings on the external hair cells of the guinea pig cochlea as studied by serial sections. *J. Ultrastruct. Res.*, **5**, 523–556.

Spoendlin, H. H. (1962). Ultrastructural features of the organ of Corti in normal and acoustically stimulated animals. *Ann. Otol. Rhinol. Lar.*, **71**, 657–677.

Tanaka, Y. and Katsuki, Y. (1966). Pharmacological investigations of cochlear responses and of olivo-cochlear inhibition. *J. Neurophysiol.*, **29**, 94–108.

Tasaki, I. (1954). Nerve impulses in individual auditory nerve fibers of guinea pig. *J. Neurophysiol.*, **17**, 97–122.

Tasaki, I. (1960). Afferent impulses in auditory nerve fibers and the mechanism of impulse initiation in the cochlea. In G. L. Rasmussen and W. F. Windle (Eds.) *Neural mechanisms of the auditory and vestibular systems.* pp. 40–47. Thomas, Springfield, Illinois.

Tasaki, I. and Davis, H. (1955). Electric responses of individual nerve elements in cochlear nucleus to sound stimulation (guinea pig). *J. Neurophysiol.*, **18**, 151–158.

Tasaki, I. and Fernández, C. (1952). Modification of cochlear microphonics and action potentials by KCl solution and by direct currents. *J. Neurophysiol.*, **15**, 497–512.

Tasaki, I. and Spyropoulos, C. S. (1959). Stria vascularis as source of endocochlear potential. *J. Neurophysiol.*, **22**, 149–155.

Tasaki, I., Davis, H., and Legouix, J.-P. (1952). The space-time pattern of the cochlear microphonics (guinea pig), as recorded by differential electrodes. *J. Acoust. Soc. Am.*, **24**, 502–519.

Tasaki, I., Davis, H., and Eldredge, D. H. (1954). Exploration of cochlear potentials in guinea pig with a microelectrode. *J. Acoust. Soc. Am.*, **26**, 765–773.

Teas, D. C., Eldredge, D. H., and Davis, H. (1962). Cochlear responses to acoustic transients. *J. Acoust. Soc. Am.*, **34**, 1438–1459.

Tonndorf, J. (1962). Time/frequency analysis along the partition of cochlear models: a modified place concept. *J. Acoust. Soc. Am.*, **34**, 1337–1350.

Tonndorf, J. and Tabor, J. R. (1962). Closure of the cochlear windows. *Ann. Otol. Rhinol. Lar.*, **71**, 5–29.

Tonndorf, J., Hyde, R. W., and Brogan, F. A. (1955). Combined effect of sound and oxygen deprivation upon cochlear microphonics in guinea pigs. *Ann. Otol. Rhinol. Lar.*, **64**, 392–405.

Vosteen, K. H. (1963). New aspects in the biology and pathology of the inner ear. *Transl. Beltone Inst. Hear. Res.*, **16**.

Weille, F. L. (1955). The significance of the arteriovenous arcades of the spiral ligament of the cochlea. *Ann. Otol. Rhinol. Lar.*, **64**, 173–180.

Weiss, T. F. (1964). A model for firing patterns of auditory nerve fibers. *M. I. T. Res. Lab. Electron. Tech. Rep. 418*.

Wever, E. G. and Bray, C. W. (1930a). Action currents in the auditory nerve in response to acoustical stimulation. *Proc. Natn. Acad. Sci. U.S.A.*, **16**, 344–350.

Wever, E. G. and Bray, C. W. (1930b). Auditory nerve impulses. *Science*, **71**, 215 (L).

Wever, E. G. and Vernon, J. A. (1956). The sensitivity of the turtle's ear as shown by its electrical potentials. *Proc. Natn. Acad. Sci. U.S.A.*, **42**, 213–220.

Wever, E. G. and Vernon, J. A. (1960). The problem of hearing in snakes. *J. Aud. Res.*, **1**, 77–83.

Wever, E. G., Vernon, J. A., Peterson, E. A., and Crowley, D. E. (1963). Auditory responses in the Tokay gecko. *Proc. Natn. Acad. Sci. U.S.A.*, **50**, 806–811.

Chapter Eight

Enlarged Mechanical Model
of the Cochlea with Nerve Supply

FOREWORD

Models of any complex system are necessarily imperfect unless, like a map that is exactly the same size as the country it represents, they become perfect replicas instead. Lloyd Jeffress used to ask students how large they imagined a computer would have to be in order to perform all the functions of a white rat. His answer was that it would be about the size of a white rat. Models of the ear may ultimately be replaced by real ears (or by replicas of them), but for now, that seems too impractical. The model maker who does not restrict himself to replication, though, does have to restrict himself in other categories. A most important restriction is common to mechanical and electrical models, and to most computer simulations: the ways in which a nervous system can interpret the signals produced in the ear have to be ignored. Georg von Békésy, after developing most of the data we have about the mechanical properties of the auditory system, began to look for models that might overcome this ultimate perceptual problem. He has made analogies between auditory and olfactory properties, between auditory and visual processes, and, in fact, has made comparisons and parallels with many other sensory phenomena. His most successful general approach has been in making models that use the skin receptors as part of the "cochlea."

Enlarged Mechanical Model of the Cochlea with Nerve Supply

Georg von Békésy*

I. MODELS IN PHYSICS AND BIOLOGY

The cochlea is extremely small and delicate, so it is natural to look for an enlarged model that permits observations to be made without micromanipulators. A model also avoids the rush and the care necessary in handling living tissue.

Mechanical models, as analyzed by Newton, Froude, Cauchy, and Reynolds (Bridgman, 1931), have been used extensively during the last half century and have been essential to the development of ships and of the wings of modern airplanes. As a matter of fact, scale models have been so successful that much work has been done to generalize tha laws governing them (Bridgman, 1931; Duncan, 1953) and to extend these laws from physics into the field of living matter (see the reviews by Stahl, 1963; Baldwin, 1964; Beament, 1960). Most of these models are of a mechanical or electrical nature, but recently mathematical models have been used and digital computers, because of their tremendous storage capacity and speed of operation, will probably lead to new applications of modeling (Hawthorne, 1964).

I have long been interested in models constructed by means of dimensional analysis. Because a little paper work often led to the same results as time-consuming experiments, it seemed like getting something for almost nothing. I learned later that the very successful

*Laboratory of Sensory Sciences, University of Hawaii, Honolulu, Hawaii.

models of earlier times were what I should like to call functional models. These models were kept as close to the original system as possible and therefore conserved many features of the original system. The improved visibility of the model made it possible to observe unexpected details which could then be verified on the original system. It seemed to be a good principle to stay as close as possible to the original system and to proceed step by step to simpler models, always checking the phenomena of interest by direct observation. This approach, though extremely tedious, makes it possible to determine which variables of the original system are vital to the phenomena under observation, and it suggests which variables can be omitted in the further simplification of the model. Sometimes there may even emerge a clear borderline beyond which further simplifications would change the original features of the system. Models thus provide a method for separating the important variables in a system under observation from the unimportant ones.

Beyond functional models are models of a kind that are better called analogues. They can go so far that they are nothing more than a form of description that is simpler or more familiar than the original phenomenon. Because there is a continuum between the functional model and the analogue, one will sometimes deduce from an analogue findings that are peculiar to it but that have little to do with the original system. In some extreme cases, especially for quantitative analogues, the model may be so oversimplified that it serves for nothing more than curve-fitting. Then it can give only what information is already explicit or implicit in the curve to which the model was fitted. Since the curve and the model express the same thing, although in different languages, the possibilities of misunderstanding are sometimes considerable.

Whereas findings based on a functional model stay the same, descriptions may change radically. A good example is the mechanical model of electrical induction described by Maxwell in 1892 (Vol. 2, p. 228), illustrated in Fig. 1. In Maxwell's time, electricity was something new, and to make it more understandable, the phenomena were translated into the more familiar terms of mechanics. Today, this approach seems outdated; since the introduction of Ohm's law, we have become so familiar with electric circuitry that, in complicated systems like an electrodynamic microphone, we prefer to visualize masses and elasticities as condensers and inductances. Therefore, as in Fig. 2, we may produce an electrical model of the mechanical parts of the microphone and study on this model how the microphone can be improved (Firestone, 1938). It is a dramatic reversal of our habits.

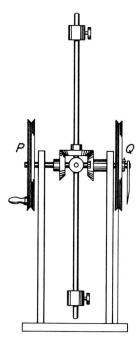

Figure 1 Maxwell's model of electrical induction. A differential gear is used to move two large masses.

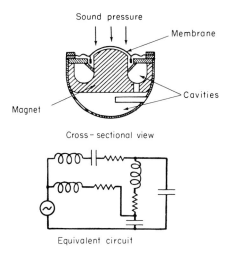

Figure 2 Cross section of an electrodynamic microphone and the corresponding electrical model. Today the electrical model is more familiar and is considered easier to evaluate than the original.

We have to conclude that a model of the cochlea should be as similar to the original system as possible. Thus I was led to the construction of a mechanical model with a nerve supply.

II. CONSTRUCTION OF THE MODEL OF THE COCHLEA WITH NERVE SUPPLY

The history of the development of hearing theories is a good example of the fact that models that are only analogues can hardly be used to test the functioning of the original system. Several analogues can usually be devised for the same property of a system, often quite differently. To explain pitch discrimination in the cochlea, several analogues have been proposed. Budde (1917a,b) made models of Helmholtz's resonance theory of hearing in which the resonating elements were the elasticity of the basilar membrane and the mass of U-shaped threads of fluid within the perilymph. Wilkinson and Gray (1924) went so far as to place a series of metallic resonators in their model of the cochlea. In contrast, Ewald (1899) used a very thin rubber membrane to represent the basilar membrane, so instead of resonance phenomena, he obtained standing waves along the rubber membrane, waves which changed their pattern with the frequency of the driving forces. Several models which showed traveling waves along the basilar membrane are well summarized in a review by Waetzmann (1926, pp. 667–700).

The patterns of vibration among these models are so different that it is extremely difficult to decide which one comes closest to nature. If statistics had been applied in deciding which theory of hearing is the most probable, preference would have been given to the traveling wave theories. As Fig. 3 shows, almost any material of longitudinal shape or with a large surface under stroboscopic illumination shows traveling waves when one point is touched with a vibrating tip. The waves always travel away from the vibrator.

A model will withstand the corrosion of time quite well if the number of explicit and implicit statements is reduced to a minimum. In this respect, geometric and mathematical models have certain advantages. As an example, the classically simple "single place" theory of hearing of Gildemeister (1930) should be mentioned. To explain the exquisite frequency discrimination of the ear for pure tones, Gildemeister assumed that a pure tone produces its activity in one small section of the basilar membrane, as shown by the knot of

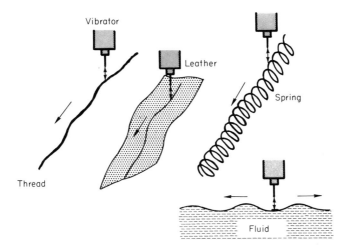

Figure 3 Traveling waves observed on different objects brought in contact with a vibrator.

lines in Fig. 4. For higher tones, the place of this activity moves toward the stapes, but for lower tones in the direction of the helico- trema as indicated by the arrow. This type of model is nothing but a geometric restatement of the question, how does the ear differentiate the frequencies of pure tones so well? In Fig. 4, the question is con- tained in the knot. Nevertheless, the theory must be valid since the ear has the qualities described. Newer experiments have not shown the activity on the *basilar membrane* to be so sharply located. But if we look instead at the higher nervous system (Katsuki *et al.*, 1958), we find the activity sharply located at certain spots for certain fre- quencies of tone or for narrow bands of noise.

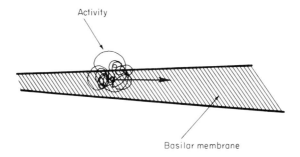

Figure 4 The "one-place" theory of hearing.

Making a model of the cochlea is, therefore, the art of stripping the real structure to its essentials and thus simplifying it, yet retaining enough more than an analogue to be sure to have a functional model.

The first step in the investigation of how far the cochlea can be simplified was to determine whether the elastic properties are the same in a fresh human preparation as in a living person (Békésy, 1960a). Fortunately, it turned out that there is only a very small change in the first day under proper cooling and humidity conditions; the eardrum impedance of a cat or guinea pig does not change when the animal is killed by an overdose of anesthetic. An even more important finding was that opening the top of a cochlear canal does not influence the vibration pattern of the basilar membrane very much when the whole cochlea is submersed in a fluid. Thus, observations with a water immersion microscopic objective are easy.

It seemed especially difficult to duplicate the lateral stress of the basilar membrane since (*a*) it is difficult to measure the lateral tension in the cochlea itself, and (*b*), in the model, such lateral tension has to be applied evenly. Any break in continuity naturally produces distortion in the vibration pattern.

The decisive experiment is shown in Fig. 5. It represents a cross section of the cochlear duct with the two canals separated by the basilar membrane and Reissner's membrane. On the left, the basilar membrane is attached to bone, but on the right side, it is attached to the ligamentum spirale, a gelatine-like substance. If the earlier assumption that the basilar membrane is under lateral tension were correct, then loosening the attachment of the ligament to the bony capsule should change the vibration pattern of the basilar membrane. When sinusoidal pressure was applied to the opening of the lower

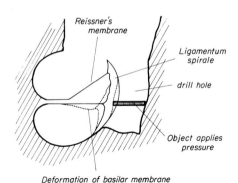

Figure 5   Relaxation of tension on the basilar membrane.

cochlear canal to put the membrane in vibration, even lateral compression of the basilar membrane by a small rod between the ligament
and the bony wall (Fig. 5) did not change the vibration pattern.
Furthermore, it was possible to brush away Reissner's membrane and
the organ of Corti without changing the vibration pattern of the
basilar membrane. So the basilar membrane can be replaced by an
elastic sheet that is not under any tension but that is fixed on both
sides. It is the deformation perpendicular to the plane of the membrane that is important.

To define the elasticity of the longitudinal membrane, the concept
of volume elasticity was used. When hydrostatic pressure is applied to
the lower side of the membrane (Fig. 6), the membrane bulges out

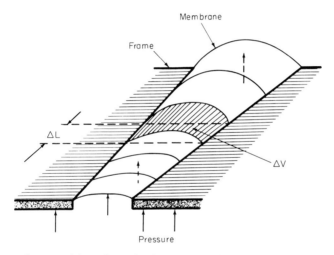

Figure 6   Definition of the volume displacement ΔV for the length ΔL of a membrane
subjected to a pressure on one side.

and a volume displacement of ΔV per mm length of the membrane
(for a hydrostatic pressure of 1 cm water column) was observed. The
value is small near the narrow end of the membrane close to the
stapes, but much larger near the helicotrema where the membrane is
softer and wider. The change from one end to the other is about 1:100
(Fig. 7).

When the volume elasticity of a model basilar membrane is kept
constant relative to the normal human cochlea, the other cochlear

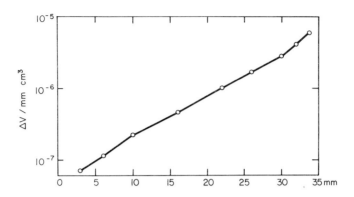

Figure 7 Volume displacement of the basilar membrane along its length for a unilateral pressure of 1 cm water.

variables can be varied to a surprising degree without changing the vibration pattern of the model membrane. It is possible to change the width of the membrane; it can even be reversed relative to the normal situation if the volume elasticity stays the same along the partition. Figure 8 shows variations that were made in the structure of the cochlea without changing the vibration pattern. Perhaps the most interesting observation is that changes in the location of the stapes or the round window do not seem to influence the vibration pattern.

For the purpose of developing a model of the cochlea with nerve supply, it was an important discovery that taking out the fluid from one canal — the scala tympani — produced only a small change. The vibration pattern remained the same, but the location of the place of maximal vibration amplitude moved a little. Thus I could use a model that still remained functional but that consisted of only one canal, a driving stapes, and a basilar membrane along the canal. In this model, one side of the basilar membrane is on the surface of the tube and can be observed and touched very easily. This half-cochlear model has the same vibration patterns as a model with the membrane completely surrounded by fluid.

In Fig. 8, a small eddy is drawn on each side of the vibrating membrane. These eddies locate the place of maximal vibration amplitude.

Now we know that a functional model of the cochlea can consist of a single tube with a membrane on its surface. Besides being easier to experiment with, this membrane can be brought into immediate contact with the skin, thereby forming a model with nerve supply.

Since the difference limen for distance sensation on the skin is

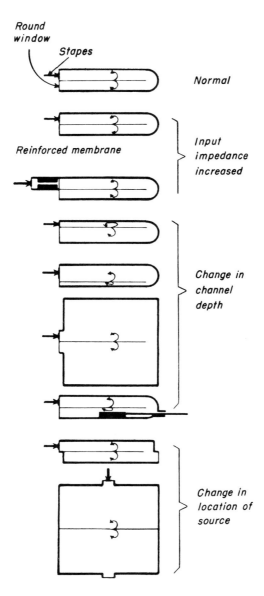

Figure 8 In order to determine the place of maximum vibration amplitude along the cochlear partition, the position of the center of the eddy produced by the vibration was observed. A series of measurements made in an ear model with the same elastic properties as the human ear showed that the vibration pattern and the center of the eddy do not change if the length of the canal is increased, if the depth of the canal is increased, or if the location of the stapes introducing the vibrations into the ear model is changed. This great stability of the vibration pattern of the cochlear partition is responsible for the fact that, in a middle-ear infection, even when the middle ear is filled with fluid, frequency discrimination in the inner ear is not altered.

large, the model was enlarged by applying the laws of hydrodynamic dimensional analysis (Diestel, 1954). The final construction is shown in Fig. 9 (Békésy, 1955). A metal tube forms a core that fits in a soft plastic tube. The core is slit and above the slit the plastic tube is

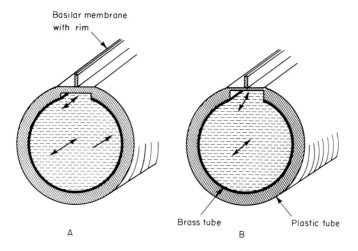

Figure 9 Cross section of a dimensional model of the cochlea. Around a brass tube a plastic mantle of vinylite was cast, forming a membrane along a slit in the brass tube. The thickness of the membrane along the slit varies to correspond to the stiffness of the human cochlea. In (a) and (b) the increase in the thickness of the membrane near the stapes can be seen. The membrane was provided with a ridge on which the arm rested. This ridge made it possible to adjust the coupling between the membrane and the tissues of the arm.

thinned to represent the basilar membrane. The membrane is thick near the stapes section of the tube (Fig. 9a) and becomes regularly thinner as it approaches the other end (Fig. 9b). The membrane has a ridge made from the same plastic as the tube. When the arm is placed on the ridge, it transmits the vibrations to the surface of the skin. Since just the edge of the ridge contacts the arm, only a small part of the vibratory energy of the membrane is transmitted to the skin. This coupling can be adjusted by changing the thickness of the ridge. Thus it is practical to prevent the damping of the vibrations of the basilar membrane when it is loaded with the arm (stroboscopic observations showed that there was no change in the vibration pattern of the membrane when the arm was placed on the edge of the ridge).

Figure 10 is a photograph of the model. On the right is a rod to which an electrodynamic driving unit is attached. The rod ends in a plate, representing the footplate of the stapes, and produces fluid vibrations in the cochlea. A bellows of thin metal is used to couple the metal plate to the tube without leakage. The whole tube is filled with water,

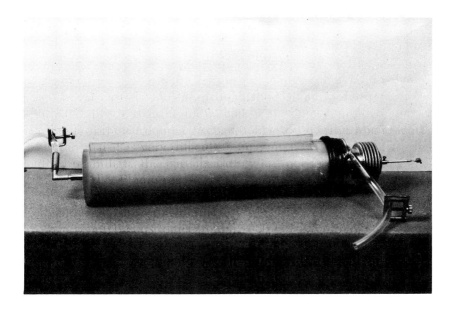

Figure 10 Photograph of the model of the cochlea. On the top of the cylinder the membrane with the ridge can be seen. On the right of the photograph is a metal bellows with a driving rod which served as stapes footplate. The model is filled with water through two tubes. The length of the model is 30 cm.

and it is naturally very important that there be no air bubbles present in the tube since they change the impedances. The small tubes on the left and right ends of the model are used to fill the cochlea. The basilar membrane with its ridge is visible. It is stiff near the bellows and much softer at the other end of the tube. Figure 11 shows how the arm is placed on the edge of the membrane. When the arm lies firmly on the ridge, it is not necessary to pull up the shirt-sleeve since the vibrations are transmitted through thin tissue without much loss.

When sinusoidal vibrations are transmitted to the rod, traveling waves are formed on the membrane; they are similar in pattern to the ones observed in the human cochlea. For high frequencies, they have a maximal amplitude near the stapes plate, and for low frequencies,

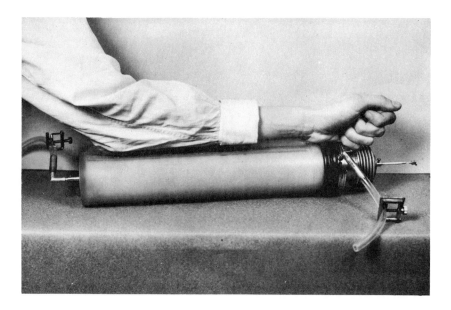

Figure 11 An arm resting on the ridge of the membrane. Localization of the vibrations is easily observed even through heavy garments.

near the other end of the tube. The speed of the traveling waves is high in the beginning and slows down later just as in the normal cochlea. One of the interesting findings is that after only two cycles of a sinusoidal vibration the place of maximal vibration amplitude is already determined. Figure 12 shows this phenomenon with the amplitude maximum at a distance of 15 cm from the model's stapes footplate. If the frequency is higher, the maximum is closer to the footplate. A comparison of the vibration amplitudes at different distances indicates clearly that the onset of vibration is delayed with the distance from the stapes.

Since the mechanical part of the cochlear model seems to be functional, the question now arises, can the nerve supply also be modeled in a way that comes close to the natural situation, and can a similarity be shown between the sensations in hearing and the ones on the skin?

III. PERCEPTION OF SKIN VIBRATIONS

The vibrations of the basilar membrane are transmitted to the organ of Corti, which contains the receptors of the auditory nerve track. The

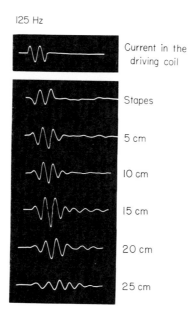

125 Hz

Current in the driving coil

Stapes

5 cm

10 cm

15 cm

20 cm

25 cm

Figure 12 Transients in the cochlear model are very short. From the top down, it can be seen that the length of the transients increases but little and that the two full waves are recognizable until the waves are as much as 20 cm away from the stapes. The longer transients at 25 cm are probably due to reflection from the end of the tube. The amplitude of the traveling wave increases somewhat until it reaches 15 cm, when it drops. The traveling time of the maximal amplitude can be seen from the displacements of the maximal amplitudes to the right.

organ of Corti consists of neat rows of cells along the whole length of the basilar membrane. It is a sense organ with a large surface area. There are other sense organs with large surface areas, such as the skin, the tongue, the retina. The assumption was made that all these sense organs must have many features in common in spite of their adaptation to different tasks. Some experiments on the lateral inhibition of taste, of smell, and of skin sensations (Békésy, 1963, 1964) not only showed *similarities* in inhibition, but also almost the same numerical values. It seemed reasonable, therefore, to try to substitute the vibratory sense organs of the skin for the organ of Corti. Naturally, there are differences, since the nerve endings in the skin are much less dense than those in the organ of Corti, and the vibratory nerves seem to act about six to eight times slower than the auditory nerves. When a continuous vibration with a constant amplitude is presented to the skin, it takes the sensation about 1.2 sec to reach its full magnitude

(Békésy, 1939), whereas for hearing the full magnitude is obtained in about 0.2 sec (Békésy, 1929). On the other hand, this slowing down of the nervous processes makes it possible to investigate some processes that are hard to observe in hearing.

When the skin is exposed to vibrations just above threshold, electrophysiological observations show nervous discharges in synchrony with the vibrations, but often omitting two or three cycles (Fig. 13a). An increase in amplitude may make the nervous system fire for every cycle (Fig. 13b). A still further increase brings about an irregular firing, as is illustrated in Fig. 13c.

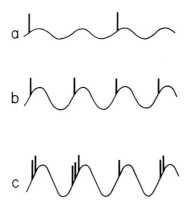

Figure 13 Schematic drawing to show how, according to electrophysiological findings, a time relation exists between neural discharges and a sinusoidal vibration amplitude. Near threshold (a) some cycles of the vibration may be omitted between the discharges. At large amplitudes (c) several discharges may occur in bursts. According to the usual conception, we would expect the pitch of a weak vibration to be lower than that of a strong one.

Peculiarly enough, we can discriminate these changes in the discharge pattern by observing the roughness of the vibratory sensation. Figure 14 shows how, for 10 Hz vibrations, the pitch sensation becomes higher as the amplitude is increased from threshold to 12 dB, corresponding to the drawings in Figs. 13a and 13b. But for higher amplitudes something new happens and the pitch drops; the nervous discharges are no longer able to follow the periodicity of the vibrations.

The same phenomenon can be shown more easily for electrical stimulation of the skin. When we double the number of electrical pulses, as illustrated in Fig. 15 for a pulse rate below 300 Hz on the finger tip, we observe a very precise roughness-pitch shift which

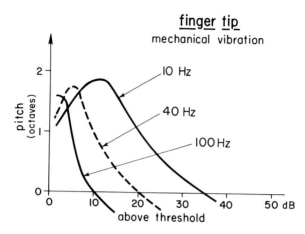

Figure 14   Vibratory "pitch" as a function of the vibration amplitude above threshold. A 100-Hz vibration 10 dB above threshold was presented to one finger and its pitch compared with that of a vibration applied to the corresponding finger on the other hand, at different amplitudes. The same procedure was repeated with the standard vibration at 40 and 10 Hz, and 20 and 35 dB above threshold.

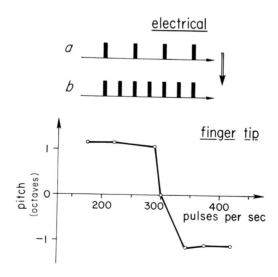

Figure 15   Drop in vibratory pitch sensation with increasing number of pulses, for electrical stimulation.

we define as an octave. For about 300 pulses per second, a doubling of the pulse rate does not produce any change in the roughness, and for even higher frequencies, doubling does not produce any rise in pitch, but a definite drop. About 300 electrical pulses per second on the finger tip is the maximum rate that can still be recognized as being in synchrony with the stimulus.

Since increasing the loudness reduces the pitch so effectively for skin sensations, it is possible to lower the pitch of a series of 50-Hz clicks to such a degree that subjects have the impression that they can almost count the clicks, i.e., that the clicks occur below the flicker limit. An experiment followed from these observations. A continuous series of clicks presented to the skin was also visible on an oscilloscope with nonpersistent screen. The sweep frequency on the oscilloscope was continuously variable and the subject adjusted it so that it seemed to agree with the apparent frequency of the clicks, i.e., both seemed to have the same flicker frequency. The adjustment of the sweep frequency to match the apparent click frequency was quite reproducible. After making the adjustment, the subject counted the number of pulses on the oscilloscope during one sweep. For vibration amplitudes 30 dB above threshold presented to the finger and the arm, this number was always greater than one. These observations were repeated by several observers with clicks at 100 and at 50 Hz. Figure 16 shows how many clicks per sweep were found for the differ-

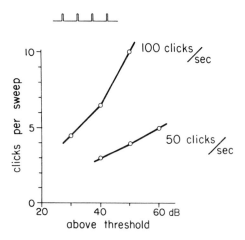

Figure 16 For low frequencies, the pitch sensation may drop so low that we have a feeling of flicker. This flicker frequency can be compared with the sweep frequency on an oscilloscope. It was found that during one flicker several clicks were presented to the skin but were not recognized as such.

ent vibration amplitudes. It is clear that, as the vibration amplitude and loudness increase, the number of clicks per sweep increases, and therefore the pitch of the vibration seems to decrease. For an amplitude change of 20 dB, the decrease is almost a full octave.

These experiments indicate strongly that, for high loudness levels, the nerve center that determines the pitch sensation for vibrations probably fires at a lower rate than the cells connected to the end organs.

These preliminary experiments seem to indicate that synchrony of the vibrations is transmitted to the higher nervous levels, but that, near threshold and for high stimulus intensities, the frequency is "demultiplied." Therefore, in the model of the cochlea with nerve supply, direct observations of the frequency of the vibrations cannot play an important role, since there is no useful correlation between the sensation and the frequency of the stimulus. The same situation is probably present in the auditory nervous system, but with higher critical frequencies.

Besides demultiplication, lateral inhibition makes the greatest contribution to the difference between the stimulus pattern and the sensation pattern. Lateral inhibition was once considered unimportant, but now it is clear that it can explain many otherwise puzzling phenomena. We can discriminate two types of inhibition: (a) that between simultaneously presented stimuli and (b) that produced by a time difference.

When we press simultaneously and with equal force on two neighboring points of the skin (Fig. 17), the result is a single sensation

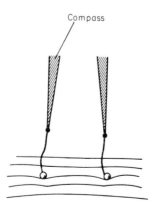

Compass

Figure 17   Each tip of a compass can be connected to a small ball with a nylon thread. The nylon thread limits the maximum pressure and the balls reduce the effect of local variations of the skin.

located halfway between the two stimuli. When the distance is increased, the magnitude may increase and spread out toward the sides, as is indicated in Fig. 18. But for a certain distance (e.g., 2.5 cm in Fig. 18), the sensation magnitude decreases radically, and one stimulus seems to cancel out the other. A further increase in the distance

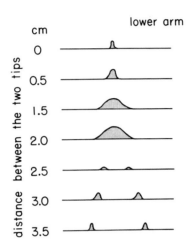

Figure 18 Summation and inhibition on the surface of the skin. When the distance between the two tips of a compass pressed against the surface of the skin is smaller than 2.5 cm, the two stimuli reinforce each other. The shaded areas represent schematically the magnitude and spread of the sensation as drawn by the observer. When the distance between the two tips is 2.5 cm, the magnitude of the sensation of the two points together is smaller than for one point alone. When the distance is larger than 3.5 cm, the two stimuli produce two separate sensations.

between the stimuli makes them separately recognizable. Therefore, by increasing the distance between the two stimuli, we first have summation, then inhibition, and finally no interaction at all. From these experiments it was concluded that every stimulus produces an area of sensation (indicated in Fig. 19 by vertical shading) surrounded by an area of inhibition. Outside the inhibitory ring there is no further interaction. When sections of skin are simultaneously stimulated with different vibratory amplitudes, they produce local sensations which summate or inhibit each other. Added together, they may produce a sensation pattern quite different from the stimulus pattern (Békésy, 1960b) but in agreement with observations in the field of localization and of the so-called enhancement of edges. It also points to a "funneling" phenomenon. Stimuli spread out over large areas on the sense organ are sharpened to much more narrowly localized sensations. Both the edge effect, known as Mach bands, and the funneling effect are illustrated in Fig. 20.

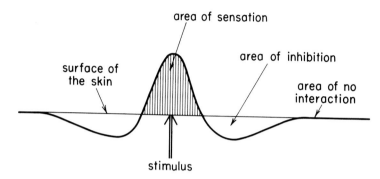

Figure 19 Since sensation magnitude decreases near the difference limen for distance perception, it seems likely that a local pressure or vibration on the surface of the skin produces, at the same time, both a sensation and an area of inhibition around the sensitive area.

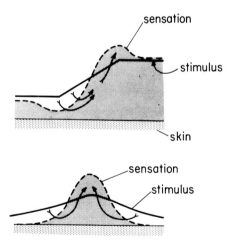

Figure 20 According to Mach's law of contrast in vision, when light density is distributed (as shown by the solid line in the upper drawing) along the retina, with two discontinuities, the sensation intensity shows a different distribution, given by the dotted line. The arrows show how this type of sensation pattern is produced by the assumed funneling action of the nervous tissue. The lower drawing shows how the law of contrast can sharpen the sensation distribution relative to the stimulus distribution when the maximum of the stimulus is flat.

Inhibition produced by time delay, though, probably plays a much more decisive role in the final shaping of the sensation pattern along the cochlear model. This pattern is quite different from the stimulus pattern along the vibrating basilar membrane. Inhibition by time delay is not a small effect, since strong stimuli can cancel out one another if one of them is delayed. When the delay is too large, there is again no more interaction and the two sensations appear separately.

To show the effect of a delay on the sensation pattern, we touch a vibrator to the arm. Stroboscopic observations show traveling waves moving away from the vibrator with a speed that depends strongly on the frequency of the vibration. These surface waves on the skin are, however, damped very little, especially at lower frequencies. Although the arm sometimes has waves along the whole surface, they can only be felt within a half wavelength of the vibrator. In Fig. 21 the

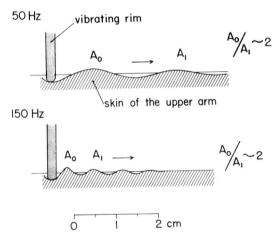

Figure 21 Stroboscopic observations show traveling waves on the skin of the arm resting on the ridge of the membrane. The waves spread out several centimeters, but are not recognized by the observer because of a type of nervous inhibition.

waves on the surface of the arm are illustrated. None of the waves at or beyond 0.5 cm from the vibrator produces any sensation that is localized at the place where the vibration occurs. But they do contribute to the sensation magnitude in the area under the vibrator. The delay produced by the traveling wave therefore has an important inhibitory effect in sense organs with large surfaces.

IV. SOME ANALOGIES BETWEEN HEARING
AND THE SKIN MODEL

The combined effect of the funneling phenomenon and the inhibition produced by time delay can be recognized when we compare the stimulus distribution along the membrane of the model with the sensation magnitude distribution produced along the surface of the arm. The upper drawing in Fig. 22 illustrates the vibration amplitude

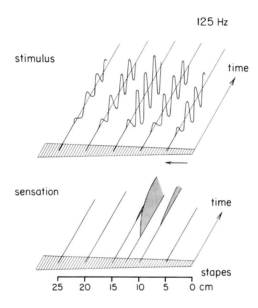

Figure 22 Inhibition on the skin model. The upper drawing shows the development of vibrations along the membrane during the onset of a continuous tone of 125 Hz. The lower drawing shows how widely these vibrations are suppressed by the skin so that only a small section of the membrane is felt as vibrating.

of the membrane at five different points when a vibration is suddenly transmitted to the artificial stapes footplate. The vibrations were sinusoidal and had a frequency of 125 Hz. The onsets of vibration at the different points of the membrane show the time delay, and, in addition, they show that the vibration amplitude has a very flat maximum about 15 cm from the stapes. From the previous discussion, it follows that vibration beyond the point of maximal amplitude occurs later and is inhibited because of the time delay relative to the vibrations of maximal amplitude. Since the traveling speed in the softer section is relatively low, the delays come into full action here. It is therefore not surprising that we have no sensation at all in the sections beyond the maximal amplitude (as can be seen in the lower drawing of Fig. 22 which represents the local sensation magnitude distribution along the membrane). Furthermore, there is also an inhibition near the stapes, presumably as an effect of the funneling action.

The combination of these two types of inhibition produces the unexpected phenomenon that the sensation is only felt in a very limited area of the membrane in spite of the fact that the whole membrane is in vibration. In the 30-cm model, the sensation produced by 125-Hz sinusoidal vibration is felt only along a 1 cm section. When the vibration frequency is increased, the sensation moves nearer the stapes; for lower frequencies, it moves away.

It is fascinating, when the frequency is continuously changed from high to low, to feel the corresponding movement of the locus of vibration from the stapes to the other end of the tube. There is a clear correlation between frequency and sensation. It was more surprising to find that frequency can be shifted quite rapidly and sensation will follow it just as rapidly. The experiments showed that only two full cycles of sinusoidal vibration are required to produce a sharp localization. In the shaded areas of Fig. 23 the local sensation magnitude

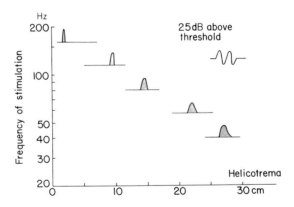

Figure 23 The length of the membrane which *seems* to vibrate is very short and remains surprisingly short even when the tone is presented for a period of only two full waves.

distribution is drawn for various frequencies of the stimulus. The lateral spread is a little larger for the low frequencies but it is still very sharp. The distribution of the local sensation magnitudes is a subjective observation and the only training that can be given to an observer is to ask him to draw the local sensation magnitudes for different light-density distributions projected on the retina. They are generally easily reproducible. Since the experiments of Savart, we have known that two cycles of a tone are enough to determine its pitch. Therefore, our model with nerve supply duplicates this aspect of hearing quite well.

There are many other phenomena that can be duplicated. Skin has the advantage over the real basilar membrane and organ of Corti that its sensitivity can be easily changed. It is possible, for instance, to produce a pronounced decrease in sensitivity by warming it with an infra-red light beam.

We tried to imitate nerve deafness on the model. In hearing it is generally assumed that in the case of nerve deafness the number of active nerve units is decreased. This produces two phenomena: *(a)* it decreases the sensitivity of the organ and *(b)* the sensation no longer increases slowly with an increase in stimulus intensity; instead it jumps suddenly from threshold to full magnitude. This phenomenon is called recruitment. If there were only a single nerve unit active, then the jump from nothing to maximal sensation magnitude would occur in a very small amplitude region of the stimulus, since in this case the well known all-or-nothing law of neurology would be active. That this assumption is correct can be shown on the skin (Fig. 24). If

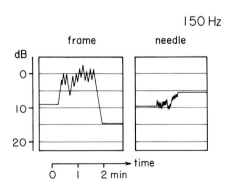

Figure 24 The just noticeable amplitude variation may become very small when a needle tip is used in place of a frame as stimulator on the skin.

we vibrate a large frame on the surface of the skin, a large number of nerve units will be stimulated. But when we exchange the frame for a needle tip, only a few nerve units will be activated; therefore, the threshold will be worse and the sensation magnitude will increase much more rapidly. To observe the rapidity of the increase in sensation magnitude, we can use a device which permits us to raise the vibration amplitudes slowly until they are perceived, and then to decrease them again by pressing a button till they are no longer perceived. The wobbling between "no perception" and "just perceptible" is a measure of the rapidity of the increase of the sensation magnitude. Figure 24 shows that the wobbling for a frame (left) is much larger than the wobbling for a needle tip (right). The ordinates represent the loss of perception in decibels. The threshold for the needle is worse. The needle shows recruitment relative to the frame stimulation.

We can produce a model of a cochlea with nerve deafness simply by warming a section of the skin touching the membrane with an infrared light or a heating pad. An "audiogram" of this model is similar to that obtained on patients with nerve deafness. Warming the whole arm produces more recruitment for the higher frequencies than for the low, since the area of vibration on the membrane is much smaller for high frequencies than for low ones. So a reduction in the number of activated nerve units is more effective for higher frequencies.

From the point of view of ear pathology, it is interesting to find that a local mechanical disturbance in one section of the basilar membrane has very little effect on the vibration pattern of the other sections. Certainly a hole in the membrane reduces vibration amplitudes, but it has little influence on the general pattern as a consequence of the traveling waves, which move along the membrane undisturbed by changes over small areas.

The model is relatively short. It should be at least 1.5 to 2 meters long to represent the whole cochlea. In its present state it only covers about two octaves in the frequency range. But in spite of this limitation it can answer some of the more complex questions, such as those raised by the Seebeck (1841) phenomenon. When we present a series of sharp clicks (Fig. 25a), the vibrations are localized near the elbow, as the drawing on the left side indicates. If we now place between every pair of clicks another single click (Fig. 25b), the pitch sensation in hearing still contains a strong component of the pitch produced by the series in Fig. 25a. The low component is stronger than would be concluded from a Fourier analysis of the series in Fig. 25b. The same thing can be observed with the model; the series in Fig. 25b still produces a strong sensation in the lower-frequency section near the elbow. When the distances between the clicks in the series in Fig. 25b become equal (Fig. 25c), then the low component disappears in the model as it does in hearing, and we localize the vibrations only near the stapes.

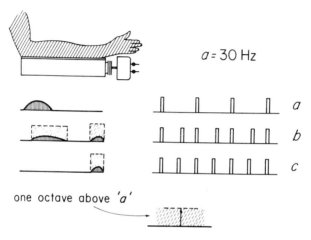

Figure 25 Seebeck's phenomenon repeated on the cochlear model with nerve supply. The click series (b) produces, at the place corresponding to the residue in hearing, a locally circumscribed stimulus. But interestingly enough, the pitch of this series is almost as high as the pitch produced by click series (c).

We can also ask how the performance of the model changes with changes in the elasticities of the membrane. When we make a membrane with the same elasticity along its whole length that the normal one had in the middle of the tube, then a change of a few cycles in frequency can move the sensation along the entire length of the tube. It is really a hypersensitive cochlea for pitch perception. But it is not very stable. It is also possible to compress the length of the cochlea by changing the volume elasticity per centimeter of length of the membrane. In this case it is much more difficult to separate frequency changes by localization of the sensation. I think the normal cochlea in the ear is very well matched to the inhibitory effects of the nervous system to produce a maximal sharpening of the localization.

V. PROBLEMS IN THE CONSTRUCTION OF A MODEL OF THE ORGAN OF CORTI

The described cochlear model is incomplete. It is only a model of the movements of the basilar membrane and their actions on a nerve system similar to the auditory nerve. But the receptors of the auditory nerves do not sit directly on the basilar membrane; instead they are imbedded in a very complicated system, the organ of Corti. The purpose of this system seems to be twofold: (*a*) to transmit the vibrations of the basilar membrane to the receptors in such a way that maximal sensitivity is obtained, and (*b*) to sharpen the stimulus localization to improve pitch discrimination in complex sounds.

The cochlear partition with the basilar membrane and the organ of Corti is, roughly speaking, a sort of gelatinous mass. The purpose of the organ of Corti is to concentrate the forces produced by the movements of the partition on the very well defined small sheet where the end organs are located. Mechanically, it transforms the large but less forceful movements of the partition into small but more forceful pressures that are able to deform the stiff cells of the end organ. It is a transformation from a weak but widespread force to a larger but more sharply localized force. The upper drawing of Fig. 26a shows how a hydraulic pressure on one side of a membrane can produce a large lateral tension in the membrane, sharply localized in the membrane itself. A membrane is a very good mechanical transformer and if it is

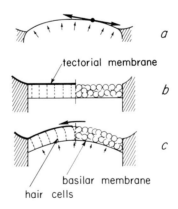

Figure 26 The organ of Corti represented as a device to match the mechanical impedance differences between the perilymph and the stiffer tissues of the organ. The matching is made for shearing forces.

completely flat, the transformation is very high (as in a drumhead stretched over the edge of its frame). Figure 26b shows schematically the construction of the organ of Corti. The basilar membrane is covered with a layer of cells. Half of the layer consists of sensitive hair cells and the other half of cells probably for the nutrition of the organ. Above the hair cells and attached to them is the tectorial membrane. It is a stiff, inelastic membrane fixed to the bony wall on the left side and floating free on the right side. A fluid pressure on the lower side of the basilar membrane produces shearing forces between the stiff tectorial membrane and the hair cells lying beneath it (Fig. 26c). Thus, the whole force acting on one side of the basilar membrane is concentrated on the borderline between the hair cells and the tectorial membrane, at exactly the place where the sense organs are found.

The second action of the organ of Corti is much more difficult to evaluate at present. Looking down on the organ of Corti (Fig. 27), we see a transition in the direction of the vibrations along its length during stimulation with a pure tone. Near the stapes there is a radial movement; then for a very short distance there is a vertical movement; and at the end there is a longitudinal movement. It is hard to tell how this change in direction influences the shearing forces produced between the tectorial membrane and the upper ends of the hair cells.

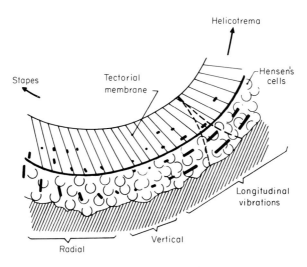

Figure 27 The distribution of radial and longitudinal vibrations along the organ of Corti for stimulation with a tone, seen through Reissner's membrane.

The difficulty in evaluating the movements of the organ of Corti is a consequence of the fact that the organ can be considered as a gelatinous band lying on the basilar membrane. In such a band there are at least five different types of waves possible (Berger, 1913): compression waves, shearing waves, dilatation waves, Rayleigh waves, and bending waves (Fig. 28). And what happens during the traveling of the waves along the membrane is a continuous exchange of energy among the different types. One type of wave can easily be damped out because its energy is taken over by another type, making it clear that a full description of the movements of the organ of Corti needs a great deal of work.

Naturally there is no difficulty in setting up a theory on this subject. I think at least five of them could be substantiated with different

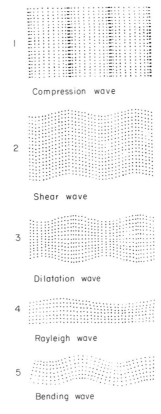

1

Compression wave

2

Shear wave

3

Dilatation wave

4

Rayleigh wave

5

Bending wave

Figure 28 The possible traveling waves in an elastic pad (R. Berger, 1913. By permission from *Gesundheits-ingenieur.*)

models and analogues. It is the same situation as with the vibrations of the basilar membrane. The correct approach here is the same as before: first measure the elasticities of the parts of the organ of Corti, and then try to strip the organ to its essential parts and make a dimensional model. Finally the synthesis can be made more complete by combining the model with a nervous system, perhaps like the skin.

By just looking at the anatomical construction of the organ of Corti, it is possible to make a few statements concerning the transmission of vibration from the basilar membrane to the border between the tectorial membrane and the hair cells. Such statements do not represent models but only analogues; they indicate which types of phenomena may be involved.

The traveling wave along the basilar membrane is very fast near the stapes and slows down considerably after the vibration amplitude reaches its maximum. Therefore, the wavelength is long near the stapes and becomes shorter after the place of maximal vibration is passed. For the funneling action of the system, it seems important to damp out these short waves after the maximum. The analogue in Fig. 29 demonstrates how this damping is achieved in the organ of Corti.

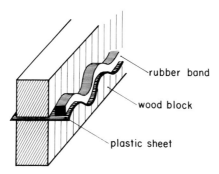

Figure 29   Mechanical model to show that the small waves along the basilar membrane are not transmitted to the part of the organ of Corti just below the tectorial membrane.

In the analogue, there is a plastic sheet representing the basilar membrane on which a rubber band of a certain thickness is glued. When, with the help of two wooden blocks, the plastic sheet is pressed into an undulating shape, analogous to waves on the basilar membrane, the free-standing rubber band is also bent. The important phenomenon is that, as the wavelength becomes smaller, the upper surface of the rubber band shows less deformation than the plastic sheet (Fig. 30). In Fig. 30a, the shape of the wave on the upper surface of the

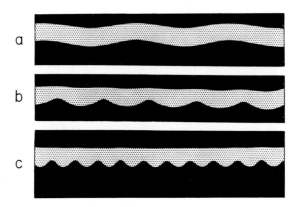

Figure 30   If one side of a foam rubber band is deformed sinusoidally, the other free side of the rubber band does not follow this deformation for short wavelengths.

rubber band is almost exactly the same as that of the plastic sheet. But when the wavelength becomes shorter, the amplitude of the wave on the surface becomes smaller than the one on the plastic sheet (Fig. 30b) and almost disappears when the wavelength of the plastic sheet becomes the same or smaller than the height of the rubber band (Fig. 30c). We may conclude that the waves on the basilar membrane, beyond the place of maximal vibration amplitude, reach the border of the hair cell and tectorial membrane in a diminished form, so the sharpening is improved by the organ of Corti on the side facing the helicotrema.

Here is another important problem based purely on anatomical considerations. In the organ of Corti, the hair cells are arranged in two separate groups (Fig. 31), namely inner and outer hair cells. The question is, what is the advantage? All that we can say with certainty is that the inner hair cells are less sensitive than the outer ones, partially because the outer hair cells outnumber them. On a skin model we can simulate this situation to find out what happens (Fig. 32). We attach to a vibrator a large frame made from tubes so as to be light in weight, and stable enough so that the vibration of the square frame is the same on all sides. The finger tips are placed on one side of the frame, the palm on the opposite side. Previous measurements showed that the tips of the fingers are much more sensitive than the skin on the palm, so the outer hair cells are represented by the finger tips and the inner hair cells by the palm. If we now start increasing the vibration amplitude from below threshold, then the first vibratory sensation is on the more sensitive finger tips (Fig. 33). When we increase the amplitude further, the locus of the sensation moves toward

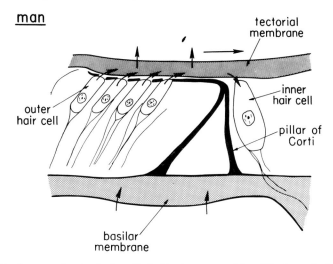

Figure 31 Inner and outer hair cells in the human cochlea. The inner hair cells are less sensitive.

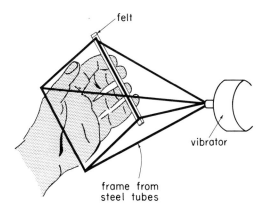

Figure 32 The finger tips touch one side of the vibrating frame, and the palm the opposite side. As the vibration amplitude is increased from threshold to strong values, the locus of the sensation moves from the finger tips to the palm.

the palm, and for vibration 25 dB above threshold, the whole sensation is in the palm. Nothing is felt on the finger tips despite their greater sensitivity at the beginning. The shifting from the finger tips to the palm can sometimes be improved by changing the threshold of the finger tips a little. This change is effected by putting some felt under the finger tips so that the transmission from the vibrating frame is reduced.

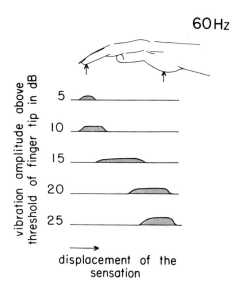

Figure 33 Displacement of the locus of the sensation from the finger tips to the palm as the vibrating amplitude of the frame shown in Fig. 32 is increased.

This shift of localization as a function of stimulus amplitude may be an important feature in discriminating pitch from loudness in hearing. At the moment, electrophysiologically, there is no clear concept of how loudness (and sensation magnitudes of other stimuli) is transmitted to higher nervous levels; it may be mediated by the number of nervous discharges per second, the number of activated neural units, or both.

Many more analogues can be constructed, and they may lead to more of the principles that play roles in the functioning of the organ of Corti. But without some numerical values for the organ of Corti, a model cannot be made and thus the model of the cochlea with nerve supply is not finished.

VI. SOME LIMITATIONS OF THE MODEL
WITH NERVE SUPPLY

The auditory nerve track is not the same as the nerve track for vibratory sensations on the skin. They seem to have more features in common than was expected, but there are some differences, too. One of the biggest is that the nerve density of the organ of Corti is much larger than that of the skin, and therefore the range of sensation magnitudes is not as great for the vibration sense as for hearing. The skin model works in an amplitude range of only about 30 dB rather than 140. This limitation becomes important when two vibrations of different frequencies must be separated by the model. It is difficult (or impossible) to pick the harmonics out of a series of clicks; the amplitudes are too low. In Fig. 34, a click train produces a sensation corresponding to the lowest component and another sensation for a

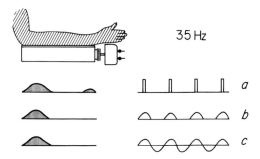

Figure 34 In the cochlear model with nerve supply, only a series of sharp clicks produces separate areas of sensation for the first and second harmonics. With a half-sine wave the second harmonic is below the threshold of skin sensation.

higher partial, as shown on the left side of the figure. But there is no possibility of discriminating between a sinusoidal vibration and a rectified form of it (Fig. 34c) because the harmonics in the rectified form are too weak to be recognized. Thus, the skin model as described is not suited for frequency analysis of complex sounds. A modification using two basilar membranes, one touching normal skin and the other touching warmed skin, is more adequate since it offers a partial representation of the effect of inner and outer hair cells.

Another limitation is the short length of the model. There should be no difficulty in making a model 150 cm long to be touched from the foot to the neck. Preliminary experiments with shorter models show that it will work, but it will not help us to findings beyond those obtained with the short model.

Still, despite all these limitations, the production of a model of the cochlea in which the skin represented the organ of Corti proved that sense organs with large surfaces — eye, skin, tongue — have many more common features than were expected. In some ways we have brought the different sense organs together and emphasized their common features rather than their differences. With time, I am sure this demonstration will change some of the attitudes in general physiology.

ACKNOWLEDGMENT

This research was supported in part by a grant (B–2974) from the National Institutes of Health, and in part by a grant from the American Otological Society (Report PPR–302).

I should like to acknowledge that Figures were taken from the following sources:
The Journal of the Acoustical Society of America
Annals of Otology, Rhinology and Laryngology
Rasmussen and Windle (1960).

REFERENCES

Baldwin, R. D. (1964). A model simulating some properties of living matter: a contribution in abstract biology. *Perspect. Biol. Med.*, **7**, 219–226.

Beament, J. W. L. (Ed.) (1960). *Models and analogues in biology.* (Symposia of the Society for Experimental Biology, No. 14.) Academic Press *and* Cambridge Univ. Press, New York *and* Cambridge, England.

von Békésy, G. (1929). Zur Theorie des Hörens. *Phys. Z.*, **30**, 115–125.

von Békésy, G. (1939). Über die Vibrationsempfindung. *Akust. Z.*, **4**, 316–334.

von Békésy, G. (1955). Human skin perception of traveling waves similar to those on the cochlea. *J. Acoust. Soc. Am.*, **27**, 830–841.

von Békésy, G. (1960a). *Experiments in hearing.* McGraw-Hill, New York.

von Békésy, G. (1960b). Neural inhibitory units of the eye and skin. Quantitative description of contrast phenomena. *J. Opt. Soc. Am.*, **50**, 1060–1070.

von Békésy, G. (1963). Interaction of paired sensory stimuli and conduction in peripheral nerves. *J. Appl. Physiol.*, **18**, 1276–1284.

von Békésy, G. (1964). Olfactory analogue to directional hearing. *J. Appl. Physiol.*, **19**, 369–373.

Berger, R. (1913). Über Erschütterungen. *Gesundheits-ingenieur,* **36**, 433–441.

Bridgman, P. W. (1931). *Dimensional analysis.* (Rev. ed.) Yale Univ. Press, New Haven, Connecticut.

Budde, E. (1917a). Über die Resonanztheorie des Hörens. A. Die Wahrnehmung des stationären einfachen Tones. *Phys. Z.*, **18**, 225–236.

Budde, E. (1917b). Über die Rosonanztheorie des Hörens. B. Unterbrechungstöne, Phasenwechseltöne, Reflexionstöne, Kombinationstöne. *Phys. Z.*, **18**, 249–260.

Diestel, H.-G. (1954). Akustische Messungen an einem mechanischen Modell des Innenohres. *Acustica*, **4**, 489–499.

Duncan, W. J. (1953). *Physical similarity and dimensional analysis*. Arnold, London.

Ewald, J. R. (1899). Zur Physiologie des Labyrinths. *Pflügers Arch. Ges. Physiol.*, **76**, 147–188.

Firestone, F. A. (1938). The mobility method of computing the vibration of linear mechanical and acoustical systems: Mechanical-electrical analogies. *J. Appl. Phys.*, **9**, 373–387.

Gildemeister, M. (1930). Probleme und Ergebnisse der neueren Akustik. Z. *Hals-Nasen- u. Ohrenheilk.*, **27**, 299–328.

Hawthorne, G. B., Jr. (1964). Digital simulation and modelling. *Datamation*, **10** (10), 25–29.

Katsuki, Y., Sumi, T., Uchiyama, H., and Watanabe, T. (1958). Electric responses of auditory neurons in cat to sound stimulation. *J. Neurophysiol.*, **21**, 569–588.

Maxwell, J. C. (1892). *A treatise on electricity and magnetism*. (3rd ed.) Clarendon Press, Oxford.

Rasmussen, G. L. and Windle, W. F. (Eds.) (1960). *Neural mechanisms of the auditory and vestibular systems*. Thomas, Springfield, Illinois.

Seebeck, A. (1841). Beobachtungen über einige Bedingungen der Entstehung von Tönen. *Annln Phys.*, **53**, ser. 2, 417–436.

Stahl, W. R. (1963). Similarity analysis of physiological systems. *Perspectives Biol. Med.*, **6**, 291–321.

Waetzmann, E. (1926). Hörtheorien. In A. Bethe, G. von Bergmann, G. Embden, and A. Ellinger (Eds.) *Handbuch der normalen und pathologischen Physiologie*. Vol. 11, pp. 667–700. Springer, Berlin.

Wilkinson, G. and Gray, A. A. (1924). *The mechanism of the cochlea*. Macmillan, London.

Chapter Nine

Monaural Processing

FOREWORD

Once a signal enters the central nervous system, its relation to the original sound is tenuous. An observer might recognize some similarities between an acoustic waveform and the pattern of basilar-membrane flapping that is consequent to it. He could easily see the connection between that original sound and its cochlear microphonic. For a few kinds of simple signals, he might be able to see a kind of relation between the sound and its earliest neural representations. But, for the most part, one pattern of auditory-nervous-system behavior is pretty much like any other. To match a fiber's response to the specific signal that triggered it is usually nearly impossible unless one is making cause-and-effect observations at the instant that the response is found. Collecting such responses while making the cause-and-effect observations is a tedious and exasperating chore, and only rarely can one get more than a few data from a given day's experimentation. Blair Simmons has organized several families of these rare and scattered data into a chapter that describes the basic neural transmission processes and their properties.

Monaural Processing

F. Blair Simmons*

I. INTRODUCTION

Sound is "processed" within the central nervous system, and this chapter should describe *how*. But such a description presumes a complete knowledge of how output differs from input, knowledge that will somehow provide a physiological basis for understanding why sounds are perceived, acted upon (if action appears appropriate), suppressed, or remembered. We should also have some clue as to how, for instance, absolute pitch can be learned, say before the age of eight or nine, but never again (Ward, 1963). Even to pretend that a reasonable start toward this goal could be made at this time would be deceptive, just as it would be to promote a certain mode of processing as fundamental and specific to any small or anatomically localized group of cells within the auditory brain.

It is, as a matter of fact, becoming increasingly difficult to define the boundaries of the auditory system in the precise manner possible in the early 1950s. The conceptual dimensions of the auditory brain are changing. For example, compare Woolsey's two diagrams of the cortical areas excited by auditory stimulation (Fig. 1)—one prepared in 1951 (from earlier data) and the other in 1959 (Woolsey, 1960). Even the 1959 version can be considerably enlarged (not only at the cortex, but in subcortical and brainstem regions) if the auditory electrical events in unanesthetized animals during learning, habituation, arousal, and so on are included (Galambos and Sheatz, 1962). To

---

*Division of Otolaryngology, Stanford University, Stanford, California.

confuse matters further, complete interruption of the main brainstem auditory pathway (brachium of the inferior colliculus) in the un-anesthetized animal causes very little if any change in the cortical electrical activity evoked by a click (Galambos *et al.*, 1961).

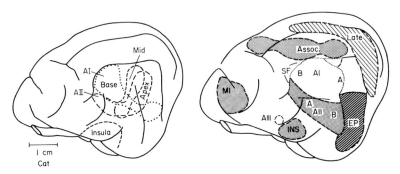

Figure 1 Areas of cortex responding to acoustic stimulation. The diagram on the left shows the response areas obtained by Woolsey and Walzl in 1942 (cited by Woolsey, 1960) by electrical stimulation of the cochlear nerve. The more detailed and considerably extended diagram on the right, compiled by Woolsey (1960), shows "four central areas with cochlea represented anteroposteriorly from apex (A) to (B) in the suprasylvian fringe sector (SF), from base to apex in AI; from apex to base in AII. In E_p representation is base above, apex below. AIII is Tunturi's third auditory area. 'Association' cortex (ASSOC) and precentral motor cortex gave late responses to click with 15-msec latencies under chloralose. Visual area II(LATE) gave responses with 100-msec latency, also under chloralose." (Woolsey, 1960. From Rasmussen, G. L. and Windle, W. F., 1960. *Neural mechanisms of the auditory and vestibular systems.* Courtesy of Charles C. Thomas, Publisher, Springfield, Illinois.)

Such observations force a conclusion that there are several "auditory systems," one piled on another. None is completely separate in the normal organism, but some are capable of partial isolation through phylogenetic, ablation, pharmacologic, or electrophysiologic techniques. To describe processing, it is convenient to recognize two such systems. The first and older is a medially positioned, *diffuse auditory system*, usually identified as part of the reticular formation, extending the length of the brainstem, and eventually reaching a number of forebrain and cortical structures.* The second is the classical *lemniscal*

---

*The vagueness with which this system is delineated is intentional. Although it is generally agreed that elements of the reticular formation, certain thalamic nuclei, and several groups of cortical radiation fibers are involved, there is no clear anatomical boundary that adequately limits its scope. The reader who wishes to consider this organization further may find several summaries helpful: Jasper *et al.* (1958), Nauta and Kuypers (1958), Galambos *et al.* (1959), French (1960), Jasper (1960), Magoun (1963), Thompson *et al.* (1963).

auditory system, more laterally placed and more discretely defined (Galambos, 1954). Within its fiber tracts, the tonotopic (arranged according to frequency) organization of the cochlea is maintained and multiplied in an orderly manner at all levels from eighth nerve to cortex. Tones of different frequencies continue to produce their maximum excitation at different places, though such places may be multiple in any one nuclear mass (Lorente de Nó, 1933; Rose, 1960). The anatomical substrate also has two general types of connections between individual neurons: some are largely specific—they contact one or a few neurons—and some supply an abundance of collaterals to many neurons. Both are necessary to explain discrete and diffuse interactions between neural populations.

This provision for diffuse and specific interactions at both the single-cell and the system level of auditory organization is in turn necessary to any understanding of that everyday intracranial miracle we call auditory processing. Sounds are perceived, then suppressed, re-membered, or acted upon, as the occasion demands. Exactly how, and, in particular, what structures are involved remain largely matters for speculation and for the increasingly popular armchair sport of model building. Although it is easy to criticize models, they do have one undisputed function as organizers of data. There is an avalanche of isolated facts about inputs and outputs, but very few really clear ideas about which features may be critical for perception and which are merely 'neural noise.' In a broad sense, two types of models are offered to help define the critical features: those that emphasize "wiring" and other engineering aspects of processing—models to help understand stimulus resolution (Wiener, 1948; Licklider, 1959)— and models to clarify the mind-body problem or the relation of the whole organism to its environment (Galambos, 1959; Pribram, 1960).

Models of the first type and basic data from many sources seem to agree on one fundamental point: *the basic pattern of neural activity produced by simple sounds consists of a core of active fibers or cells surrounded by a halo of inhibited units* (Allanson and Whitfield, 1956; Békésy, 1958; Galambos, 1961; Greenwood and Maruyama, 1965).

As illustrated in Fig. 2, *this pattern may change its center of activity according to stimulus frequency, its contrasts or sharpness according to intensity, or both as a function of time.* Further, such patterns, islands of activity surrounded by zones of neural silence, may describe combinations of sounds by other shifts in their geometry. However, the precise nature of these more intricate patterns is not yet known for acoustic stimuli. In fact, one must borrow heavily from studies of other sensory systems to justify the assumption of their existence (Hartline *et al.*, 1952; Kuffler, 1953; Mountcastle and Powell, 1959).

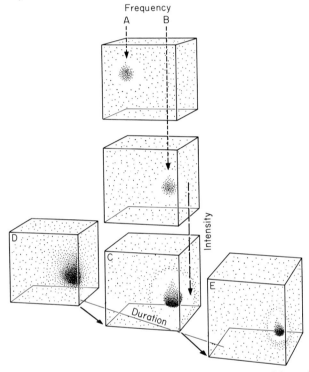

Figure 2 Patterns of neural activity within a hypothetical section of the auditory brain during acoustic stimulation with a simple sound. The pattern may change its location according to frequency (A to B), its contrast according to intensity (B to C), or both according to stimulus duration (D to C to E).

Even though this basic organization is recognized and some neural correlates for discrimination have been demonstrated, the problems of processing are just beginning. It is important to ask other questions about coding. For instance, some features of the frequency code differ at the cortex and the brainstem, and pitch perception ordinarily utilizes the cortical code. Yet after decortication and a period of re-learning, an organism may just as conveniently utilize the brainstem code (Raab and Ades, 1946; Maruyama and Yoshinobu, 1961; Neff, 1961). These and other types of ablation studies have demonstrated that processing does not necessarily require delivery of information to a specific locus within the auditory system. In fact, impressive amounts of tissue may be missing or destroyed in early life without total devastation of complex auditory perceptions (Landau *et al.*, 1960; Scharlock *et al.*, 1963). Another example is the occasional individual with only one ear who can localize the source of a sound with impressive accuracy, probably using "processing" quite different from that used by the normal person with his elegant neural arrangements for processing binaural sounds.

Thus our view of auditory processing must not be limited to a convenient but unrealistic notion of one mechanism for one parameter; nor can we assume that one method of processing is applicable to all individuals, or that emphases are exactly the same in all species. Indeed, Galambos (1952) suggested that some degree of caution be exercised in interpreting electrophysiological data obtained from acoustically naive animals, for whom, say, a 1000-Hz tone has no meaning.

Barlow (1961) made an eloquent appeal for another way of looking at the goals of sensory processing. In his model, he first pointed out that the primary effect of a sensory message is not to enrich an organism's sensory environment, but to modify its behavior in such a way that it will have a greater chance of survival. He therefore proposed that, "Sensory relays are for detecting, in the incoming messages, certain 'passwords' that have a particular key significance for the animal. . ." Such stimuli act as "releasers," evoking specific responses, and they must be distinguished from all other stimuli.

Second, he proposed that sensory relays are "filters" whose pass characteristics can be controlled according to the requirements of other parts of the nervous system. And even the passwords for a particular relay may be changed from time to time, according to the organism's subsequent experience or learning.

Barlow's third hypothesis for sensory relays is that neural messages are recoded according to their redundancy; the relays pass those messages that are "news," but reject those that have either been said before or are being transmitted by other means. The coding sets priorities for the input messages. Input differs from output partially according to what messages are expected on the basis of past experience: few outputs are available for expected inputs, but many outputs or impulses are alloted for unusual or unexpected stimulus inputs. According to Barlow, such a code should produce output patterns corresponding to complex features of the inputs, not to properties that are physically or anatomically simple.

At the current level of understanding there is neither the insight nor usually the data to decide finally upon such matters, nor is it absolutely necessary to do so. As a matter of fact, one can choose to emphasize those aspects of processing that seem likely to be related to *both* concepts — models or wiring diagrams (Fig. 2), and Barlow's experimental view — and that is the choice made here.*

II. SPONTANEOUS ACTIVITY

Most auditory neurons are spontaneously active, discharging intermittently in the absence of sound. The rate and regularity of this activity varies considerably in different regions or between individual units in the same region, and for a variety of reasons (Eccles, 1964). In a general way, the rate (and regularity) of spontaneous discharges is highest in the eighth nerve and cochlear nucleus (Tasaki, 1954; Tasaki and Davis, 1955; Rodieck *et al.*, 1962; Moushegian *et al.*, 1962; Kiang, 1963), and gradually decreases in more cephalad locations (Galambos *et al.*, 1952; Katsuki, 1961). The exact decrement in spontaneous activity remains unclear, since most observations have been made on drugged animals which frequently show altered spontaneous activity and spread of electrical excitability (Erulkar *et al.*, 1956; Katsuki *et al.*, 1959a; Starr and Livingston, 1963).

In the few observations from awake animals, the level of spontaneous activity was found to depend also upon the alertness of the organism (Starr and Livingston, 1963). Increased spontaneous discharging in single cells may herald the appearance of stimulus-related activity where none was previously observed (Hubel *et al.*, 1959; Galambos, 1960).

Spontaneous activity can be diminished, but not eliminated, by cutting the eighth nerve. The most severe decrements occur in the cochlear nucleus, and less severe ones at ascending levels (Starr and Livingston, 1963).

A single fiber's spontaneous activity may, in some instances, be related to its auditory response characteristics. For example, cochlear and brainstem units with high spontaneous activity usually respond to sounds with high rates of discharge. Kiang (1963) noted that the eighth-nerve fibers with the shortest interspike intervals during the multiple discharges after a click have the highest characteristic fre-

---

*The reader should consult the recent reviews by Wever (1962), Small (1963), Elliott (1964), and Hawkins (1964) for a more complete list.

quencies. However, he found no correlation between rates of spontaneous activity and a fiber's most sensitive response frequency (Kiang, 1963), nor did he feel that the organism's physiological condition or level of anesthesia affects spontaneous discharging. According to Katsuki *et al.* (1958), units with high spontaneous-discharge rates are most sensitive to high tones; those with low rates of spontaneous activity respond best to low-frequency sounds. This pattern is not always the case further cephalad. In the ventral cochlear nucleus, at least, some units with little spontaneous activity can be driven by high-frequency tones (Moushegian *et al.*, 1962).

Perhaps the most important consideration about spontaneous activity is that it provides a variable background against which neural responses to sound are displayed. Excitation, no-change, and suppression of activity — or more likely all three — each reflect the pattern of processing. One has, of course, a natural tendency to devote the most attention to analyzing excitatory responses to sound. The brain is under no obligation to do likewise. Suppression of spontaneous activity is clearly a major contributor to the repertoire of neural processing at all levels of the classical auditory pathway, including the eighth nerve (Katsuki *et al.*, 1962; Rupert *et al.*, 1963), and is a predominant feature of response to acoustic stimulation in such diverse locations as the visual association cortex and certain reticular-formation neurons (Katsuki, 1961; Bental and Bihari, 1963). Within the classical auditory areas, suppression of spontaneous activity provides a means for sharpening contrasts (Allanson and Whitfield, 1956). And suppression of, or perhaps even lack of change in, spontaneous activity is as precisely controlled as the more dramatic excitation (Nelson and Erulkar, 1963).

III. TEMPORAL PATTERNS

The auditory system's response to sound is not static — processing requires many times the duration of a simple impulsive stimulus. The pattern produced by a single click, for example, continues to develop for at least 100 msec and patterns for steady tones continue to change appreciably for many seconds (or minutes) after their initiation.

At first, limitations in observational techniques confined the majority of electrophysiological investigations to the first few milliseconds of this response to sound — to the so-called "on" responses and evoked potentials produced by sudden synchronous excitation of a great many single fibers or cells (Chang, 1959). Of these, the cochlear N_1 (the first neural-response peak) and cortical evoked response are the best known examples in the auditory system. More recently, response-averaging techniques have given increasing degrees of resolving power to the analysis of these "slow waves." Studies of the later portions of the human EEG response to sounds should eventually yield long-sought electrophysiological correlations between stimulus magnitude, vigilance, etc. (Davis, 1964a, 1964b; Haider et al., 1964; Keidel and Spreng, 1965).

Observing temporal behavior with microelectrodes on single fibers or cells is a technique that has also undergone considerable refinement. A summary of characteristic patterns of single-fiber responses to sustained stimulation is shown in Fig. 3, beginning with primary neurons (designated A and B). Surprisingly little has been written about adaptation in individual eighth-nerve fibers. Katsuki et al. (1958) mentioned only that the response to a continuous tone is "tonic" (continuing as long as the tone remains on), but a slight degree of declining activity shortly after stimulus onset can be seen in his illustrations (Katsuki et al., 1962). A relatively very slow rate of adaptation is further indicated by a number of observations of the decline in amplitude of whole-nerve (synchronized), gross-electrode-recorded responses to repetitive stimuli (Derbyshire and Davis, 1935; Peake et al., 1962a,b). The adaptation curve of Fig. 3A represents an inference in the absence of specific data and is presented for comparison. The curve of Fig. 3B, showing suppression of spontaneous activity by acoustic stimulation, is similarly tentative. Nothing firm can be said about how these rates may differ for basal or apical fibers, even though one suspects that fibers with high characteristic frequencies ought to adapt more rapidly.

Rose et al. (1959) described the temporal behavior of units within the cochlear nucleus and noted two basic types of cell. One type (Fig. 3C) "... is characterized by high sensitivity to small differences in tone intensity, by high initial discharge rate, and by long times required before a unit reaches a steady discharge rate." The second type (Fig. 3D) "... is characterized by low sensitivity to stimulus strength, by relatively low initial discharge rate, and by quick attainment of the equilibrated rate which is maintained without change for a long time." These investigators also provided convincing evidence that this second type of unit may in fact be a partially adapted form of the first type.

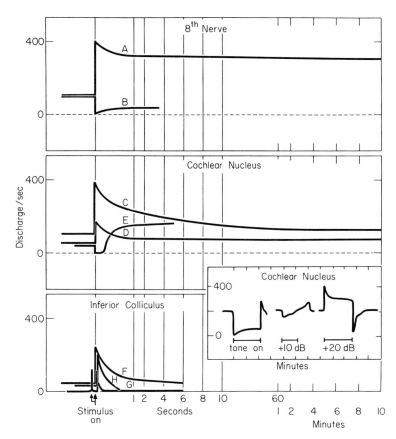

Figure 3 Temporal patterns of some single fiber discharges during sustained tonal stimulation. Eighth-nerve fibers (A,B) are hypothetical. Cochlear nucleus data (C, D, E) from Rose *et al.* (1959), and the insert from Moushegian *et al.* (1962). Inferior colliculus curves (F, G, H) are modified from Erulkar (1959), and from Rose *et al.* (1963). Medial geniculate patterns (not shown) are probably similar to those of the inferior colliculus, but even shorter in duration of response. All of these patterns should only be regarded as examples. Numerous variations occur.

The other response patterns observed in the cochlear nucleus appear to represent interaction between excitation and inhibition. The insert in Fig. 3 shows an example of this mixture obtained from the same neuron at three intensities of the same tone (Moushegian *et al.,* 1962). At the lowest intensity, the initial response is suppression of spontaneous activity followed by an overshoot before the return to the baseline. Restimulation at a 10-dB-higher intensity first causes suppression and then poststimulation excitation of neural activity. An additional 10 dB increment results in an initial excitatory response that is almost a mirror image of the first pattern. In still other units, the time course of inhibitory-excitatory interactions may be quite different, as in Fig. 3E. Here, there is a brief but complete inhibition before excitation. Rose *et al.* (1959) found such responses most easily in units showing decreased activity with increases in stimulus intensity.

Goldberg *et al.* (1964) saw no drastic differences in simple adaptation characteristics between the cochlear nucleus and the superior olivary complex (primarily the trapezoid body and the medial pre-olivary nuclei). Again, adaptation rates of both types of units depend chiefly upon stimulus intensity, not frequency. These investigators further subdivided the rapid-discharge units (Fig. 3C) into those with regular and those with irregular interspike intervals. They postulated that irregular discharge reflects a changing input to that cell, whereas regular discharge indicates that the rate is principally controlled by the refractory period of that neuron. This matter is of some interest since Allanson and Whitfield (1956) emphasized that considerably more irregularity and slower firing rates in unit discharges have been recorded in the trapezoid body than in "first-order neurons."

From studies of the inferior colliculus, Erulkar (1959) described two basic types of responses to tones at a unit's best frequency. At stimulus onset, a unit may discharge several times, then remain silent — suppressing spontaneous activity — for the duration of the stimulus (Fig. 3G); or the pattern may be one of initial rapid firing followed by a decrement that usually approaches spontaneous activity levels within 4 sec, but may be sustained as long as 30 min (Fig. 3F). Rose *et al.* (1963) confirmed and extended the dimensions of these findings, but limited the stimulus duration to several hundred milliseconds. About 50 percent of the units they examined showed almost pure onset responses. In many units showing sustained responses, "on" responses were also frequently obtained toward the edge of the unit's frequency or intensity response area. Thus, for some fibers, responses near threshold are characterized by an irregular, sustained discharge pattern : (... ....). As sound intensities increase, patterns are characterized by an initial brief burst of activity, a silent interval, and resumption of firing (Fig. 3H): (.... ....). Further intensity increments decrease the duration of the silent interval; an increase in stimulus frequency, toward the fiber's upper sensitivity limit, can cause this pattern to change abruptly to a pure "on" response: (...... .   ). In this study, and in others at different brainstem loci, it was also noted that minute differences in the response characteristics of individual neurons are often retained during stimulation by several different sounds, or even by sounds delivered to the opposite ear.

Nelson and Erulkar (1963) elegantly demonstrated that a sizable portion of the inhibitory-excitatory interactions that produce such patterns in the inferior colliculus develop at lower auditory levels. They also showed that the "on" response characteristic of a large percentage of inferior colliculus units is as precisely controlled as are the discharges of fibers with a more prolonged response time.

The proportion of units that respond only to the onset of a stimulus increases in the medial geniculate body (Gross and Thurlow, 1951; Galambos, 1952; Katuski et al., 1959a; Aitkin et al., 1966). Some of these units, in their initial responses, make very little distinction between clicks and wide bands of tones (Galambos, 1952). A few fibers respond only after the stimulus has been turned off, but they are rare compared to the "off" response units in the lateral geniculate. A few neurons continue to respond to continuous stimulation over longer periods of time (4–6 sec), others are characterized best as abbreviated versions of inferior colliculus units (Fig. 3H), and a few respond by an inhibition of spontaneous activity.

With the exception of the excellent electroanatomical study of the medial geniculate by Rose and Woolsey (1959), the number of observations (a total of about 400 fibers) hardly justifies any further statements about its responses. Studies on undrugged animals have yet to be reported in any detail. Such studies may clear up at least one puzzling point: investigators typically comment upon the relatively slow discharge rates (spontaneous or stimulus-evoked) of medial-geniculate units, yet the metabolic activity of this region is unquestionably high (Windle, 1963). If these slow rates are not caused by drugs, then the most parsimonious explanation may be that there is an almost equal balance between excitation and inhibition a few moments after the beginning of auditory stimulation.

In contrast to the state of investigation in the medial geniculate, an accurate description of cortical response patterns suffers more from conflict of observations than from lack of them. For example, what proportion of cells responds at all to an auditory stimulus? Erulkar et al. (1956), reporting on 402 units in anesthetized animals, found 34 percent totally unresponsive and another 53 percent so markedly insecure in their response that quantitative observations were impossible. Galambos (1960), reporting on 96 units in unanesthetized animals, found only 18 percent totally unresponsive, and were able to categorize the type of pure-tone response in 70 percent. On the matter of response patterns themselves, Katsuki *et al.* (1962) insisted that cortical neurons respond very briefly at stimulus-on, or stimulus-off, or both, but only very rarely with any sustained activity beyond perhaps 200 msec. These cortical units did not change their discharge characteristics as a function of stimulus frequency or of intensity, either. Both Erulkar *et al.* (1956) and Galambos (1960), on the other hand, found a smaller percentage of such unit patterns (and some of them changed with frequency or intensity), as well as a significant (perhaps equal) number of neurons that discharged (or whose occasionally rapid spontaneous activity was suppressed) for *at least* several seconds during continuous stimulation. Similar patterns were also reported by Whitfield and Evans (1964).

In seeking order in the variety of response patterns in the auditory cortex and at other levels, it is first of all important to consider differences in observational techniques. Patterns of activity in the ventral cochlear nucleus, for instance, are not appreciably affected by general anesthesia (Moushegian *et al.*, 1962), but cortical activity definitely is. Erulkar *et al.* (1956) discussed this point in some detail. An anecdotal account of cortical units may also prove illuminating (Katsuki *et al.*, 1959a): "Recordings of responses were more successful immediately before complete recovery from anesthesia than after the animal had aroused completely from it. After complete awakening, remarkable spontaneous discharges were observed while the responses to sound stimulation were often scarcely encountered." In general, drugs tend to suppress those response patterns that require time to develop or those that spread more diffusely throughout the brain, though exceptions do exist (Vernier and Galambos, 1957).

There is considerable macroelectrode evidence, and some single-cell evidence for the long-held suspicion that the distribution of response patterns is not homogeneous throughout the auditory cortex. Sustained DC shifts can be recorded from some areas of AI in the cat cortex only during continuous stimulation (Gumnit and Grossman, 1961). Individual cells that respond with a relatively high degree of regularity and sustained activity are also found most often in AI. Units whose responses to sounds are frequently irregular, or may demand unusual stimulus programming, are found more frequently in the E_p region of the cat's primary auditory cortex (Galambos, 1960). There is very little such evidence for similar specialization at lower levels. However, only the cochlear nucleus has received even a sizable fraction of the effort so far expended on uncovering these specialized regions in the primary cortex.

I have given a large amount of space to temporal patterns in order to stress their significance. An organism allows a signal to develop (and persist) in a certain manner only as it may contribute to the significance of the neural mosaic. One that continues to be "important" in the eighth nerve one or two seconds after a tone is introduced may not be so critical at the level of the inferior colliculus or the medial geniculate body. Patterns vary according to experimental conditions, and indeed, according to the temperament of the observer; a different emphasis is likely to be made after an examination of the first few milliseconds of a response than from observations a few hundred milliseconds later. These factors complicate and occasionally confound any attempt to proceed step by step from one report on processing to another with some assurance that the same nervous system is always at work.

IV. FREQUENCY

The examination of neural processing of frequency is classically divided into observations of tonotopic organization (Ades, 1959; Rose and Woolsey, 1959; Rose, 1960; Woolsey, 1960), studies of intensity-frequency response areas of single fibers, and observations (both by macroelectrode and by microelectrode) of temporal patterns, some of which are relevant to pitch resolution in "place-sensitive" unit populations, and others of which are relevant to the determination of the boundaries of synchronous discharging or "volley coding."

Response areas typical of individual neurons at various auditory locations are shown in Fig. 4. According to Kiang et al. (1962), the response areas of eighth-nerve fibers show a high-frequency cutoff characteristic that is nearly vertical and a low-frequency cutoff characteristic that gradually accepts more and more frequencies as the intensity level increases (Figs. 4A and B). Minor differences in the sharpness of high- and low-frequency cutoff characteristics (skirts) have been reported, but they now appear to have resulted more from arbitrary selection criteria than from real differences in the response areas (Tasaki, 1954; Katsuki et al., 1958). It is generally believed that the shape of such tuning curves reflects the cochlear-partition traveling-wave characteristic. No specific information is yet available on the degree to which the highly organized dendritic complex of these nerves may further sharpen this tuning to what is finally observed in

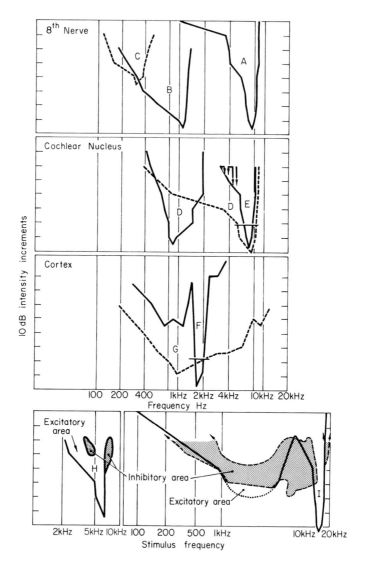

Figure 4 Frequency-intensity response areas of "typical" units. Eighth nerve (A,B,C) redrawn from Kiang (1963). Cochlear nucleus (D,D,E) redrawn from Rose *et al.* (1959). Auditory cortex (F,G) redrawn from Hind (1960). Unit H at lower left, redrawn from Moushegian *et al.* (1962), illustrates one pattern of several in the cochlear nucleus wherein spontaneous activity is inhibited, rather than enhanced by stimulation. Unit I at right, redrawn from Galambos and Davis (1944) is also probably from the cochlear nucleus. The heavy line shows the unit's response area. Within this area, discharges were inhibited when a second tone was added at any of the frequencies and intensities indicated by the shaded area.

eighth-nerve axons. Although response areas of the type shown in Fig. 4A and B are unquestionably the dominant pattern, there may also be a significant group of fibers with low characteristic frequencies and more symmetrical response areas (Fig. 4C). Katsuki (1961) suggested that the presence of such fibers indicates different patterns of innervation for the apical and basal portions of the cochlea. Yet even considering this finding, it is more than a little surprising to find neural response areas so homogeneous in form over nearly the entire length of the cochlear partition.

In the dorsal and ventral cochlear nuclei and elsewhere along the classical pathway, two types of fiber response areas are found: narrow-band and broad-band (Hilali and Whitfield, 1953; Rose et al., 1959; Hind, 1960; Katsuki, 1961). In Fig. 4D, E, F, and G, only units from the cochlear nucleus and primary cortex are illustrated; there do not yet appear to be any striking deviations from these basic patterns in other portions of the pathway. Comparisons of the response areas of the narrow-band units (Figs. 4E and F) with those of eighth-nerve fibers (Fig. 4A and B), show a major difference in "sharpening" only at low frequencies. Between the cochlear nucleus and the cortex there is very little further resolution in response-area tuning. At stimulus intensities only 20 dB above threshold sensitivity in either location, the frequency response area is much too wide to account for known pitch resolution or DL size. As intensity continues to increase, resolution becomes still poorer. One is thus forced to conclude that response-area tuning in single neurons is not the ultimate mechanism of frequency processing. In fact, most such tuning is already nearing completion in the cochlear nucleus.*

The further resolution of frequency must be sought elsewhere. One possibility, temporal patterning, was previously mentioned—abrupt changes in discharge characteristics result even from modest changes in stimulus frequency.†

---

*It would, however, be injudicious to assume that the similar shape of cochlear-nucleus, inferior-colliculus, medial-geniculate, and cortical neuron response areas means no change in the underlying neural processing. Erulkar's (1959) observations of single units (within the inferior colliculus) that show two different frequency response areas, one for each ear, ought to discourage even the most rabid advocate of a brainstem composed only of relays to the cortex.

†Such sharp temporal contrasts appear primarily at a fiber's upper frequency limit. This characteristic complements one aspect of brainstem auditory frequency processing—it offers a very precise definition of the upper edge of a unit's frequency-response area.

Another mode of pitch resolution is presumably contained within the details of the spatial patterns developed by tonotopic organizations of the primary pathways. Yet all efforts to discover the full implication of such multineuron patterns at subcortical levels have so far been unsuccessful. At the cortical surface, the gross tonotopic organization repeatedly demonstrated by various macroelectrode techniques (e.g., Fig. 5) has received only indifferent confirmation when microelectrodes have been lowered into place. Observations have failed to resolve the single fiber's relation to the overall low-to-high frequency organization. Most investigators who have sought to clarify such single-cell activity patterns have ended their analyses with something like: "Although this study tends to support an organization of best frequencies from low to high (posterior to anterior in the AI region of the cat), it did not always turn out that way. During a single penetration, for instance, fibers with best frequencies of 2000, 7000, 23000, and 6000 Hz were found, and in that order." However, Hind (1960) found that, during a single microelectrode penetration, the majority of units (71 percent) do have their most sensitive response frequencies contained within one octave. More information about the organization of the auditory cortex is clearly needed before the codes of frequency patterning can be broken.

The pitch discrimination abilities of decorticated animals make it seem unlikely that the cortical patterns are necessary for the resolution of single-frequency tones, or perhaps of *any* steady-state stimulus (Neff, 1961; Dewson, 1964). It is therefore equally unlikely that such sounds will prove to be the most rewarding tools with which to seek the key to cortical and subcortical patterns of pitch. The potentially infinite number of combinations of acoustic stimuli precludes an adequate summary of even the comparatively meager data available on responses to complex sounds. However, it may be profitable to describe one example—an analysis of the responses of 164 cortical auditory units recorded from awake cats by Galambos (1960); the analysis will also illustrate the importance of the experimenter's imagination in dealing with cortical processing. Of the units studied, 82 percent of area AI and 60 percent of area E_p units responded to some acoustic stimulus, but with response latencies varying between 8 and 80 msec (or even longer); only 62 percent in AI and 31 percent in E_p did so on more than half of the stimulus presentations. Pure tones produced some type of response (sustained driving or suppression, "on-off," "on," or "off") 70 percent (AI) and 44 percent (E_p) of the time. Of these, 10 percent (AI) and 74 percent (E_p) responded over a wide range of frequencies. Consistent responses to single clicks were obtained in 26 percent (AI) and 8 percent (E_p) of the units, or to broad-band noise for 66 percent (AI) and 20 percent (E_p) of the units. Six (AI) and 13 (E_p) units responded best to odd sounds such as paper tearing, jingling keys, etc.

Compared to other studies of cortical neurons, these percentages of acoustically active units are impressively high. That some degree of imagination is required to obtain this proportion is suggested in Galambos's (1960) further description of this population of cells. He noted that a pattern of inconsistent responses to standard stimuli could occasionally be bettered when the animals' attention was gained either by presenting a "novel" (unadapted) sound or by awakening a drowsy animal. Slow warbling tones, rapid frequency sweeps, small rather than large intensity changes, or new stimulus repetition rates were found to create optimal stimuli for still other units. Of those units that responded to a wide range of frequencies (broad-band units of the type shown in Fig. 4G), the majority were outside the AI area of the primary auditory cortex. Their responses were characterized by rapid adaptation to standard stimuli and by occasional unexplained changes in character.

Katsuki et al. (1959b) and Katsuki (1961) extended the behavioral cataloguing of these broad-band-unit responses to two simultaneous tones. No combination of tones ever reduced the response area produced by one tone alone. Such a failure of two tones to interact is almost never found in narrow-band units. In fact, one of the few methods for driving a cortical unit with a steady-state stimulus for an extended period employs two tones that are harmonically related or are adjusted to beat at a rate between 50 and 200 Hz.*

Simultaneous two-tone stimuli or other complex sounds have marked effects on the response areas of sharply tuned cortical neurons, and indeed upon a high percentage of neurons at all subcortical levels.

Though two examples are shown in Fig. 4H and I, a detailed description of these interactions can only be obtained if read within the context of the original publications (Galambos and Davis, 1944; Rose et al., 1959; Moushegian et al., 1962); only the most general view can be provided here. It is quite clear that a sizable segment of the auditory system, even at the cochlear nucleus, is geared for the processing

---

*The findings of Gumnit and Grossman (1961) are of considerable interest in further exploring the curiously transient nature of cortical activity to sustained sounds. From DC recordings (macroelectrode), they showed a continuing negative shift during long-duration acoustic stimulation for large areas of auditory cortex.

of complex sounds — that two or more frequencies often can produce exquisite resolution by a neuron otherwise only sluggishly sensitive to a single tone.

How excitation by different types of complex sounds may prove to be pertinent in terms of significance for different organisms is completely unknown. It would be tempting, for instance, to attribute some special significance to fibers that are especially responsive to frequency modulation when they are described in the inferior colliculus of the bat if it were not for the sobering observation that FM-sensitive units are also present in other auditory nervous systems (Thurlow *et al.*, 1951; Grinnell and McCue, 1963; Whitfield and Evans, 1965).

The role of volley or periodicity coding of frequency information is equally unresolved either for simple or for complex sounds. Wever's 1949, 1964) views on the general nature of synchrony in the eighth nerve are at least approximately correct. At very low frequencies, synchronous discharging is quite likely the major component of coding. As stimulus frequency increases from 400 Hz to 4000 Hz, synchrony diminishes and the *place* of excitation predominates. However, when one is forced to examine closely the electrophysiological observations at hand, it is apparent that important details about magnitudes, central-nervous-system processing, and synchrony in primarily place-sensitive fibers are absent or only anecdotally described. Maximum rates for synchronous discharges are, however, available. In the eighth nerve, a sizable degree of synchronous discharging is observed at stimulation rates up to at least 800 Hz, and some synchrony is detectable by macroelectrodes at 3500 to 4000 Hz (Derbyshire and Davis, 1935; Peake *et al.*, 1962b). Yet all evidence of such macroelectrode-recorded synchrony gradually disappears at higher brain levels. In secondary neurons (presynaptic connections in the trapezoid body), the maximum synchronous frequency is about 2500 Hz (Kemp *et al.*, 1937). Slow-wave activity above 2000 Hz decreases markedly in the region of the accessory superior olive (Tsuchitani and Boudreau, 1964). The maximum synchrony decreases to about 1000 Hz in the region of the inferior colliculus (Kemp *et al.*, 1937). At and beyond the medial geniculate body,* a generous estimate would be 200 Hz (Goldstein *et al.*, 1959). Single-fiber observations confirm these

---

* In some cases, these estimates are conservative, since they ignore synchrony that is detectable only at very intense levels of stimulation.

measurements. That is, units discharged at intervals related to the stimulus frequency or submultiples of that frequency at maximum rates between 2000 Hz and 4000 Hz in the eighth nerve (Tasaki, 1954; Rupert *et al.*, 1963), at 2000 Hz in the accessory superior olive (Moushegian *et al.*, 1964b), and at 200 Hz in the medial geniculate body* (Vernier and Galambos, 1957).

The mechanics of the cochlea force the consideration of two types of synchrony — one occurs during low-frequency, steady-state stimulation; the other occurs at higher stimulus frequencies and represents the detection of the envelope in a predominantly place-sensitive population of fibers. In the eighth nerve, the high rates (2000 Hz and above) of repetitive discharging observed by macroelectrodes originate in fibers of the basal turn. The tonotopic characteristics of these fibers is therefore higher than their synchronous response to repetitive clicks or bursts of noise (Peake *et al.*, 1962a,b). At the inferior colliculus, the waveform and amplitude of slow-wave activity evoked by rapidly repetitive clicks can be altered by filtered noise. The nature of these changes indicates that fibers within the tonotopic organization continue to participate in synchronous discharging (Kemp *et al.*, 1937). At the medial geniculate body, click-evoked electrical activity may be suppressed by discrete bands of continuous tones, predominately those below 2000 Hz. This suppression is not likely due to masking since the transition from no effect to complete suppression may often depend upon changes in the tone as small as 6 dB or 100 Hz (Galambos, 1952). At the primary cortex, when repetitive clicks are presented in a background of steady tones between 400 and 8000 Hz, evoked activity is enhanced. This activity increase does not occur in a background of noise (Gumnit and Grossman, 1961). On the other hand, Kiang and Goldstein (1959) examined the possibility that the gradual disappearance of synchronous discharging in place-sensitive neurons at higher brainstem levels might be accompanied by a recoding in terms of tonotopic organization. Within the limits of their techniques, they were unable to find evidence for such recoding. They pointed out, however, that the final resolution of this question should be examined by other techniques.

Meanwhile, the other, more classical type of neural synchrony

---

*This rate is, incidentally, not appreciably different from maximum repetitive discharge rates of other sensory-system fibers within the thalamus (Poggio and Mountcastle, 1963).

needs to be examined for new developments.* Single-fiber responses recorded from the eighth nerve and the brainstem have in general confirmed Wever's (1949) ideas. He was, in fact, able to restate his 1949 conclusions in 1964 without major modifications. Of the many single-unit studies reporting the presence of synchronous discharges at low frequencies, three are especially interesting: Katsuki *et al.* (1962), Rupert *et al.* (1963), and Moushegian *et al.* (1964a). Each study described units that discharge in synchrony with stimuli somewhat below a unit's most sensitive response frequency. There are *asynchronous* discharges immediately below, at, and above that best frequency. For example, Moushegian *et al.* (1964a) reported a superior-olivary unit with a 3000 Hz best frequency; the unit demonstrated marked synchrony at 752 Hz and some synchrony up to 2006 Hz, but none at 2505 Hz. These three studies also mentioned that all fibers responding to low frequencies do not do so in the same manner. Some units may be completely insensitive to the periodicity of the stimulus tone over a wide range of frequencies and intensities. Katsuki *et al.* (1962) also described a population of eighth-nerve fibers whose frequency-response contours are much less sharply tuned at higher frequencies than the majority of units. Such fibers were the only ones found with best frequencies below 400 Hz. About equal numbers of sharply and diffusely tuned units were found with best frequencies between 300 and 1000 Hz, and no diffusely tuned fibers were observed with best frequencies above 6000 Hz. However, Katsuki *et al.* (1962) did not specifically describe the synchronous discharge behavior of these units, nor has confirmation yet been obtained from other laboratories. In the other report on eighth-nerve synchrony, Rupert *et al.* (1963) pointed out that some units are at times "poor responders" to acoustic stimuli, changing their spontaneous rate of discharge only slightly, if at all, immediately after a stimulus is introduced. However, if stimulation continues, the spontaneous activity may become synchronous with the tone and may occasionally gradually or abruptly revert to asynchrony. At other stimulus frequencies, that same unit may promptly and continuously respond synchronously.

---

*The reader interested in pursuing other routes of study has his choice of several different types of investigations: selective destruction of the auditory nerve (Dandy, 1934, 1960) or of the apical cochlea (Schuknecht, 1960), selective electrical stimulation of the spiral lamina in animals (Woolsey, 1960), or more diffuse stimulation of the eighth nerve in man (Simmons *et al.*, 1964; Simmons, 1966). And there is a voluminous literature on pitch defects in clinical cases and on discrimination in lower vertebrates.

Nothing further can be said about frequency-related synchrony in units either at higher brainstem or cortical locations. There is, of course, no axiom that demands that both tonotopic and temporal pitch cues be either processed or discriminated at the same places within the nervous system. Still, unless one postulates two completely different sets of fibers within the brainstem, it is difficult to see how synchrony could completely avoid modulating the timing patterns of primarily place-sensitive neurons. Computer-analyzed data from single fibers will undoubtedly give us a more precise picture of both types of synchrony, or the lack of it, at several levels of the auditory brain.

V. INTENSITY

The nervous system's response to increasing stimulus intensity is generally described in terms of increasing synchrony, increasing discharge rates, spreading activity, and decreasing stimulus-response latencies. Such descriptions are well documented at all levels of the auditory system, not only by macroelectrode observation, but also by inference from the tuning curves and from some of the temporal characteristics of most single fibers. Further study of temporal patterns (Fig. 3), however, suggests that although this simple arrangement may suffice for an overview, it is inadequate to explain why a given stimulus magnitude may continue to sustain electrical activity in, say, the cochlear nucleus but not in the medial geniculate. A stubborn perplexity also remains when one tries to reconcile most of these overview observations to the fact that increasing loudness usually also means improving discrimination, a problem already mentioned in connection with frequency processing.

In the eighth nerve, intensity coding has traditionally been discussed according to one of two basic concepts. The earlier concept emphasized the *summation* of neural activity caused by spreading excitation along the cochlear partition as stimulus intensity increases (Steinberg and Gardner, 1937; Stevens and Davis, 1938). At almost the same time, however, observations on loudness defects in damaged ears (Fowler, 1928, 1937) and histological studies in animals (Lurie, 1940) served to focus and hold attention on the *place* theory of loudness coding: nerve fibers innervating the outer rows of hair cells are excited by less intense sounds than are fibers innervating the inner hair cells. There have since been several variations on both the *place* and *summation* themes, including a movement marked *duo* by general agreement, but giving the burden to the *place* theme in spite of the fact that more than one type of loudness defect can be demonstrated in damaged end organs (Palva, 1957).

Single-fiber analysis of eighth-nerve fibers has not appreciably clarified the situation. At frequencies below about 1000 Hz, a clear bimodal distribution of response thresholds appears (Katsuki *et al.*, 1962). At higher frequencies, the thresholds of the majority of fibers are about evenly distributed over a range in excess of 80 dB. Once excited, an individual fiber is generally able to reflect further intensity increases by a sigmoid-shaped increase in discharge rate over a range of about 40 dB. Katsuki noted that the slope of this sigmoid is not constant and that some fibers (usually those with low best frequencies and asymmetrical tuning curves) reach their maximum firing rate over less than a 40 dB range.

Although Katsuki's observations are the most extensive, two minority reports are pertinent. Tasaki (1954) noted that two populations of intensity-sensitive neurons exist in the basal turn of the guinea pig cochlea, but could not demonstrate a similar bimodal distribution of apical (low-frequency) fibers. In the pigeon, where no inner-outer division of hair cells exists, Stopp and Whitfield (1961) were unable to find differences in fiber responses from those observed in the mammalian cochlea.

Stimulus intensity has been studied in the cochlear nucleus, the superior olive, and the trapezoid body by several investigators. Rose *et al.* (1963) mentioned two types of discharge patterns, one reflecting vastly greater sensitivity to intensity change than the other. Their further observations on converting sensitive fibers to relatively insensitive ones by prior stimulation may have some relevance for the occasionally divergent findings in the eighth-nerve fibers. Most cochlear-nucleus fibers respond over a range of intensities similar to those observed in the eighth nerve. Typically, that range is slightly wider (20 to 50 dB) and more varied (at a unit's best frequency). Only Tasaki and Davis (1955) mentioned a bimodal distribution of threshold sensitivities. The traditional concept of intensity coding is clearly in trouble when it comes to explaining unit behavior of the sort illustrated in Fig. 3E and the insert on the cochlear nucleus (also in Fig. 3).

If these minority discharge patterns observed in the cochlear nucleus, the superior olive, and elsewhere are being interpreted correctly, a major step in intensity processing takes place between the cochlear nucleus and the inferior colliculus. This transition strongly suggests that intensity coding ceases to be a matter of spreading excitation and becomes a matter of increasingly sharp signal resolution in temporal patterns.

In the inferior colliculus, some units continue to respond to changes in intensity in the same manner as eighth-nerve and cochlear-nucleus units – there is a more or less simple increment in discharge rate from threshold through intensities of 40 to 50 dB above threshold (Erulkar, 1959). In a larger percentage (over 50 percent), responses are characterized by one or more of the following: major abrupt changes in pattern near threshold intensities or near the margins of the effective range of stimulus frequencies, progressive or abrupt inhibition of discharges at intensities perhaps only 20 dB above the unit's threshold at all or some few effective frequencies, precise changes in the relation between the initial "on" response and the silent interval that follows (Rose et al., 1963). The orderliness of such changes constitutes an embarrassing wealth of potential information about intensity. It is not inconceivable, for example, that individual elements transmit intensity increments as progressively longer silent intervals, or eventually as no response at all.

Macroelectrode observations suggest that some fundamental transformation of neural response also occurs cephalad to the inferior colliculus (Starr and Livingston, 1963). Single-fiber analysis within the medial geniculate is still inadequate to define clearly whether the marked diminution in gross electrical activity observed there represents a further refinement in inhibitory processing or (most unlikely) a lack of affect toward intensities of simple sounds. Katsuki (1961) emphasized that changes in intensity produce only slight changes in medial-geniculate single-unit discharge rates (compared to the changes at lower levels). Galambos (1952) was impressed by the specificity of interaction between simultaneous tones and clicks, which seems to indicate that suppression of unit firing may play a prominent role in the resolution of stimulus intensity. However, he also carefully pointed out that similar interactions are obtainable from fibers in the brachium of the inferior colliculus.

Cortical management of stimulus intensity has mainly been described within the classical concepts of the activity spreading over larger areas, and of the changing character of the initial "on" response (Ades, 1959; Tunturi, 1960). Figure 5 shows Tunturi's diagrammatic representation of the intensity-frequency pattern of the primary auditory cortex in the dog. As stimulus intensity increases from threshold, excitation spreads outward from a small strip at the most sensitive (superior) edge of the cortex. At intensities 20 to 80 dB above threshold, the response area spreads until virtually the entire iso-frequency strip is excited. The anterior-posterior location of maximum activity is determined by the stimulus frequency.

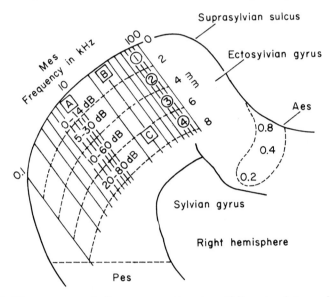

Figure 5 "Arrangement of afferent connections to middle ectosylvian auditory area (MES) of the dog brain and relation of intensity for ipsilateral ear along iso-frequency contours" (Tunturi, 1952. By permission from *American Journal of Physiology*.) The dashed lines indicate arbitrary 2-mm-wide zones in which the indicated difference in intensity level was found between the thresholds for the two ears.

Within this very general scheme, no single recording site seems able to reflect a change in the amplitude of the "on" response over more than about a 20-dB range of stimulus intensities. Sandel and Kiang (1961) found a wider range of "on" response amplitude changes, but perhaps more interesting was their analysis of the "off" response —another slow-wave electrical event sometimes seen after an abrupt discontinuation of a stimulus and once thought to result from the ensuing acoustic transients. Instead, they showed, this response reflects a finer pattern of ongoing suppression of surrounding cortical or subcortical activity during stimulation; the pattern requires 100 msec or more to develop completely, and is sensitive to changes in stimulus magnitude or frequency. On casual inspection, the variety of input-output curves for "on" and "off" responses bear a resemblance to some of the medial geniculate slow-wave patterns mentioned by Galambos *et al.* (1952).

The individual cortical units so far described do not appreciably clarify this pattern's detail. Two groups of units are recognized: one is relatively insensitive to low-level sound or to specific frequency (Fig. 4G) and is perhaps predominantly located outside of the AI area; the other group (Fig. 4F) may be sensitive to near-threshold stimuli. Both groups demonstrate considerable reluctance to discharge more than a short burst of spikes at any magnitude of simple intensity change.

This apparently indifferent behavior of single cortical units toward simple intensity increments should come as no surprise, since the cortex and medial geniculate are not required for this type of discrimination (Raab and Ades, 1946). These areas nevertheless *do* respond to stimulus magnitude. We are thus once again forced to seek first a perceptual parameter more appropriate for the task before the pursuit of its processing can continue.

Meanwhile, there are other questions on stimulus magnitude worth exploring at several levels within the auditory system. Starr and Livingston's (1963) observations on electrical activity during sustained acoustic stimulation have rather forcefully revived the long-standing problem of relating single-cell responses to collective activity recorded by macroelectrodes. In contrast to single-cell data, average electrical activity in the cochlear nucleus, the superior olive, and the inferior colliculus *increases* during the first 30 to 60 min of stimulation. Middle-ear muscle relaxation during this period is the major cause for the increasing amplitude, but Galin (1964) demonstrated that these amplitudes can also be modified by learning. Even in anesthetized animals, slow-wave activity does not show a decrement that can be considered to reflect absolutely the nature of single-cell discharges.

These findings are not isolated ones. Several other investigators have had cause to question seriously the wisdom of assuming that such volume-conducted electrical activity is always related to synchronous discharging of large numbers of single fibers or cells in that same tissue population (Purpura, 1959; Katsuki, 1961; Mountcastle, 1961). Relating the various methods of sampling electrical activity in the brain is, of course, one of the classical problems of neurophysiology and involves many more variables than just stimulus magnitude.

Returning briefly to the coding of loudness, one final question still needs an answer. Do two (or more) codes exist simultaneously within the brain, one for *place*, and another for *summation?*

VI. DIFFUSE OR CHANGING ELEMENTS IN PROCESSING

Though the majority of the electrical events so far described have been observed in cell populations generally associated with the lemniscal system, there is no good reason to assume that all such interactions take place or are exclusively controlled from within that system.* In fact, considerable information suggests that the type of sensory processing envisioned by Barlow (1961) is heavily influenced by components of the diffuse auditory and poly-sensory systems of the brainstem and cortex. Let me offer one example among many. If an animal is exposed to repetitive clicks that are presumably without significance for him, the electrical activity evoked within the brain by those clicks will be principally within the lemniscal auditory system. If the clicks are somehow made significant, say by association with a mildly noxious stimulus, click-evoked electrical activity begins to appear at several sites in the reticular and limbic systems, and in widely separated nonauditory cortical areas; it is also markedly increased and changed in the lemniscal system. As the association continues, this additional electrical activity may diminish in amplitude in some of these regions, and may completely disappear *if* the association is discontinued *or if* the animal learns to avoid the noxious stimulus (Hearst *et al.*, 1960; Galambos and Sheatz, 1962).

In Fessard's (1961) view, the main function of the lemniscal system is to develop a fine degree of stimulus resolution. This focusing is not likely to be accomplished without sacrificing plasticity for precise and predictable organization. The diffuse system, on the other hand, is ideally suited for the job of insuring that plasticity is retained, to be used as needed to modify or abstract from lemniscal processing. However, admitting a diffuse system into partnership with lemniscal neurons explains little about the specifics of processing. In fact, we are now forced to re-examine every one of the many input-output functions so far described within the lemniscal system, to try to discover those dimensions that are innate (if any) and those that are outside modifications (for surely those modifications are the key to data significance). The types of modifications to be expected are completely unknown, but perhaps responses of units within the diffuse system will provide suggestions.

---

*The reader wishing to pursue the details of such control in other sensory systems will find the reports by Wall (1959, 1960), Wall and Cronly-Dillon (1960), Galin (1963), Wilson *et al.* (1964), and the review by Rose and Mountcastle (1959) helpful.

The responses of single units within these diffuse or association areas do not appear to be concerned with the spectrum of the acoustic stimulus. Characteristically, units within the reticular brainstem respond, over a wide range of frequencies and intensities, with a slow rate of discharge that is usually maintained as long as the stimulus continues. Other units may respond only at stimulus onset, may continue to discharge after the sound ceases, may be inhibited by an acoustic stimulus, or may occasionally demonstrate more complex temporal patterns (Scheibel et al., 1955; Fessard 1961; Katsuki, 1961). Reticular, thalamic, and cortical units that respond to visual, somesthetic, and auditory signals may or may not respond to each stimulus identically, and responses to ongoing stimulation in one modality may be strikingly modified by introduction of a second sensory stimulus (Buser and Imbert, 1961; Fessard, 1961; Bental and Bihari, 1963). Information on changes in these discharge characteristics, which may be presumed to accompany stimulus-oriented behavior of the organism, are not yet available except as they are reflected in reports of cortical "attention units" that respond according to the novelty of the sound and environment rather than to the physical characteristics (Hubel et al., 1959).

Other techniques (direct-current recording and brain stimulation) promise to yield insight not only into the behavior of the diffuse and poly-sensory systems, but also into their influence upon sensory-specific pathways. In several cortical and subcortical areas, sustained and transient shifts in the DC potentials accompany changes in the amplitude of the AC evoked response to acoustic or other sensory stimulation (Brown, 1959; Hind, 1960; Adey, 1963; Rowland, 1963). Also, DC stimulation of the motor cortex allows an ambient sound (or light, or touch) to cause movement of a limb when that reaction is ordinarily expected only when a stronger (suprathreshold) sensory stimulus is applied. Furthermore, this effect lasts for several minutes after discontinuation of the current (Rusinov, 1953, 1960). Morrell (1961, 1963) applied the same polarization technique but also recorded from single cells in the motor cortex. Before polarization, tones produced no discharges. During polarization, tones regularly produced discharges in cells of several different types. In another experiment, rabbits were conditioned with a single 500-Hz tone and with a repetitive 200-Hz tone. Both tones were previously habituated but both produced discharges during cortical polarization. However, the 200-Hz tone continued to produce discharges for 20 min afterward; the 500-Hz tone failed to do so.

It is still not possible to assign exact roles to either the diffuse or the lemniscal system. The best that can be said at the moment is that auditory activities within the brain are capable of expanding beyond the limits· of the classical pathways, that behavioral events or artificially induced electrical events can control this distribution, and that this control originates within the diffuse and poly-sensory systems. The observations so far mentioned deal mainly with transient events, those for which it has been popular to emphasize the probable importance of efferent innervations or feedback loops that exercise control over sensory inputs. It remains to be pointed out that even if such circuits are initially in control, the affected sensory input may eventually encompass that regulator's effect within its own repertoire of responses. At times, the altered response may be temporary, subject to revision if circumstances change; at other times, and perhaps at earlier ages, the alteration may be permanently imprinted into sensory behavior (Hess, 1964). The now classic studies of Hydén and Egyházi (1962) on brainstem vestibular nuclei suggest that the effects of learning can be demonstrated in the most fundamental of sensory nuclei. Hydén measured differences in the RNA content and in the composition of the RNA itself in secondary vestibular neurons (Deiter's nucleus from three groups of rats; the changes depended upon the animals' previous experiences with balance and motion. One group (control) received no special vestibular stimulation. The second group (passive stimulation) were regularly rotated on a turntable. The third group (learning) were obliged to obtain their food by developing skill at walking a tightly stretched wire.

Such experiments utilize a considerably different type of input-output measurement from those that occupy the majority of this chapter. Hydén and Egyházi's experiments particularly look like an important step toward a molecular basis of memory (Dingman and Sporn, 1964), and it is not inconceivable that certain of the DC observations may also reflect a biochemical basis for another type of shorter term memory.

These last few paragraphs are a very superficial tribute to some major and relatively new developments in the study of sensory processing. With these developments, or more realistically *because* of them, some drastic and occasionally inconvenient changes in conceptual organization of the brain have been forced upon us. Not the least of these is that when an important auditory decision is to be made by an organism, it "consults" at length the nonauditory areas of the brain before assigning the acoustic event its niche. This changing conception is perhaps most pertinent for those whose professional and creative interests are intimately tied to an understanding of a single sense modality. Too often our studies have taken place only *in vitro*. Perhaps it is time to seek again those aspects of sound and its perception that are not so easy to assign numbers to. If real progress is to continue, future investigators of auditory physiology are clearly committed to exploring sensory modifications as they involve the entire organism, its environment, and its ability to change it.

REFERENCES

Ades, H. W. (1959). Central auditory mechanisms. In J. Field (Ed.) *Handbook of Physiology.* Vol. 1, pp. 585–613. American Physiological Society, Washington.

Adey, W. R. (1963). Aspects of brain physiology in the space environment. In M. A. B. Brazier (Ed.). *Brain function.* (Proceedings of the first conference.) pp. 321–345. Univ. of California Press, Berkeley *and* Los Angeles.

Aitkin, L. M., Dunlop, C. W., and Webster, W. R. (1966). Click-evoked response patterns of single units in the medial geniculate body of the cat. *J. Neurophysiol.,* **29,** 109–123.

Allanson, J. T. and Whitfield, I. C. (1956). The cochlear nucleus and its relation to theories of hearing. In C. Cherry (Ed.) *Information theory.* pp. 269–286. Academic Press *and* Butterworths, New York *and* London.

Barlow, H. B. (1961). Possible principles underlying the transformations of sensory messages. In W. A. Rosenblith (Ed.) *Sensory communication.* pp. 217–234. M.I.T. Press *and* Wiley, New York.

von Békésy, G. (1958). Funneling in the nervous system and its role in loudness and sensation intensity on the skin. *J. Acoust. Soc. Am.,* **30,** 399–412.

Bental, E. and Bihari, B. (1963). Evoked activity of single neurons in sensory association cortex of the cat. *J. Neurophysiol.,* **26,** 207–214.

Brown, G. W. (1959). Electrical impedance variation within the hypothalamus associated with learning. *Fedn Proc. Fedn. Am. Socs Exp. Biol.,* **18,** 19(A).

Buser, P. and Imbert, M. (1961). Sensory projections to the motor cortex in cats. In W. A. Rosenblith (Ed.) *Sensory communication.* pp. 607–626. M.I.T. Press *and* Wiley, New York.

Chang, H.-T. (1959). The evoked potentials. In J. Field (Ed.) *Handbook of physiology.* Vol. 1, pp. 299–313. American Physiological Society, Washington.

Dandy, W. E. (1934). Meniere's disease: Symptoms, objective findings, and treatment in forty-two cases. *Archs Otolar.,* **20,** 1–30.

Dandy, W. E. (1960). As cited in W. F. Windle (Chairman), Discussion of anatomy and physiology of peripheral auditory mechanisms. In G. L. Rasmussen and W. F. Windle (Eds.) *Neural mechanisms of the auditory and vestibular systems.* pp. 95–98. Thomas, Springfield, Illinois.

Davis, H. (1964a). Enhancement of evoked cortical potentials in humans related to a task requiring a decision. *Science,* **145,** 182–183.

Davis, H. (1964b). Some acoustic relations of the slow cortical-evoked response. *J. Acoust. Soc. Am.,* **36,** 1997 (A).

Derbyshire, A. J. and Davis, H. (1935). The action potentials of the auditory nerve. *Am. J. Physiol.,* **113,** 476–504.

Dewson, J. H., III (1964). Speech sound discrimination by cats. *Science,* **144,** 555–556.

Dingman, W. and Sporn, M. B. (1964). Molecular theories of memory. *Science,* **144,** 26–29.

Eccles, J. C. (1964). *The physiology of synapses.* Academic Press, New York.

Elliott, D. N. (1964). Review of auditory research. In P. R. Farnsworth (Ed.) *Annual review of psychology.* Vol. 15, pp. 57–86. Annual Reviews, Palo Alto.

Erulkar, S. D. (1959). The responses of single units of the inferior colliculus of the cat to acoustic stimulation. *Proc. R. Soc.,* **150,** *ser. B,* 336–355.

Erulkar, S. D., Rose, J. E., and Davies, P. W. (1956). Single unit activity in the auditory cortex of the cat. *Bull. Johns Hopkins Hosp.,* **99,** 55–86.

Fessard, A. (1961). The role of neuronal networks in sensory communications within the brain. In W. A. Rosenblith (Ed.) *Sensory communication.* pp. 585–606. M.I.T. Press *and* Wiley, New York.

Fowler, E. P. (1928). Marked deafened areas in normal ears. *Archs Otolar.,* **8,** 151–155.

Fowler, E. P. (1937). Measuring the sensation of loudness. *Archs Otolar.,* **26,** 514–521.

French, J. D. (1960). The reticular formation. In J. Field (Ed.) *Handbook of physiology.* Vol. 2, pp. 1281–1305. American Physiological Society, Washington.

Galambos, R. (1952). Microelectrode studies on medial geniculate body of cat. III. Response to pure tones. *J. Neurophysiol.,* **15,** 381–400.

Galambos, R. (1954). Neural mechanisms of audition. *Physiol. Rev.,* **34,** 497–528.

Galambos, R. (1959). Electrical correlates of conditioned learning. In M. A. B. Brazier (Ed.) *The central nervous system and behavior.* pp. 375–415. (Transactions of the first conference.) Josiah Macy, Jr. Foundation, New York.

Galambos, R. (1960). Studies of the auditory system with implanted electrodes. In G. L. Rasmussen and W. F. Windle (Eds.) *Neural mechanisms of the auditory and vestibular systems.* pp. 137–151. Thomas, Springfield, Illinois.

Galambos, R. (1961). Processing of auditory information. In M. A. B. Brazier (Ed.) *Brain and behavior.* Vol. 1, pp. 171–203. American Insitute of Biological Sciences, Washington.

Galambos, R. and Davis, H. (1944). Inhibition of activity in single auditory nerve fibers by acoustic stimulation. *J. Neurophysiol.,* **7,** 287–303.

Galambos, R. and Sheatz, G. C. (1962). An electroencephalograph study of classical conditioning. *Am. J. Physiol.,* **203,** 173–184.

Galambos, R., Rose, J. E., Bromiley, R. B., and Hughes, J. R. (1952). Microelectrode studies on medial geniculate body of cat. II. Response to clicks. *J. Neurophysiol.,* **15,** 359–380.

Galambos, R., Schwartzkopff, J., and Rupert, A. L. (1959). Microelectrode study of superior olivary nuclei. *Am. J. Physiol.,* **197,** 527–536.

Galambos, R., Myers, R. E., and Sheatz, G. C. (1961). Extralemniscal activation of auditory cortex in cats. *Am. J. Physiol.,* **200,** 23–28.

Galin, D. (1963). Modification of evoked responses in auditory nuclei with conditioning in the cat. *Fedn Proc. Fedn Am. Socs. Exp. Biol.,* **22,** 678 (A).

Galin, D. (1964). Effects of conditioning on auditory signals. In W. S. Fields and B. R. Alford (Eds.) *Neurological aspects of auditory and vestibular disorders.* pp. 61–76. Thomas, Springfield, Illinois.

Goldberg, J. M., Adrian, H. O., and Smith, F. D. (1964). Response of neurons of the superior olivary complex of the cat to acoustic stimuli of long duration. *J. Neurophysiol.*, **27**, 706–749.

Goldstein, M. H., Jr., Kiang, N. Y-s., and Brown, R. M. (1959). Responses of the auditory cortex to repetitive acoustic stimuli. *J. Acoust. Soc. Am.*, **31**, 356–364.

Greenwood, D. D. and Maruyama, N. (1965). Excitatory and inhibitory response areas of auditory neurons in the cochlear nucleus. *J. Neurophysiol.*, **28**, 863–892.

Grinnell, A. D. and McCue, J. J. G. (1963). Neurophysiological investigations of the bat, *Myotis lucifugus*, stimulated by frequency modulated acoustical pulse. *Nature, Lond.*, **198**, 453–455.

Gross, N. B. and Thurlow, W. R. (1951). Microelectrode studies of neural auditory activity of cat. II. Medial geniculate body. *J. Neurophysiol.*, **14**, 409–422.

Gumnit, R. J. and Grossman, R. G. (1961). Potentials evoked by sound in the auditory cortex of the cat. *Am. J. Physiol.*, **200**, 1219–1225.

Haider, M., Spong, P., and Lindsley, D. B. (1964). Attention, vigilance, and cortical evoked-potentials in humans. *Science*, **145**, 180–182.

Hartline, H. K., Wagner, H. G., and MacNichol, E. F., Jr. (1952). The peripheral origin of nervous activity in the visual system. *Cold Spring Harbor Symp. Quant. Biol.*, **17**, 125–141.

Hawkins, J. E., Jr. (1964). Hearing. In V. E. Hall (Ed.) *Annual review of physiology*. Vol. 26, pp. 453–480. Annual Reviews, Palo Alto.

Hearst, E., Beer, B., Sheatz, G. C., and Galambos, R. (1960). Some electrophysiological correlates of conditioning in the monkey. *Electroenceph. Clin. Neurophysiol.*, **12**, 137–152.

Hess, E. H. (1964). Imprinting in birds. *Science*, **146**, 1128–1139.

Hilali, S. and Whitfield, I. C. (1953). Responses of the trapezoid body to acoustic stimulation with pure tones. *J. Physiol., Lond.*, **122**, 158–171.

Hind, J. E. (1960). Unit activity in the auditory cortex. In G. L. Rasmussen and W. F. Windle (Eds.) *Neural mechanisms of the auditory and vestibular systems*. Pp. 201–210. Thomas, Springfield, Illinois.

Hubel, D. H., Henson, C. O., Rupert, A. L., and Galambos, R. (1959). "Attention" units in the auditory cortex. *Science*, **129**, 1279–1280.

Hydén, H. and Egyházi, E. (1962). Nuclear RNA changes of nerve cells during a learning experiment in rats. *Proc. Natn. Acad. Sci. U.S.A.*, **48**, 1366–1373.

Jasper, H. H. (1960). Unspecific thalamocortical relations. In J. Field (Ed.) *Handbook of physiology*. Vol. 2, pp. 1307–1321. American Physiological Society, Washington.

Jasper, H. H., Proctor, L. D., Knighton, R. S., Noshay, W. C., and Russell, T. C. (Eds.) (1958). *Reticular formation of the brain*. Henry Ford Hospital International Symposium. Churchill *and* Little, Brown, London *and* Boston.

Katsuki, Y. (1961). Neural mechanism of auditory sensation in cats. In W. A. Rosenblith (Ed.) *Sensory communication*. pp. 561–583. M.I.T. Press *and* Wiley, New York.

Katsuki, Y., Sumi, T., Uchiyama, H., and Watanabe, T. (1958). Electric responses of auditory neurons in cat to sound stimulation. *J. Neurophysiol.*, **21**, 569–588.

Katsuki, Y., Watanabe, T., and Maruyama, N. (1959a). Activity of auditory neurons in upper levels of brain of cat. *J. Neurophysiol.*, **22**, 343–359.

Katsuki, Y., Watanabe, T., and Suga, N. (1959b). Interaction of auditory neurons in response to two sound stimuli in cat. *J. Neurophysiol.*, **22**, 603–623.

Katsuki, Y., Suga, N., and Kanno, Y. (1962). Neural mechanism of the peripheral and central auditory system in monkeys. *J. Acoust. Soc. Am.*, **34**, 1396–1410.

Keidel, W. D. and Spreng, M. (1965). Computed audio-encephalograms in man (a technique of "objective" audiometry). *Int. Audiol.*, **4** (1), 56–60.

Kemp, E. H., Coppée, G. E., and Robinson, E. H. (1937). Electric responses of the brain stem to unilateral auditory stimulation. *Am. J. Physiol.*, **120**, 304–315.

Kiang, N. Y-s. (1963). Spontaneous activity of single auditory nerve fibers in cats. *J. Acoust. Soc. Am.*, **35**, 793 (A).

Kiang, N. Y-s. and Goldstein, M. H., Jr. (1959). Tonotopic organization of the cat auditory cortex for some complex stimuli. *J. Acoust. Soc. Am.*, **31**, 786–790.

Kiang, N. Y-s., Watanabe, T., Thomas, E. C., and Clark, L. F. (1962). Stimulus coding in the cat's auditory nerve. *Ann. Otol. Rhinol. Lar.*, **71**, 1009–1026.

Kuffler, S. W. (1953). Discharge patterns and functional organization of mammalian retina. *J. Neurophysiol.*, **16**, 37–68.

Landau, W. M., Goldstein, R., and Kleffner, F. R. (1960). Congenital aphasia. *Neurology*, **10**, 915–921.

Licklider, J. C. R. (1959). Three auditory theories. In S. Koch (Ed.) *Psychology: a study of a science.* Vol. 1, pp. 41–144. McGraw-Hill, New York.

Lorente de Nó, R. (1933). Anatomy of the eighth nerve. *Laryngoscope*, **43**, 327–350.

Lurie, M. H. (1940). Studies of acquired and inherited deafness in animals. *J. Acoust. Soc. Am.*, **11**, 420–426.

Magoun, H. W. (1963). *The waking brain.* (2nd ed.) Thomas, Springfield, Illinois.

Maruyama, N. and Yoshinobu, K. (1961). Experimental study on functional compensation after bilateral removal of auditory cortex in cats. *J. Neurophysiol.*, **24**, 193–202.

Morrell, F. (1961). Effect of anodal polarization on the firing pattern of single cortical cells. *Ann. N.Y. Acad. Sci.*, **92**, 860–876.

Morrell, F. (1963). Information storage in nerve cells. In W. S. Fields and W. Abbott (Eds.) *Information storage and neural control.* pp. 189–229. Thomas, Springfield, Illinois.

Mountcastle, V. B. (1961). Duality of function in the somatic afferent system. In M. A. B. Brazier (Ed.) *Brain and behavior.* Vol. 1, pp. 67–93. American Institute of Biological Sciences, Washington.

Mountcastle, V. B. and Powell, T. P. S. (1959). Neural mechanisms subserving cutaneous sensibility, with special reference to the role of afferent inhibition in sensory perception and discrimination. *Bull. Johns Hopkins Hosp.*, **105**, 201–232.

Moushegian, G., Rupert, A. L., and Galambos, R. (1962). Microelectrode study of ventral cochlear nucleus of the cat. *J. Neurophysiol.*, **25**, 515–529.

Moushegian, G., Rupert, A. L., and Whitcomb, M. A. (1964a). Brain-stem neuronal response patterns to monaural and binaural tones. *J. Neurophysiol.*, **27**, 1174–1191.

Moushegian, G., Whitcomb, M. A., and Rupert, A. L. (1964b). Neuronal periodicities to tones in feline auditory medulla. *J. Acoust. Soc. Am.*, **36**, 1996 (A).

Nauta, W. J. H. and Kuypers, H. G. J. M. (1958). Some ascending pathways in the brain stem reticular formation. In H. H. Jasper (Ed.) *International symposium: Reticular formation of the brain.* Henry Ford Hospital International Symposium. Churchill *and* Little, Brown, London *and* Boston.

Neff, W. D. (1961). Neural mechanisms of auditory discrimination. In W. A. Rosenblith (Ed.) *Sensory communication.* pp. 259–278. M.I.T. Press *and* Wiley, New York.

Nelson, P. G. and Erulkar, S. D. (1963). Synaptic mechanisms of excitation and inhibition in the central auditory pathway. *J. Neurophysiol.*, **26**, 908–923.

Palva, T. (1957). Self-recording threshold audiometry and recruitment. *Archs Otolar.*, **65**, 591–602.

Peake, W. T., Goldstein, M. H., Jr., and Kiang, N. Y-s. (1962a). Responses of the auditory nerve to repetitive acoustic stimuli. *J. Acoust. Soc. Am.*, **34**, 562–570.

Peake, W. T., Kiang, N. Y-s., and Goldstein, M. H., Jr. (1962b). Rate functions for auditory nerve responses to bursts of noise: Effect of changes in stimulus parameters. *J. Acoust. Soc. Am.*, **34**, 571–575.

Poggio, G. F. and Mountcastle, V. B. (1963). The functional properties of ventrobasal thalamic neurons studied in unanesthetized monkeys. *J. Neurophysiol.*, **26**, 775–806.

Pribram, K. H. (1960). The intrinsic systems of the forebrain. In J. Field (Ed.) *Handbook of physiology.* Vol. 2, pp. 1323–1344. American Physiological Society, Washington.

Purpura, D. P. (1959). Comments in F. Morrell, Electroencephalographic studies of conditioned learning. In M. A. B. Brazier (Ed.) *The central nervous system and behavior.* pp. 357–358. (Transactions of the first conference.) Josiah Macy, Jr. Foundation, New York.

Raab, D. H. and Ades, H. W. (1946). Cortical and midbrain mediation of a conditioned discrimination of acoustic intensities. *Am. J. Psychol.*, **59**, 59–83.

Rodieck, R. W., Kiang, N. Y-s., and Gerstein, G. L. (1962). Some quantitative methods for the study of spontaneous activity of single neurons. *Biophys. J.*, **2**, 351–368.

Rose, J. E. (1960). Organization of frequency sensitive neurons in the cochlear nuclear complex of the cat. In G. L. Rasmussen and W. F. Windle (Eds.) *Neural mechanisms of the auditory and vestibular systems.* pp. 116–136. Thomas, Springfield, Illinois.

Rose, J. E. and Mountcastle, V. B. (1959). Touch and kinesthesis. In J. Field (Ed.) *Handbook of physiology.* Vol. 1, pp. 387–429. American Physiological Society, Washington.

Rose, J. E. and Woolsey, C. N. (1959). Cortical connections and functional organization of the thalamic auditory system of the cat. In H. F. Harlow and C. N. Woolsey (Eds.) *Biological and biochemical bases of behavior.* pp. 127–150. Univ. of Wisconsin Press, Madison.

Rose, J. E., Galambos, R., and Hughes, J. R. (1959). Microelectrode studies of the cochlear nuclei of the cat. *Bull. Johns Hopkins Hosp.*, **104**, 211–251.

Rose, J. E., Greenwood, D. D., Goldberg, J. M., and Hind, J. E. (1963). Some discharge characteristics of single neurons in the inferior colliculus of the cat. *J. Neurophysiol.*, **26**, 294–320.

Rowland, V. (1963). Steady potential shifts in cortex. In M. A. B. Brazier (Ed.) *Brain function.* pp. 136–148. (Proceedings of the first conference.) Univ. of California Press, Berkeley *and* Los Angeles.

Rupert, A. L., Moushegian, G., and Galambos, R. (1963). Unit responses to sound from auditory nerve of the cat. *J. Neurophysiol.*, **26**, 449–465.

Rusinov, V. S. (1953). An electrophysiological analysis of the connecting function in the cerebral cortex in the presence of a dominant area. *Proc. XIX Int. Physiol. Congr.*, 152–156. Akademia Nauk SSR *and* Izdatelbstvo, Moscow.

Rusinov, V. S. (1960). General and localized alterations in the electroencephalogram during the formation of conditioned reflexes in man. *Electroenceph. Clin. Neurophysiol.*, *Suppl.* **13**.

Sandel, T. T. and Kiang, N. Y-s. (1961). Off-responses from the auditory cortex of anesthetized cats: effects of stimulus parameters. *Archs. Ital. Biol.*, **99**, 105–120.

Scharlock, D. P., Tucker, T. J., and Strominger, N. L. (1963). Auditory discrimination by the cat after neonatal ablation of temporal cortex. *Science*, **141**, 1197–1198.

Scheibel, M., Scheibel, A., Mollica, A., and Moruzzi, G. (1955). Convergence and inter-action of afferent impulses on single units of reticular formation. *J. Neurophysiol.*, **18**, 309–331.

Schuknecht, H. F. (1960). Neuroanatomical correlates of auditory sensitivity and pitch discrimination in the cat. In G. L. Rasmussen and W. F. Windle (Eds.) *Neural mechanisms of the auditory and vestibular systems.* Pp. 76–90. Thomas, Springfield, Illinois.

Simmons, F. B. (1966). Electrical stimulation of the auditory nerve in man. *Archs Otolar.*, **84**, 2–54.

Simmons, F. B., Mongeon, C. J., Lewis, W. R., and Huntington, D. A. (1964). Electrical stimulation of acoustical nerve and inferior colliculus. *Archs. Otolar.*, **79**, 559–567.

Small, A. M. (1963). Audition. In P. R. Farnsworth (Ed.) *Annual review of psychology.* Vol. 14, pp. 115–154. Annual Reviews, Palo Alto.

Starr, A. and Livingston, R. B. (1963). Long-lasting nervous system responses to pro-longed sound stimulation in waking cats. *J. Neurophysiol.*, **26**, 416–431.

Steinberg, J. C. and Gardner, M. B. (1937). The dependence of hearing impairment on sound intensity. *J. Acoust. Soc. Am.*, **9**, 11–23.

Stevens, S. S. and Davis, H. (1938). *Hearing.* Wiley, New York.

Stopp, P. E. and Whitfield, I. C. (1961). Unit responses from brain-stem nuclei in the pigeon. *J. Physiol., Lond.*, **158**, 165–177.

Tasaki, I. (1954). Nerve impulses in individual auditory nerve fibers of guinea pig. *J. Neurophysiol.*, **17**, 97–122.

Tasaki, I. and Davis, H. (1955). Electric responses of individual nerve elements in cochlear nucleus to sound stimulation (guinea pig). *J. Neurophysiol.*, **18**, 151–158.

Thompson, R. F., Johnson, R. H., and Hoopes, J. J. (1963). Organization of auditory, somatic sensory, and visual projection to association fields of cerebral cortex in the cat. *J. Neurophysiol.*, **26**, 343–364.

Thurlow, W. R., Gross, N. B., Kemp, E. H., and Lowy, K. (1951). Microelectrode studies of neural auditory activity of cats. I. Inferior colliculus. *J. Neurophysiol.*, **14**, 289–304.

Tsuchitani, C. and Boudreau, J. C. (1964). Wave activity in the superior olivary complex of the cat. *J. Neurophysiol.*, **27**, 814–827.

Tunturi, A. R. (1952). A difference in the representation of auditory signals for the left and right ears in the iso-frequency contours of the right middle ectosylvian auditory cortex of the dog. *Am. J. Physiol.*, **168**, 712–727.

Tunturi, A. R. (1960). Anatomy and physiology of the auditory cortex. In G. L. Ras-mussen and W. F. Windle (Eds.) *Neural mechanisms of the auditory and vestibular systems.* pp. 181–200. Thomas, Springfield, Illinois.

Vernier, V. G. and Galambos, R. (1957). Response of single medial geniculate units to repetitive click stimuli. *Am. J. Physiol.*, **188**, 233–237.

Wall, P. D. (1959). Repetitive discharge of neurons. *J. Neurophysiol.*, **22**, 305–320.

Wall, P. D. (1960). Cord cells responding to touch, damage, and temperature of skin. *J. Neurophysiol.*, **23**, 197–210.

Wall, P. D. and Cronly-Dillon, J. R. (1960). Pain, itch, and vibration. *A. M. A. Archs. Neurol.*, **2**, 365–375.

Ward, W. D. (1963). Absolute pitch. *Sound*, **2** (3), 14–21.

Wever, E. G. (1949). *Theory of hearing.* Wiley, New York.

Wever, E. G. (1962). Hearing. In P. R. Farnsworth (Ed.) *Annual review of psychology.* Vol. 13, pp. 225–250. Annual Reviews, Palo Alto.

Wever, E. G. (1964). The physiology of the peripheral hearing mechanism. In W. S. Fields and B. R. Alford (Eds.) *Neurological aspects of auditory and vestibular disorders.* pp. 24–50. Thomas, Springfield, Illinois.

Whitfield, I. C. and Evans, E. F. (1964). Unit responses in the unanesthetized cortex to steady and varying acoustic stimuli. *Electroenceph. Clin. Neurophysiol.,* **16,** 623 (A).

Whitfield, I. C. and Evans, E. F. (1965). Responses of auditory cortical neurons to stimuli of changing frequency. *J. Neurophysiol.,* **28,** 655–672.

Wiener, N. (1948). *Cybernetics.* Wiley, New York.

Wilson, V. J., Talbot, W. H., and Kato, M. (1964). Inhibitory convergence upon Renshaw cells. *J. Neurophysiol.,* **27,** 1063–1079.

Windle, W. F. (1963). Neuropathology of certain forms of mental retardation. *Science,* **140,** 1186–1189.

Woolsey, C. N. (1960). Organization of cortical auditory system: a review and a synthesis. In G. L. Rasmussen and W. F. Windle (Eds.) *Neural mechanisms of the auditory and vestibular systems.* pp. 165–180. Thomas, Springfield, Illinois.

Chapter Ten

Functional Manifestations of Lesions of the Sensorineural Structures

FOREWORD

When a clinician meets a research scientist from his own field of specialization, he sometimes shows a little awe, and sometimes shows a little displeasure—the former because the researcher knows some things that the clinician does not; the latter because that knowledge is not often enough applied to the practical problems of the clinician's daily existence. The researcher, in turn, responds in the same ambivalent ways toward the clinical worker. He is impressed by the practitioner's talents—talents of a sort that the theorist usually lacks—but he is distressed that the talents are sometimes applied in ways that are counter to currently accepted theory. Too often, these ambivalences seem excessively one-sided, with the clinician getting too much blame and too little credit. In *this* field of study, based as it is in a physiological system, auditory science meets otological and audiological practice daily. This field has one broad advantage over many, though, in that the laboratory worker and the clinic worker usually recognize that they can't do without each other. Many of the insights into complex auditory processes have come about because of the investigation of the causes of a pathological condition. And many of the therapeutic procedures now in use stem from an ivory-tower inquiry. Harold Schuknecht is one of the rare students of hearing who is known for both kinds of work.

Functional Manifestations of Lesions of the Sensorineural Structures

Harold F. Schuknecht[*]

I. INTRODUCTION

The relation between measured changes in hearing and pathological alterations in the auditory systems of man and animals leads to improved understanding of the functional role of the anatomical structures, and to more precise clinical diagnoses. New methods for the prevention and alleviation of deafness also evolve. Concepts concerning the pathophysiology of the auditory system certainly must be amended too as clinical and pathological findings are accumulated. And, of course, knowledge of the ways in which auditory structures can fail cannot help leading to a better understanding of the operation of the normal auditory system.

II. LESIONS OF THE SENSE ORGAN

Only the organ of Corti is ordinarily considered in discussions of the auditory sense organ; however, it is more correct to include all the structures of the cochlear duct. Alterations in the inner ear fluids as well as structural changes in the organ of Corti, stria vascularis,

[*] Harvard Medical School and Massachusetts Eye and Ear Infirmary, Boston, Massachusetts.

tectorial membrane, Reissner's membrane and basilar membrane interfere with sensory function.

The important cytological elements in the organ of Corti are (a) the hair cells; (b) the supporting cells (the pillars of Corti, Deiters's cells, Hensen's cells, and sulcus cells); (c) the tectorial membrane; and (d) the basilar membrane. In animal specimens fixed by arterial perfusion, it is possible to evaluate the extent of change in individual cells, but in human specimens, postmorten autolysis makes it impossible to determine more than the presence or absence of cells. Alterations in the inner-ear fluids appear to produce the same type of dysfunction as that created by structural changes in the organ of Corti. Changes in the fluids may consist of alterations in volume, in biochemistry (electrolytes, proteins, and enzymes), or in bioelectric potentials. Representative clinical entities in this group of disorders are Ménière's disease, deafness due to atrophy of the stria vascularis, and tumors of the internal acoustic canal.

Some auditory phenomena are significant in the diagnosis of sensory lesions. They include elevated auditory thresholds, loudness recruitment, lowered speech-discrimination ability, and diplacusis.

A.   Elevation of Auditory Thresholds

Microscopic studies demonstrated a close relation between hair-cell population and the magnitude of the threshold elevation (Schuknecht, 1953), but such relations are significant only in ears in which the hair-cell loss extends over several millimeters and is uniform. The experimental findings show that a partial loss of the outer hair cells results in a threshold elevation of less than 50 dB; the magnitude of the elevation depends upon the number of cells missing (Fig. 1). A loss of the outer hair cells together with some of the inner hair cells creates hearing losses greater than 50 dB. These relations apply to lesions involving frequencies up to 4000 Hz; for higher frequencies, the threshold elevations are greater. A complete loss of hair cells throughout the cochlea creates total deafness. There is no evidence that nerve endings in the cochlea can be excited acoustically without hair cells.

Atrophy of the stria vascularis (Figs. 2 and 3) of the middle and apical turns in the human cochlea creates threshold elevations that are nearly equal for all frequencies (Schuknecht and Igarashi, 1964). There appears to be no close relation between the extent of strial atrophy and the magnitude of threshold elevation. However, only the presence or absence of strial tissue can be determined with a light microscope; maybe varying amounts of the remaining tissue are non-functional. In these cochleae, there is a normal volume of endolymph, but presumably some quality of the fluid is altered as a result of the strial atrophy, which in turn adversely affects the sensitivity of the sense organ throughout the cochlea.

There is one other interesting possible source of threshold elevation—cochlear conductive deafness. At this time, though, such a hearing loss is a strictly hypothetical concept.

B. Loudness Recruitment

The recruitment phenomenon was described by Fowler (1937) as occurring in patients with "perceptive deafness." Simply stated, a patient with loudness recruitment responds to increased stimulus intensity with an abnormally rapid rise in loudness. Even though the listener's threshold is elevated, a high stimulus intensity may produce loudness equal to that in a normal ear. Another manifestation of the recruitment phenomenon may be an increased ability to detect small changes in stimulus intensity (a decreased intensity difference limen) (Lüscher, 1950).

Dix *et al.* (1948) were the first to note the absence of loudness recruitment in patients with lesions that involve only the cochlear nerve. Audiometric data make it obvious that the recruitment phenomenon is related to dysfunction of the sense organ and may occur in cochleae with alterations in endolymph as well as in those with structural changes in the organ of Corti.

A precise neurophysiological correlate of loudness is not known. One possibility is that loudness is determined by the total number of impulses arriving at the auditory cortex per unit of time. This total would include the number of nerve fibers excited and the frequency of the impulses within these fibers.

One of the pathological correlates of loudness recruitment is partial loss of hair cells, and a disorder that typifies this condition is stimulation deafness (Davis *et al.*, 1950). The earliest structural change that results from high-intensity stimulation is injury to the outer hair cells —possibly because they are located on the basilar membrane about midway between its fixed margins, so that the amplitude of the membrane movement is greatest there. When the supporting elements of the organ of Corti are not severely injured, the innervation of the area may be preserved (Schuknecht, 1953). Apparently it is the dis-

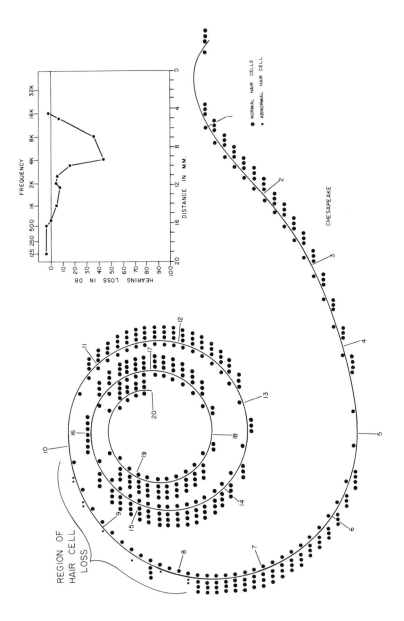

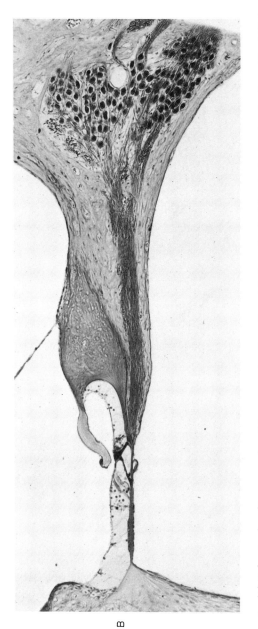

B

Figure 1 (A) Behavioral audiogram and cochlear reconstruction of a cat that received a blow to the head; animal sacrificed 22 days after injury. The circles indicate hair cells. The loss of hair cells from the 7.75–10.5 mm region is related to a hearing loss for 4000 and 8000 Hz. (B) Photomicrograph showing a loss of outer hair cells as a result of high-intensity acoustic stimulation. The inner hair cells and pillar cells appear normal, and the spiral ganglion is normal. The cat was sacrificed three months after injury.

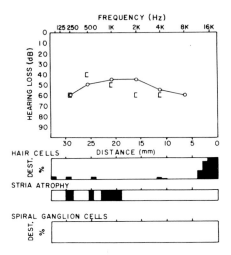

Figure 2 This 89-year-old patient complained of a slowly progressive hearing loss during the last 25 years of life. Atrophy of the stria vascularis in the apical half is the only significant structural change in the cochlea.

proportion between the population of hair cells and the population of cochlear neurons that provides the anatomical basis for loudness recruitment in stimulation deafness.

The extent of loss of cochlear neurons usually parallels the extent of injury suffered by the supporting cells of the organ of Corti, particularly Deiter's cells and the pillar cells (Schuknecht, 1953). The organ of Corti may be stripped of hair cells, but, if the pillars and Deiter's cells remain, there will usually be little or no loss of neurons. When the height of the pillar arch shortens or the outer pillars partially collapse, there probably is some decrease in innervation density. In acquired lesions, a total loss of pillar cells and Deiters's cells is commonly associated with a severe loss of cochlear neurons. But there are exceptions. Occasionally, the change that follows infectious labyrinthitis is characterized by a homogeneous eosinophilic deposit in the fluid spaces of the organ of Corti, particularly in Corti's tunnel. Such a deposit is associated with a severe loss of cochlear neurons even when the supporting cells are preserved. In hereditary dysgenesis or agenesis of the organ of Corti, on the other hand, normal innervation may exist in the presence of gross anomalies in the supporting cells (Fig. 4).

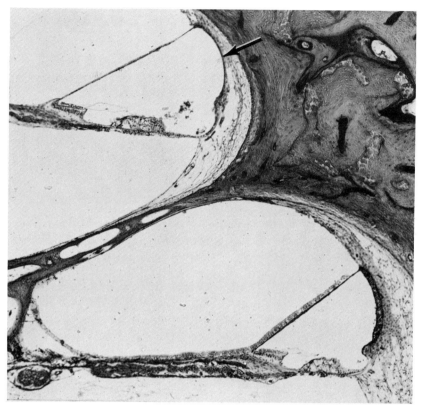

Figure 3 Photomicrograph from an elderly patient with a slowly progressive hearing loss characterized by a flat audiometric curve. Note atrophy of the stria vascularis in the middle turn (arrow).

Loudness recruitment is also found in ears with endolymphatic hydrops (Ménière's disease), and in those with atrophic changes in the stria vascularis. Both conditions are characterized anatomically by normal hair-cell and neuronal populations (Schuknecht, 1963), and functionally by flat (equal loss) pure-tone audiograms. It seems reasonable to suspect that chemical alterations in the endolymph in these ears results in the loss in sensitivity of the end-organ. The anatomical findings in "recruiting" cochleae appear to be consistent with the hypothesis that intense loudness sensation requires normal or near normal afferent innervation and a defective sense organ, but one possessing sufficient hair cells to excite these fibers (Fig. 5).

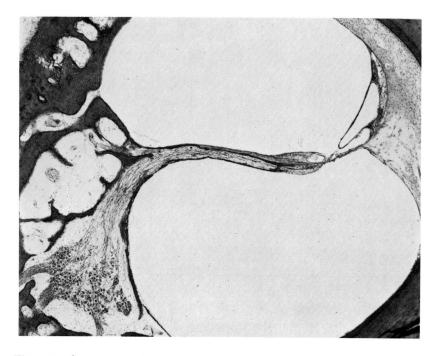

Figure 4 Photomicrograph showing dysgenesis of the structures of the cochlear duct, with severe anomaly of the organ of Corti in the presence of a normal spiral ganglion. This ten-year-old child was born deaf.

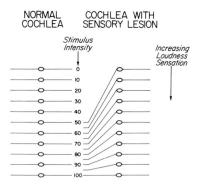

Figure 5 Model demonstrating a possible mechanism for loudness recruitment and the decreased intensity difference limen. On either side of an arbitrary stimulus intensity scale are schematically drawn sets of neurons representing populations for the normal cochlea and for the cochlea with a sensory lesion. Let us assume that, with increasing stimulus intensity, an increasing number of neurons are activated. For the normal cochlea, a full set of neurons is activated at an intensity of 100, and loudness sensation is maximum. In the cochlea with the sensory lesion, however, the level at

C. Diminished Discrimination for Speech

The ability of the cochlea to receive acoustic information and code it into appropriate patterns of neural activity determines the intelligibility of complex signals such as speech. A threshold loss, regardless of whether it involves a broad or restricted region of the auditory spectrum, leaves acoustic information unrepresented in the neural patterns that flow to the higher centers. Increasing signal intensity to optimum suprathreshold levels may improve the neural pattern, but defects can persist for several reasons:

1. When hair cells are either missing or diseased, an alteration of sensitivity will occur, and abnormal patterns of neural discharge may be expected.

2. The recruitment phenomenon produces a condition whereby the loudness scale is compressed with the effect that the neural pattern is abnormal, and speech discrimination is diminished.

3. Pitch distortion, be it the result of harmonic distortions originating in the middle or inner ear, or of a shift in response zones along the cochlear partition, results in interference with the normal neural coding process and in diminished discrimination.

D. Distortion of Pitch

Sensory lesions may result in distortion of the sense of pitch. A pure tone may be heard as noisy, rough, or buzzing. It may sound double, as though two tones were being introduced in combination. A tone may sound pure, but its pitch may be different from that perceived by the normal ear. The former distortions of pitch sensation are termed monaural diplacusis; the last is called binaural diplacusis.

One possible explanation for diplacusis is distortion. The auditory system responds unequally to different frequencies, so, when the ear is driven at high intensities, and nonlinear distortion is introduced, a cochlea with a localized area of injury (and thus with hearing loss for a restricted range of frequencies) may demonstrate diplacusis because a more responsive area of the cochlea is responding to a harmonic

---

which the first neural unit is excited is at an intensity of 50. As stimulus intensity is increased, however, additional neurons are activated at an abnormally rapid rate, so that at an intensity of 100, the full set of neurons is activated and loudness sensation equals that of the normal ear. It also is apparent from a study of the model that a smaller change in stimulus intensity is required in the pathological ear to activate more neurons than in the normal ear, the psychoacoustic manifestation of which is the decreased intensity difference limen.

tone introduced by the distortion. Studies by Békésy (1960) and by Wever and Lawrence (1954) showed frequency distortions to occur even at moderate stimulus intensities, particularly for the low frequencies.

Another explanation is based on the concept that the pitch displacement is the result of a shift, on the cochlear partition, of the location of maximum neural activity coincident with the spread of the field of excitation for the fundamental tone. This thesis gains support from the study of Davis *et al.* (1950), who investigated pitch and loudness sensation in human subjects following exposures to pure tones at high intensities. They made several pertinent observations:

1. Large amounts of diplacusis are produced only when hearing losses are restricted to a small frequency range.

2. Large displacements of pitch are always upward.

3. There is a strong tendency for many different frequencies to sound the same in pitch, with their pitches being displaced upward by varying amounts (to the same final pitch).

4. Usually, loudness increases while pitch remains constant as the frequency of the test tone is increased at constant intensity.

5. As the intensity of the test tone is increased, the displacement of pitch decreases (and loudness increases), until finally, pitch matches that for a normal ear.

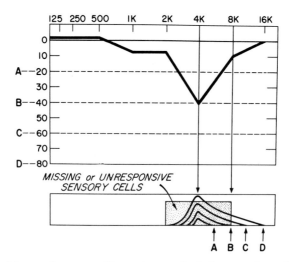

Figure 6 Model to explain a possible mechanism for diplacusis. The audiogram shows a 4000-Hz "dip" characteristic of stimulation deafness and typical of the temporary hearing losses produced by Davis *et al.* (1950). The underlying bar represents the total

Figure 6 shows a model that explains how the place theory of pitch perception and the resonance curves of displacement of the cochlear partition may interact to account for diplacusis.

III. LESIONS OF THE ACOUSTIC NERVE

Audiometric study of patients with early tumors of the acoustic nerve has uncovered a pattern of dysfunction that is characteristic of the loss of cochlear neurons (Fig. 7). Similar hearing losses occur in presbycusis (Schuknecht, 1955) (Figs. 8 and 9) and in cases of multiple sclerosis in which there is demyelinization of auditory nerve fibers.

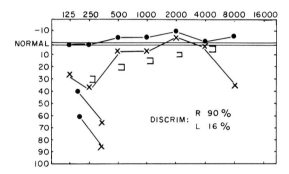

Figure 7   Audiogram of a patient with acoustic neurinoma on the left side. The pure-tone thresholds for the speech frequencies are near normal, but the speech discrimination score is only 16 percent.

population of sensory cells. The stippled area is a zone in which the outer hair cells are nonfunctional, and only the less sensitive inner hair cells are responsive. Curves A, B, C, and D represent displacement amplitudes on the basilar membrane for sensation levels of 20, 40, 60, and 80 dB for the 4000-Hz tone. The model indicates that, at a 20 dB sensation level (Curve A), the displacement pattern lies entirely within the zone of unresponsive units. At 40 dB (curve B), the displacement pattern has moved far enough in the basal direction to activate neural units in the region for which the characteristic frequency is 8000 Hz, and the pitch perceived is that for 8000 Hz, instead of that for the fundamental tone of 4000 Hz. The concept, of course, relegates a strong role to the place theory of pitch perception. At 60 dB (Curve C), the maximum neural activity still occurs at point B, and pitch is perceived as for 8000 Hz, but louder than before. At a level of 80 dB (Curve D), the displacement pattern is sufficiently intense to excite responsive sensory units, presumably inner hair cells with higher thresholds, in the 4000-Hz region, and (possibly aided by the mechanism of recruitment) pitch matches a test tone of 4000 Hz.

The auditory manifestations of a loss of some of the cochlear neurons in the presence of a normal organ of Corti are (*a*) decreased speech discrimination in the presence of a good pure-tone threshold, and (*b*) absence of loudness recruitment. Another behavioral phenomenon that sometimes occurs in such ears is abnormally rapid fatigue during sustained stimulation; however, this condition is less consistent and may result from the chemical alterations that are known to occur in the inner-ear fluids coincidental with tumors of the acoustic nerve (Schuknecht and Seifi, 1963; Schuknecht *et al.*, 1968).

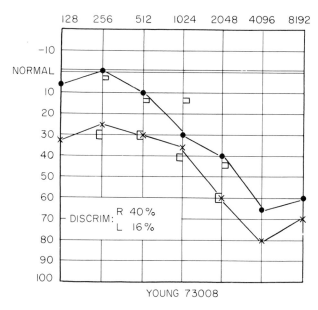

Figure 8 Audiogram of an elderly patient with a moderate high-frequency hearing loss and a severe loss of auditory discrimination. A progressive loss of speech discrimination in the presence of rather stable pure-tone thresholds in older people has as its underlying correlate a progressive loss of cochlear neurons.

Among those who have contributed information on cochlear nerve sectioning are Wittmaack (1911), who reported that the cochlear nerve could be sectioned in animals without injury to the organ of Corti, and, later, Kaida (1927–1931) and Hallpike and Rawdon-Smith (1934), who confirmed this observation and showed that, to prevent degeneration of the membranous labyrinth, it is necessary to avoid injury to the internal auditory artery.

Dandy (1934) performed partial section of the VIIIth cranial nerve for the relief of Ménière's disease, and found that frequently no

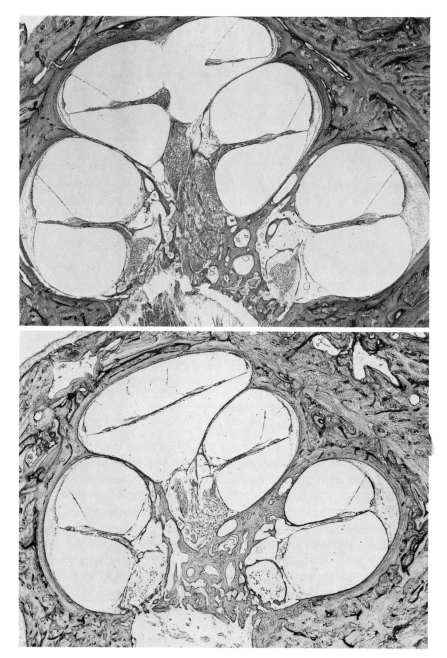

Figure 9 Top: Photomicrograph showing a normal spiral ganglion in a 54-year-old woman with normal hearing. Bottom: Severe degeneration of the spiral ganglion in an 85-year-old man with a progressive hearing loss during the later years of life.

change in auditory thresholds occurs even if large portions of the nerve are sacrificed. The hearing losses that do occur are for high frequencies.

Neff (1947) performed partial section of the cochlear nerve in conditioned cats, and found that severe neural lesions are compatible with normal auditory thresholds. He also found that hearing losses, when produced, are always for high frequencies, even though attempts were made to section different portions of the nerve.

It is now quite clear that these investigators produced high-frequency hearing losses because they selectively sectioned the afferent innervation from the basal turn of the cochlea, which has a superficial and posterior position in the cochlear nerve trunk, making it vulnerable to the surgeon approaching the nerve at the internal auditory meatus, through the posterior cranial fossa.

Before it was known that large deficits of cochlear neurons could exist without elevation of pure-tone thresholds, we performed an experiment (on cats) in which cochlear nerves were partially sectioned, after which hearing was tested behaviorally (Fig. 10). Histological studies and ganglion-cell counts revealed that up to 75 percent of the afferent innervation to a region of the cochlea can be sacrificed without creating threshold elevations for frequencies with their fields of excitation in those regions (Schuknecht and Woellner, 1955). Subsequently, Elliott (1961) determined the effect of a loss of cochlear neurons on pitch discrimination (Fig. 11). Cats with greater than 90 percent deficits have normal difference limens for frequency. The data suggest that pitch discrimination is not related to innervation density. Possibly it is related to a spatial shift of activity within the population of cochlear neurons.

A summary analysis of the data from both human observations and animal experiments leads to these conclusions:

1. The earliest manifestations of pure cochlear nerve degeneration is loss of discrimination for complex signals, which is manifested clinically as a loss in speech discrimination.

2. More than 75 percent of the cochlear neurons to a particular region of the cochlea may be missing without creating threshold losses for frequencies having their locus of importance in those regions.

3. More than 90 percent of the cochlear neurons may be missing to a particular region of the cochlea without affecting pitch discrimination for frequencies having their displacement patterns in those regions.

4. Loudness recruitment and the decreased intensity difference limen (which are characteristic of sensory lesions) do not occur with pure cochlear nerve lesions.

Despite the all-or-none law, a competent human auditory system can carry all the information required for speech intelligibility because of the great number of channels (fibers) in the communication system. In the diseased ear with a loss of auditory nerve fibers, there is a more stringent limit on the amount of information that can be transmitted to the brain. This deficiency results in an auditory system that can transmit simple signals, but cannot handle complex ones. It is well recognized that the most frequent early symptom of a lesion of the auditory nerve is a loss of speech discrimination, but only when the lesion is severe does a threshold loss for pure tones also occur.

IV. LESIONS OF THE AUDITORY CORTEX

It is a common opinion that lesions of the higher auditory pathways produce hearing disturbances that are characterized by loss of ability to discriminate and interpret the meaning of sound. The effect of unilateral temporal lobe tumors on hearing has interested clinicians for some time, but as yet, no clear diagnostic pattern of auditory loss has been established for such lesions (Henschen, 1896, Case 22; McNally *et al.*, 1936; Seiferth, 1949). Although bilateral temporal lobe lesions are uncommon, they are believed to exist in Pick's (1922) disease and in cerebro-vascular disorders. Such cases have been reported to have total bilateral hearing loss (Henschen, 1896; Mott, 1907; Bramwell, 1927). It should be understood, however, that most of these reports lack adequate audiometric and pathological documentation.

Recent studies indicate that a loss of speech discrimination also is a common early expression of a temporal lobe tumor. This observation was slow in developing because the discrimination defect does not register in commonly used tests, but becomes manifest only when more difficult test material is used. Apparently, the amount of auditory information that is provided with each phoneme in normal speech is in excess of what is necessary for intelligibility, and therefore, mild degrees of receptive aphasia (loss of auditory intelligibility) can escape detection by standard discrimination tests. Bocca *et al.* (1955) and Pietrantoni *et al.* (1956) showed, however, that if a patient with a temporal-lobe tumor is given a more difficult discrimination test consisting of distorted speech (accelerated, interrupted, limited

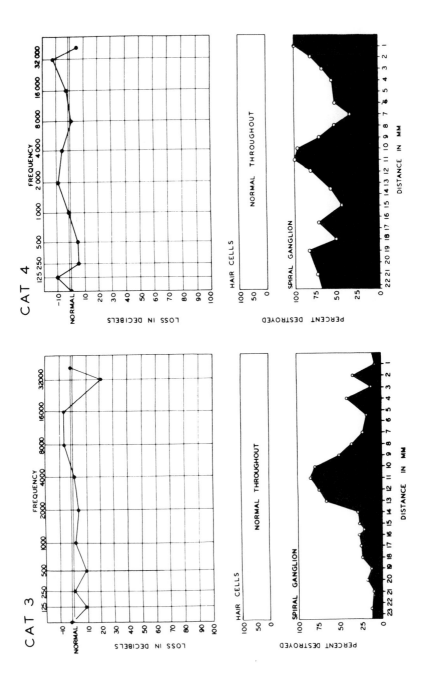

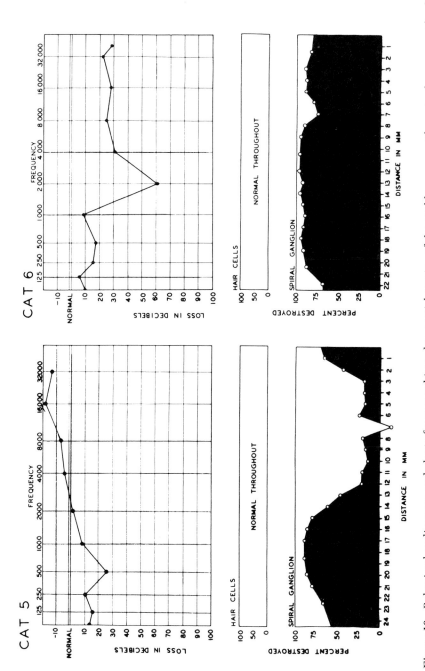

Figure 10 Behavioral audiograms and charts for cats subjected to partial section of the cochlear nerve. The animals were sacrificed about six weeks after nerve section. Note the normal auditory thresholds for cats 3 and 4 in spite of extensive loss of spiral-ganglion cells. A loss of more than 75 percent of spiral-ganglion cells results in a threshold elevation for pure tones.

in frequency range, delivered in noise), the intelligibility is diminished in the ear contralateral to the temporal lobe lesion. In patients with infantile hemiplegia, Goldstein *et al.* (1956) observed normal

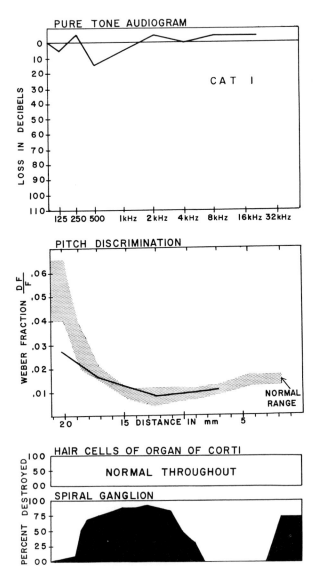

Figure 11 Normal audiogram and normal pitch discrimination in a cat with a 75 to 90 percent loss of spiral-ganglion cells in the 11 to 18 mm region. Pitch discrimination is plotted as the Weber fraction, and the stippled area indicates the normal range as determined on eight normal animals. Courtesy of Elliott.

pure-tone thresholds, but diminished speech discrimination, in the ear on the opposite side from the brain lesion.

The human cerebral cortex has been mapped according to minor variations in the pattern of gray matter. The auditory cortex of man is located in the superior temporal gyrus along the Sylvian fissure, which corresponds to topographical areas 41, 42, and 22 of Brodmann (1909). Campbell (1905) further divided this area into an audito-sensory region (41), thought to be related to auditory perception, and an audito-psychic region (42 and 22), thought to be important for auditory memory. These concepts are not established well enough to justify our thinking of these areas as discrete functional zones.

Further evidence regarding the function of the auditory cortex of man comes from the investigations of Penfield and Rasmussen (1950), who electrically stimulated the cortex during the course of intracranial operations performed under local anesthesia. They stated that (a) auditory responses are more numerous in the audito-psychic area, and less frequent in the audito-sensory area; (b) electrical stimulation results in a sensation of sound in some patients and of being deaf in others; and (c) auditory sensations resulting from cortical stimulation are most often referred to the contralateral ear. They also found that electrical stimulation close to the margins of the Sylvian fissure is more apt to produce a sensation of simple sounds, such as buzzing or ringing, but stimulation away from the fissure is more apt to introduce an element of interpretation of the sound. These observations have not been confirmed and must be interpreted with some caution.

In a series of experiments on behaviorally trained cats, Jerison and Neff (1953) found that total bilateral ablation of the cortical projection areas of the auditory system does not alter the pure-tone thresholds. They found that, after auditory cortical ablations, cats can respond to (a) the onset of a sound, (b) a change in the intensity of a stimulus, and (c) a change in the frequency of a tone, but they cannot respond to changes in (a) patterns of tones, (b) durations of sounds, or (c) localization of sound in space. In an analysis of these findings, Neff (1965) pointed out that the tasks that can be learned appear to involve the use of new neural units, when the stimulus is altered. It is not known whether these tasks are performed by other lower centers or by other parts of the higher centers.

V. COMMENTS

The enormous social and economic impact of deafness on individual people has not been appreciated generally by those who have not experienced it. The otologist, who in years past was concerned mainly with life-saving surgical procedures, can now direct more of his attention to the management of the hard-of-hearing patient (Davis, 1960). His objectives are served by closer communication with the basic scientist. In turn, the scientist needs to know the range of pathological entities that occur so that he may encompass their existence in his theoretical statements. A theory of pitch perception, for example, that ignores the existence of diplacusis is necessarily incomplete. A description of the auditory system's processing of complex signals cannot properly ignore the nature of recruitment. And the list continues in the same fashion. It is necessary for both the practitioner and the researcher to know each other's fields.

Thus, I have tried to define some of the general types of sensory and neural pathology that have been identified in animal and human ears, and have shown that they are expressed by distinct patterns of disorder in psychoacoustic function. For the diagnosis and management of otologic disorders, the intelligent interpretation of psychophysical test data is an important adjunct to the history and otologic examination. There is a continuing challenge for the otologist to seek applications for newly-gained knowledge concerning the auditory mechanisms in health and disease. The same challenge is reflected on the basic scientist to invent and modify so that our joint understanding of auditory function can grow.

REFERENCES

von Békésy, G. (1960). *Experiments in hearing.* McGraw-Hill, New York

Bocca, E., Calearo, C., Cassinari, V., and Miglivacca, F. (1955). Testing cortical hearing in temporal lobe tumors. *Acta Oto-Lar.,* **45,** 289–304.

Bramwell, E. (1927). Case of cortical deafness. *Brain,* **50,** 579–580.

Brodmann, K. (1909). *Vergleichende Lokalisationslehre der Grosshirnrinde in ihren Prinzipien dargestellt auf Grund des Zellenbaues.* Barth, Leipzig. (Reprinted 1925.)

Campbell, A. W. (1905). *Histological studies on the localization of cerebral function.* Cambridge Univ. Press, Cambridge, England.

Dandy, W. E. (1934). Effects on hearing after subtotal section of cochlear branch of auditory nerve. *Bull. Johns Hopkins Hosp.,* **55,** 240–243.

Davis, H. (1960). Contributions from deafness to neurophysiology and psychology. In H. K. Beecher (Ed.) *Disease and the advancement of basic science.* pp. 253–263. Harvard Univ. Press, Cambridge, Massachusetts.

Davis, H., Morgan, C., Hawkins, J., Galambos, R., and Smith, F. (1950). Temporary deafness following exposure to loud tones and noise. *Acta Oto-Lar., Suppl.* **88,** 1–57.

Dix, M. R., Hallpike, C. S., and Hood, J. D. (1948). Observations upon the loudness recruitment phenomenon, with especial reference to the differential diagnosis of disorders of the internal ear and VIIIth nerve. *J. Lar. Otol.*, **62**, 671–686.

Elliott, D. N. (1961). The effect of sensorineural lesions on pitch discrimination in cats. *Ann. Otol. Rhinol. Lar.*, **70**, 582–598.

Fowler, E. P. (1937). Measuring the sensation of loudness; a new approach to the physiology of hearing and the functional and differential diagnostic tests. *Archs Otolar.*, **26**, 514–521.

Goldstein, R., Goodman, A., and King, R. (1956). Hearing and speech in infantile hemiplegia before and after left hemispherectomy. *Neurology*, **6**, 869–875.

Hallpike, C. S. and Rawdon-Smith, A. F. (1934). The "Wever and Bray phenomenon," a study of the electrical response in the cochlea with especial reference to its origin. *J. Physiol., Lond.*, **81**, 395–408.

Henschen, S. E. (1896). *Klinische und anatomische Beiträge zur Pathologie des Gehirns.* Vol. 3. Almquist and Wiksell, Upsala, Sweden.

Jerison, H. and Neff, W. D. (1953). Effect of cortical ablation in the monkey on discrimination of auditory patterns. *Fedn Proc. Fedn Am. Socs. Exp. Biol.*, **12**, 73–74(A).

Kaida, Y. (1927–1931). Über das Verhalten des inneren Ohres nach Stammläsion des N. acusticus. *Jap. J. Med. Sci. Trans. Abstr., XII, Oto–Rhino-Lar.*, **1**, 237–241.

Lüscher, E. (1950). The difference limen of intensity variations of pure tones and its diagnostic significance. *Proc. R. Soc. Med.*, **43**, 1116–1128.

McNally, W. J., Erickson, T. C., Scott-Moncrieff, R., and Reeves, D. L. (1936). Brain tumors and hearing. *Ann. Otol. Rhinol. Lar.*, **45**, 797–799.

Mott, F. W. (1907). Bilateral lesion of the auditory cortical centre: Complete deafness and aphasia. *Brit. Med. J.*, **2**, 310–315.

Neff, W. D. (1947). The effects of partial section of the auditory nerve. *J. Comp. Physiol. Psychol.*, **40**, 203–215.

Neff, W. D. (1965). Auditory discriminations affected by cortical ablations. In A. B. Graham (Ed.) *International symposium: Sensorineural processes and disorders.* pp. 201–206. (Henry Ford Hospital), Little, Brown, Boston.

Penfield, W. and Rasmussen, G. (1950). *The cerebral cortex of man.* Macmillan, New York.

Pick, A. (1922). Bermerkungen zu der Arbeit von R. A. Pfeifer: Die Lokalisation der Tonskal innerhalb der kortikalen Hörsphäre, *Mschr. Psychiat. Neurol.*, **51**, 314.

Pietrantoni, L., Bocca, E., and Agazzi, C. (1956). Diagnosi delle sordità retrococleari. *Atti XLIV Congr. Soc. Ital. Lar. Otol. Rinol.* Idos, Milano.

Schuknecht, H. F. (1953). Lesions of the organ of Corti. *Trans. Am. Acad. Ophthal. Oto-Lar.*, **57**, 366–383.

Schuknecht, H. F. (1955). Presbycusis. *Laryngoscope*, **65**, 402–419.

Schuknecht, H. F. (1963). Meniere's disease: a correlation of symptomatology and pathology. *Laryngoscope*, **73**, 651–665.

Schuknecht, H. F. and Igarashi, M. (1964). Pathology of slowly progressive sensorineural deafness. *Trans. Am. Acad. Ophthal. Oto-Lar.*, **68**, 222–242.

Schuknecht, H. F. and Seifi, A. E. (1963). Experimental observations on the fluid physiology of the inner ear. *Ann. Otol. Rhinol. Lar.*, **72**, 687–712.

Schuknecht, H. F. and Woellner, R. C. (1955). An experimental and clinical study of deafness from lesions of the cochlear nerve. *J. Lar. Otol.*, **69**, 75–97.

Schuknecht, H. F., Griffin, W. L., Davies, G., and Silverstein, H. (1968). Chemical evaluation of inner ear fluid as a diagnostic aid. *Acta Oto-Lar.*, **65**, 169–173.

Seiferth, L. B. (1949). Verletzungen des Temporallappens und Otavusstörungen. *Arch. Ohr.-, Nas.- u. KehlkHeilk.*, **155**, 357–364.

Wever, E. G. and Lawrence, M. (1954). *Physiological acoustics.* Princeton Univ. Press, Princeton, New Jersey.

Wittmaack, K. (1911). Über sekundäre Degenerationen im inneren Ohre nach Akustikusstammverletzungen. *Verh. Dt. Otol. Ges.*, **20**, 289–296.

Chapter Eleven

Musical Perception

FOREWORD

For human listeners, the most important use of the auditory system is to perceive speech signals. Yet historically, the study of hearing has been occasioned more by an interest in aesthetics than in communication. Pythagoras and Aristotle, Kepler and Helmholtz, and most of the other early students of audition and acoustics began their studies because of questions about the nature of music. Today too, the student of hearing who is not also deeply interested in music is rare. Certainly, every aspect of the acoustic stimulus is important to musicians, and every aspect of the auditory response is pertinent to music. Conversely, everything we have learned about music is relevant to the search for knowledge about how the ear works. A complete theory of hearing must, for example, incorporate an explanation of why tones an octave apart sound, somehow, alike. It must encompass such problems as how absolute pitch functions, why musical instruments are indistinguishable from each other when certain short segments of their waveforms are removed, why some frequency combinations form acceptable complex tones, but slight variations do not, and so on. Dixon Ward, as both psychoacoustician and musician, has brought together the most important of the data on the perception of musical stimuli.

Musical Perception

W. Dixon Ward*

I. INTRODUCTION

The last few decades have produced important new procedures and results in regard to the physics and physiology of the auditory process. However, advances in knowledge about the perception of music during the same time have, by and large, been much less spectacular. This paradoxical state of affairs arises for two reasons.

First of all, there has been less work because there are less workers, and there are less workers because there is less money. Government research funds have been readily available since 1940 for research that provides a "practical application" to military or medical problems. But problems of musical perception, unfortunately, seldom have direct bearing on the solemn problems of national welfare. As a result there are at present no research organizations whose primary goal is the intensive study of musical perception, — organizations such as the Institute of Musical Science envisioned by Fletcher (1947). Therefore most of the recent work bearing on musical perception is either some sporadic output from research departments of certain musical instrument firms, is an incidental by-product of research on a more "important" subject, or has come from one of a scattered handful of scientists who somehow sandwich in a study or two between their teaching activities and supported research.

The second reason for the dearth of research is that musical perception is so inextricably bound up with individual preference. If a per-

---

* Department of Otolaryngology, University of Minnesota, Minneapolis, Minnesota.

son says he likes rock-and-roll and listens to it with evident pleasure, then rock-and-roll is music to him, no matter what it may be to you or me. If critics complain that a particular concert hall does not produce good music even when the New York Philharmonic is playing, then it is indeed a poor concert hall for those critics, no matter how well engineered its construction may have been. (On the other hand, critics' complaints do not tell us anything about what the average concertgoer thinks about the hall — or would have thought if he had not read the critics' comments.) Although well-planned and well-controlled preference studies are vital to musical esthetics, it is difficult to devise controls that are adequate to provide an unequivocal answer to experimental questions. Furthermore, it is easy to get completely bogged down in the nature-nurture argument in interpreting the results. Therefore, many scientists avoid the area entirely, and as Poland (1963) pointed out, too many musicians spend their time seeking a priori truths: "Instead of looking on music as a human experience and asking questions about musical behavior, they assume or search for universals" (Poland, 1963, p. 156).

The best that one can do in reviewing the facts about musical perception, therefore, is to consider the fields of controversy one by one and to point out what we do *not* know. I shall try to avoid topics that are matters of esthetic judgment only, although in some aspects of musical perception (such as vibrato and consonance for example), one cannot completely divorce the objective data from the subjective. Since the entire field of musical perception can hardly be covered in this short chapter, I shall concentrate most heavily on the perception of musical pitch.

II. THE ATTRIBUTES OF TONE

Music is, of course, an involved sequence of highly complex sounds. The complexity is so great that one must begin by simplifying the situation, even at the risk of oversimplification. The traditional method has been to study short sequences of one or two pure tones (sinusoids). If it sometimes turns out that results of experiments on pure tones are poor predictors of musical perception, it is more often the case that results with complex tones modify rather than negate those with pure tone. At any rate, the bulk of musical research has been done with pure tones.

The four attributes of auditory events having the most relevance to musical perception are pitch, loudness, timbre, and duration. Pitch and loudness are primarily functions of the physical parameters of frequency and intensity, respectively, and subjective duration is, of course, largely dependent on the physical duration, although none of these three attributes is completely independent of any of the physical dimensions listed. Timbre, which is a function of the harmonic content of the sound and hence ought not to apply to sinusoids at all, is often used as a wastebasket category; if two sounds are "different" though having the same pitch and loudness, then they must differ in timbre.

Auditory events also possess the attributes of density and volume. High-pitched sounds tend to be subjectively denser and less voluminous than low-pitched ones. Actually, sounds can be rated or scaled in terms of nearly any adjective that one wants to apply—witness the use by musicians of terms such as "dark" tones, "liquid" tones, "rounded" tones, etc. These "attributes" are linked fairly closely to timbre, and need not be considered further.

A diagram showing equal-pitch, -loudness, -volume, and -density curves over a small range of frequency and intensity (Stevens, 1934) is shown in Fig. 1. For constant loudness, only slight changes in in-

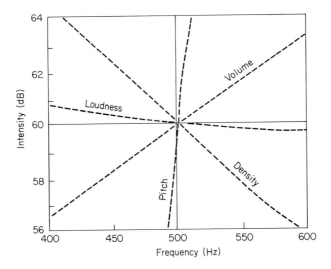

Figure 1 Equal-loudness, -pitch, -volume, and -density contours in the immediate vicinity of 500 Hz and 60 dB (Stevens, 1934. By permission from *Proceedings of the National Academy of Sciences.*)

tensity are needed as the frequency changes from 400 to 600 Hz; a similar constancy for pitch can also be seen. However, to hold volume constant, the intensity must be decreased. Figure 1 suggests that auditory density may be loudness per unit volume, just as the physical density of objects is the mass per unit volume; this hypothesis has been verified by Stevens *et al.* (1965).

A. Just-Noticeable Differences

Judgments of equality or inequality of stimuli with respect to a given attribute can be made with good reliability. The just-noticeable-difference *(jnd)* of frequency or intensity under various conditions is small, although the exact value obtained depends on the particular method employed. For example, slight changes in a sustained tone are more easily perceived than small differences between two tones presented successively (Montgomery, 1935). Under optimum conditions, changes of as little as 0.5 dB in intensity (Harris, 1963) or 0.1 percent in frequency (König, 1957) can be detected 75 percent of the time by the best listeners.

The listener's task becomes somewhat more difficult if he is required not only to detect a difference but to assign a *direction* to the change. It is a common experience that one may often have difficulty in deciding whether one is just a shade too sharp or too flat when tuning an instrument, even though it may be perfectly clear that the tuning is not correct. Difficulty in judging direction of pitch changes seems to be exaggerated for frequencies above about 4000 Hz (which, perhaps not just coincidentally, happens to be the fundamental frequency of the topmost note on the piano). This point is incidentally illustrated in what is probably the first study of the jnd for *pitch* (Henning, 1966). Henning cites Harris' (1952) argument that even though one varies only the *frequency* of the electrical signal to an earphone or loudspeaker, holding the *intensity* constant, one still has no assurance that differences in the response characteristics of the transducer or the auditory mechanism may not give rise to *loudness* differences between comparison stimuli that are in fact greater than the *pitch* differences. So Henning forced his subjects (two musicians) to listen *only* for pitch differences by randomly varying the intensities of the signal. (A better—or at least different—method would involve first determining an equal-loudness contour for the ear under test and then restricting the comparison stimuli to this contour, but no one has yet used this technique.) At any rate, Henning found that his jnds increased sharply at 5000 Hz, in contrast to the "classical" results of Shower and Biddulph (1931), who showed only a slight increase at this point. Although Henning attributes the difference to unwanted loudness changes associated with Shower and Biddulph's stimuli (their listeners' task was merely to detect a 3/sec frequency warble), it may just as well be ascribed to difficulty in assigning a *direction* to a pitch change at high frequencies.

Indeed, it may be that in some cultures, pitch is not typically regarded as having a "direction" at all. Tanner and Rivette (1964) report that 3 Indian students were unable to identify the direction of a pitch change corresponding to a frequency change of 4% (well over half a semit) at 1000 Hz.

Much greater variability is found in judgments of the *relative* loudness of two stimuli. Most of the work done in scaling loudness (as well as other intensive sensory attributes such as brightness of lights, intensity of odor, strength of handgrip, and roughness of sandpaper) has come from the Psycho-Acoustic Laboratory (now the Laboraory of Psychophysics) at Harvard. Judgments of relative loudness have been made with many different procedures (Stevens, 1959) and show conclusively that for the typical observer the loudness in "sones" is a power function of sound pressure with an exponent of about 0.6. So if one wants to double the loudness of a sound, he should raise the sound pressure level by about 10 dB. A 20-dB increase quadruples the loudness, a 30-dB increase changes it eight-fold, and so on. Armed with this knowledge, one could determine how much louder "fortissimo" is than "pianissimo" for musicians, by comparing the performed levels of passages so marked.

B. Pitch Scaling

The sone scale has become a fairly reliable and useful tool for the prediction of loudness judgments, and has therefore gained general acceptance. Not so, however, for an analogous scale for pitch, the "mel" scale. In procedures similar to those used in scaling loudness, observers can be asked to set the frequencies of a pair of stimuli so that the second is "twice as high" in pitch as the first (Stevens *et al.*, 1937); to adjust the third of three tones so that the "interval" between the second and third is the same as that between the first and second (Stevens and Volkmann, 1940); or to give a number that corresponds to the pitch of a second tone, given that the first (standard) is 100 (Beck and Shaw, 1963). In this type of pitch scaling too, the particular procedure used plays a large role in determining the results obtained, and individual differences are vast. Therefore, no one claims yet to have determined "the" mel scale. It is clear, though, that the pitch-extent involved here is quite different from what musicians mean by pitch. For example, 2000 Hz is much less than twice as "high" as 1000 Hz, and 200 Hz is much *more* than twice as high as 100 Hz, although both of these pairs of tones represent a span of one musical octave.

The fact that pitch-extent and musical pitch are *different* does not imply that one or the other is *wrong*. It is nonsense to give musical pitch a cavalier dismissal simply because an octave interval has a different size in mels depending on the frequency range, and to conclude that "these facts contradict the widespread notion that equal ratios of frequency give rise to equal intervals of pitch" (Stevens and Volkmann, 1940). Such statements alienate musicians from psychophysics. Any competent musician knows that equal ratios of frequency do indeed give rise to approximately equal intervals of pitch—as *he* defines intervals, at any rate. So when he reads such a statement, his tendency is to dismiss everything that the author says.

The fact of the matter is that pitch can be scaled in mels or in some other subjective musical interval such as semits (semitones), octaves, or fifths. When a quartet of singers is preparing to begin, only one note need be sounded on the pitchpipe in order for each voice to begin at its appropriate pitch. If the sounded tone is A4 (440 Hz), the first tenor, for example, mentally shifts a musical fifth down from this tone and comes in fairly accurately on D4. He apparently has an internal scale of relative pitch, a movable conceptual grid or template, so to speak, that specifies the pitch relations among the notes of our Western scale. When one is able to start at some arbitrary frequency and lay off equal subjective intervals higher and lower without instrumental aid, one determines a valid subjective scale whether the steps are 100-mel intervals or subjective octaves.

Measuring pitch in mels, however, especially if the subject has any musical training, is analogous to pacing off a room for wall-to-wall carpeting when a steel measuring tape is handy. Why not measure length to a fraction of an inch using the tape instead of merely determining that it is between three and four yards? Judgments of what constitutes "half-pitch" vary widely; the judgments of five observers who were to set an oscillator to "half of 2000 Hz" ranged from 508 to 1006 Hz, and the typical intrasúbject average deviation was about 10 percent (Stevens *et al.*, 1937). In contrast, the standard deviation of judgments of "octave above 1000 Hz" is less than 3 percent and that of a single observer's judgments only about 0.6 percent (Ward,

1954). Clearly, much finer measurements can be made using subjective musical intervals.

Subjective musical pitch is regarded with suspicion by the mel proponents because they look on it as an attempt to "copy" the physical musical scale and as therefore merely a deliberate commission of the "stimulus error." For example, Stevens, in discussing how one may judge loudness, has said, "With enough experience, people can *learn* the decibel scale and become fairly good at making estimates of decibel levels. At the same time, however, they can also judge apparent loudness—how the sound really sounds to them" (Stevens, 1959, p. 1002). This use of the word "really" provides insight into Stevens's metaphysics, but is of little other relevance. If a given person could make judgments of decibel levels with more precision than he could of sone levels, without any instrumental aid whatever, then the "subjective decibel" scale of this person would be just as valid as— and somewhat more useful than—his sone scale. The same thing goes, of course, for mels and subjective octaves. It can be argued that there is just as much cultural overlay involved in making "twice-as-much" judgments as in making octave judgments—one does not come equipped with an automatic internal "doubler" or "halver" (for an exchange of views in this vein, see the 1963 letters by Warren and by Stevens).

According to Revesz (1913), pitch should always be considered to have two aspects: a unidirectional *tone-height* and a cyclical *chroma*. While tone-height increases continuously as frequency is raised, chroma is repeated every octave. In his schema, then, musical pitch may be represented as a line spiralling up the surface of a cylinder, getting ever higher in tone-height as frequency increases, yet returning to the same chroma (a given chroma corresponds to all points on a particular surface line parallel to the axis of the cylinder) every time the frequency is doubled, approximately. Thus 440 Hz has the same chroma as 220 Hz although it is much higher in tone-height. An ingenious study by Shepard (1964) has demonstrated that chroma and tone-height can be studied separately.

Revesz assumed that a subjective octave corresponded exactly to a physical octave, and that all listeners would agree on this point, but these assumptions are not correct. Individual scales of musical pitch of pure tones, derived from octave judgments, show reliable individual differences (Ward, 1954). Furthermore, the subjective octave turns out to be slightly larger than the physical octave. Though most pronounced for frequencies above 1000 Hz, this enlargement holds over the entire frequency range. For example, in judging the octave of 300 Hz, the higher tone must be made 0.8 percent sharp in order for the interval to sound like a true octave, a fact ignored for the many years that have elapsed since Stumpf and Meyer (1898) first discovered it.

The usefulness of musical-pitch relations is exemplified by a study by Elfner (1964). He was interested in the effect of sleep deprivation on pitch perception. He found that the frequency separation required for a satisfactory subjective octave increased about 5 percent after 24 hours of sleeplessness. The same effect could have been measured by using judgments of half pitch, but in order to reach the same level of statistical significance, many times as many estimates would have to be made because of the larger intra- and intersubject variability.

III. TUNING AND TEMPERAMENT

If, then, our musicians have a musical-pitch template that they can use to measure pitches, what is the nature of the scale after which it is patterned? In other words, what physical scale are they trying to duplicate? Unfortunately, there are numerous claimants. The three main contenders are Pythagorean tuning, just intonation, and equal temperament (Table I).

TABLE I

COMPARISON OF THE MAJOR THEORETICAL SYSTEMS OF TEMPERAMENT
Numerical values indicate the distance in cents (1/1200 octave) between the unison and the scale step concerned.

	Solfeggio	Just intonation	Equal temperament	Pythagorean tuning
unison	do	0	0	0
minor 2nd		112	100	90
major 2nd	re	204	200	204
minor 3rd		316	300	294
major 3rd	mi	386	400	408
fourth	fa	498	500	498
tritone		590	600	612
fifth	sol	702	700	702
minor 6th		814	800	792
major 6th	la	884	900	906
minor 7th		996	1000	996
major 7th	ti	1088	1100	1110
octave	do	1200	1200	1200

In equal temperament (ET), the octave (most scales agree that a physical octave should be a frequency ratio of 2 : 1) is divided into 12 equal logarithmic steps; each interval is called a *semit* and represents a frequency range about 5.9 percent greater than the next lower. A semit is divided into 100 equal steps or cents; thus an octave is 1200 cents wide. In other words, with this hypothetical logarithmic grid, the wires all have the same separation.

The other scales have slightly irregular spacing. In one variety of just intonation (JI), the intermediate steps must be determined by the smallest whole-number ratios possible. Thus the musical fifth in JI is given by a frequency ratio of 3 : 2 (a difference in frequency level of 702 cents instead of the 700 of ET), the major third by 5 : 4 (386 cents instead of 400), and so on.

Finally, the Pythagorean system of tuning (PT) is based upon the use of successive "perfect" fifths (the 3 : 2 ratio, or 702 cents). Thus G, a fifth above C, will be 702 cents higher than C, as in JI. However, the next step is a fifth above G, which gives a D that is 702+702=1404 cents above the starting C. Subtracting an octave of 1200 cents (always permissible here) gives D, the major second, a value of 204 cents. Similarly, going on up by fifths gives a major sixth, A, of 906 cents, a major third, E, of 408 cents, and so on. The trouble is that continuation of this process culminates in a fourth, F, of 522 cents, and an octave, B sharp, that is 24 cents too sharp. One way to resolve this problem is to go *downward* by fifths for half the intervals; thus, F would be 702 cents below C, or 498 above the lower C. Similarly, B flat is 702 below that, or 996 cents, and so on. The intersection of the upward half with the downward now occurs at the tritone (F sharp or G flat—whichever you prefer), which is either 612 or 588 cents.

This discussion has considerably simplified the problem; hundreds of pages are still being printed each year in discussions of JI and its "beauty." (For anyone interested in the intricacies of tuning and temperament, Barbour's 1951 book can be highly recommended.) The main point here, though, is that all systems except ET stress that simple ratios are preferred. Although the ancients may have believed that simple ratios were inherently better *per se*, the modern justification for small ratios takes two slightly more tenable forms. The first is based mostly on the physics of the situation. If the fundamental frequencies of two simultaneous complex musical tones bear a small-number ratio to each other, then many of the partials will coincide. If the frequency of one changes ever so slightly, then beats will appear between partials that formerly coincided. Therefore, in order to minimize these beats, one performer may automatically "lock into" synchrony with the other, producing JI. Tacit here is the assumption that beats are undesirable.

The second justification is really not much different, except that the problem has been moved into the receiving organism. It is hypothesized that we prefer pairs of tones for which the frequencies of neural discharge agree. This old suggestion of Max Meyer's (1898) is championed by Boomsliter and Creel (1961).

Supporters of ET, however, are not much impressed by such arguments. They ignore the theoretical arguments and instead emphasize the practical advantage of equal temperament, namely that one need not retune an instrument every time the music changes key. And they point out that the evidence provides precious little support for the desirability of whole-number ratios. Barbour (1951, p. 201) concluded his book as follows, "This contemporary dispute about tuning is perhaps a tempest in a teapot. It is probably true that all the singers and players are singing and playing false most of the time. But their errors are errors from equal temperament. No well-informed person today would suggest that these errors consistently resemble departures from just intonation or from any other tuning system described in these pages. Equal temperament does remain the standard, however imperfect the actual accomplishment may be." There are still many music theorists who take issue with this rather strong statement. Let us, therefore, see what the evidence does indicate.

Only recently have there been devised means for measuring the frequencies of short tones accurately. Two chief methods are now in use: (a) actually measuring the number of waves per unit time from an oscillographic trace of the tone, and (b) using the chromatic stroboscope. The chromatic stroboscope is a device having twelve patterned dials whose speeds of rotation, regulated by a temperature-controlled, 440-Hz tuning fork, correspond very nearly to the steps of the equally-tempered scale. That is, each successive wheel is spinning 5.946 percent faster than the next lower one. The incoming signal from a microphone, recorder, or phonograph, amplified and clipped, controls the flashing of a light that illuminates the dials. When the frequency of the signal (or of one of its components) corresponds exactly to one of the steps of the equally-tempered scale, then the pattern on the corresponding disc appears stationary. A slight mistuning will produce a slowly rotating pattern whose speed of rotation is proportional to the mistuning. A control permits adjustment of the speed of the entire set of dials over a range of 100 cents, so that any frequency up to 4000 Hz can be accurately determined.

Greene (1937), in Seashore's laboratory, used oscillographic recording. He analyzed eleven solo performances by six violinists on three "standard musical selections," recording the difference between successive notes. In his analysis, all 2-semit changes were called major seconds, all 3-semit changes minor thirds, and so on, regardless of the actual notes involved. This procedure assumes that the pitch of each successive note is derived by the musician from the immediately preceding one rather than from its relation to the keynote. That is, sequences of F to G and C to D are lumped into the same category, since both involve a movement of 2 semits whether the piece is written in C or F or any other key. Table II shows Greene's results.

TABLE II

DISTRIBUTION OF INTERVALS IN CENTS (FROM GREENE, 1937); VIOLIN SOLOISTS

Interval	25 percentile	Mean	50 percentile
Minor 2nd	82	88	97
Major 2nd	199	206	214
Minor 3rd	289	296	301
Major 3rd	400	406	417
4th	492	498	505

Nickerson (1948) took exception to this procedure. He argued that, when one is performing a piece of music in the key of C, only the sequence C to D gives information about the major second. F and G, even when sounded in succession, indicate the intonation of the fourth and fifth, respectively, since the listener refers all tones to the keynote and thus is really judging C to F and C to G. His data were therefore analyzed from this viewpoint.

In Nickerson's study, each of the 24 members of six string quartets played the first 80 measures of Haydn's Emperor Quartet, Opus 76, N. 3 twice—first solo and then with the members of the quartet. The theme of this movement, better known as "Deutschland Über Alles," is a 20-measure tune in G that is repeated by each of the four voices in succession. Nickerson, using a film loop and chromatic stroboscope, analyzed 25 percent (randomly selected) of the As, Bs, Cs, Ds, and Es for each voice while it was carrying the theme. No harmony parts were

included in the analysis. For each performance, the interval between
the note in question and the keynote (obtained by averaging the first,
last, and two intermediate Gs) was calculated. These results are summarized in Table III. The presence of other instruments seems to
have little effect on intonation: only the major third has a different
size under solo and ensemble conditions. To the casual glance, the
range and variability figures of Table III may suggest that the performers were not very proficient, which is not at all true. Even when
tuning an instrument to the *same* pitch as a standard, the typical musician will show a standard deviation, in repeated settings, of about 10
cents (Corso, 1954).

TABLE III

DISTRIBUTION OF INTERVALS IN CENTS (FROM NICKERSON, 1948);
SIX STRING QUARTETS

Interval	N	25 percentile	Mean	75 percentile	Range
2nd; solo	30	199	201.0	206	183–214
2nd; ensemble	30	197	203.1	206	190–225
3rd; solo	60	404	411.1	418	391–435
3rd; ensemble	60	396	406.3	415	379–426
4th; solo	36	496	501.2	508	481–523
4th; ensemble	36	493	501.3	512	486–523
5th; solo	48	702	708.4	712	692–731
5th; ensemble	48	700	704.9	710	689–722
6th; solo	24	901	907.3	918	880–926
6th; ensemble	24	903	906.5	911	887–919

Next, Mason (1960) studied solo and ensemble performances of
Ravel's "Pavane pour une infante défunte" by two woodwind quin-
tets, one composed of faculty members at Brigham Young University,
the other of students. Both melodic and harmonic voices were recorded and analyzed using magnetic tape loops and chromatic stroboscope, following the definition of interval used by Nickerson. Table
IV shows Mason's results for the four performances. The row marked
"root" indicates the frequency of the keynote as it occurred in the
piece relative to the theoretical value of the keynote. The fact that the
values are all positive means that even the tonic was played sharp.
(Note, however, that the other intervals are measured relative to the
actual, not the theoretical, root frequency.) Again, only slight differences are seen between solo and ensemble performance.

TABLE IV

TABLE IV

SIZES OF MEAN INTERVALS IN CENTS (FROM MASON, 1960);
FACULTY AND STUDENT WOODWIND QUARTETS

Interval	Faculty solo	Faculty ensemble	Student solo	Student ensemble
Root	6	9	11	19
2nd	199	200	207	210
3rd	404	402	408	415
4th	504	504	500	506
5th	700	706	711	714
6th	903	904	908	912
7th	1104	1102	1111	1110

Shackford (1961, 1962a) returned to measurement of oscillographic traces in analyzing performance of three different string trios. Each trio played a set of four 30-measure pieces composed by Shackford. He was interested in harmonic as well as melodic relations, so his analysis included measurements of differences between the voices at certain places in the music. He took care to avoid open strings in his compositions (where, of course, subjective pitch no longer plays a role)—a precaution not always observed in earlier studies. Table V presents his results.

TABLE V

DISTRIBUTION OF INTERVALS IN CENTS (FROM SHACKFORD, 1961–2);
THREE STRING TRIOS

Interval	N	25 percentile	Mean	75 percentile	Range
Melodic semit	146	86	93	101	44–122
Melodic 2nd	134	199	204	209	187–228
Melodic 4th	32	494	501	510	480–525
Melodic 5th	28	692	701	708	682–723
Harmonic 2nd	51	197	204	211	179–235
Harmonic minor 3rd	15	287	305	318	275–334
Harmonic major 3rd	31	402	410	418	383–444
Harmonic 4th	22	487	506	525	485–528
Harmonic tritone; Diminished 5th	36	583	593	602	567–628
Harmonic tritone; Augmented 4th	34	601	611	619	585–637
Harmonic 5th	53	699	707	714	684–734

W. DIXON WARD

Averages obtained by these various experimenters are again tabu-
lated in Table VI together with theoretical values of the intervals in
JI and PT (the theoretical values in ET, of course, are integral multiples of 100). Among the experimenters who gathered the data in Table
VI, the consensus is that musical performance tends to conform to PT.
And of the three alternatives, the Pythagorean does fit the data most
closely. The evidence is conclusive that JI is simply not used by these
musicians. However, a closer inspection reveals that the agreement is
the best for those intervals *whose PT is appreciably sharper than ET*:
the 2nd, 3rd, 6th, and 7th (see Table I). On those few of the tested
intervals whose Pythagorean tuning is flatter than ET, only the semit
data conform to the Pythagorean prediction. The average 4th, instead
of being 498 cents, is some 5 cents higher. Even the ubiquitous 5th
itself is played, on the average, sharper than the 702 cents predicted;
indeed, in Shackford's study, it is played sharpest in a harmonic context, where the minimization-of-beat forces would be expected to be
the most active. Unfortunately, no data have been gathered on the
minor 6th and minor 7th, both of which are flatter in PT than in ET.
However, the minor 3rd in Shackford's data is also played sharp —
some 11 cents sharper than the theoretical Pythagorean value.

TABLE VI

SUMMARY OF MEAN INTERVAL SIZES FROM ALL STUDIES ON ACTUAL PERFORMANCE

Interval	Greene	Nickerson	Mason; faculty	Mason; students	Shackford; melodic	Shackford; harmonic	Predicted: just	pyth.
Semit	88				93		94	90
							112	
2nd	206	202	200	209	204	204	182	
							204	204
Minor 3rd	296					305	298	294
							316	
Major 3rd	406	409	403	411		410	386	408
4th	498	501	504	503	501	506	498	498
5th		707	703	712	701	707	702	702
Major 6th		907	903	910			884	906
Major 7th			1103	1111			1088	1110

Thus evidence indicates strongly that in musical performances the
target pitch for frequencies actually produced in response to a given
notation is one that is just a shade sharper than that called for by ET.
In the 500 to 1000 Hz region, even the subjective octave (a sacrosanct

2:1 in all theoretical systems) is about 1210 cents for pure tones (Ward, 1954). In his studies, Shackford (1962a,b) measured harmonic 10ths, 11ths, and 12ths and found that they were sharped to about the same extent as 3rds, 4ths, and 5ths.

Boomsliter and Creel (1963) too have provided striking confirmation of this theory. They constructed a reed organ with a special keyboard that provides three to six choices for each note of the chromatic scale. Trained musicians were then asked to select the specific tones they would use for a given melody. Unfortunately, the choices available for each note all represent some sort of whole-number ratio and are not equally spaced. The procedure also suffers from the fact that since the keyboard is fixed, the subject can always select the same *mi*, for example, thus being much more consistent than he otherwise might. However, even with these limitations, it is clear from the sample data they present that the preferred scale almost always is composed of tones consistently higher in frequency than those of ET. For example, in three classical numbers (the Marseillaise, a Bartok dance, and Mozart's Serenata Notturna), all notes above *do* are preferred 4 to 23 cents sharp.

That musicians "play sharp," of course, is not likely to be the whole story, although it is a good point of departure for further research. Context certainly will often play a role in determining the target pitch for a specific note. Some analysis along these lines has been done by Shackford (1962a,b), and although the number of items in his sample is generally too small to give a high level of statistical significance, certain trends can be seen. One example of the effect of context can be seen in Table IV. In the two rows next to the bottom are shown the results of two different "spellings" of the harmonic tritone. When the music is such that the tritone is presented as an augmented fourth (e.g., C to F sharp), the performed interval is significantly greater than when it occurs as a diminished fifth (C to G flat). Boomsliter and Creel (1963) also point out contextual effects; especially striking are the bizarre tunings preferred by the arranger for a popular quartet in the melody of their theme song, where tones as far off as a *sol* of 675 cents were selected.

Undoubtedly, the surface has been barely scratched in the study of intonation in performance. However, it is now clear that, on the average, the internal scale of musical pitch used by musicians corresponds fairly closely to ET, but with a slight stretch that results in a tendency toward sharping all tones relative to the tonic. It is interesting to note that Kolinski (1959) has proposed a new system of temperament in which the scale is deliberately stretched by about 3.5 cents per octave. He reports that listening tests showed that a piano thus tuned was judged superior to one tuned to strict equal temperament. However, this observation is probably irrelevant, since the tuning of pianos is always "stretched" anyhow. This stretch occurs because piano strings, not being infinitely thin, vibrate in such a manner that the partials are not exactly harmonically related (extreme examples of this principle are bells, cymbals, and other percussion instruments whose various partials have very irregular spacing). For example, the second partial of the A4 string in a good piano is 1 to 2 cents higher than an octave above the fundamental (Young, 1952). Thus when a piano tuner matches the fundamental of A5 to the second partial of A4, he automatically stretches the scale.

Perhaps the stretched scale of the piano is at least partially responsible for the fact that the internal scale of musical pitch is also stretched. Indeed, perhaps the correspondence (except for stretch) between musical pitch and ET is due to the extensive experience all musicians have had with the universal piano.

IV. VIBRATO

One of the main problems in measuring intonation in performance comes from the fact that Western musicians (particularly violinists and singers) are encouraged to produce a tone with "vibrato" — a fairly regular oscillation of frequency that causes the pattern on the chromatic stroboscope to rotate rapidly back and forth. It may or may not be coupled with a "tremolo" which is a similar cyclic variation in intensity.

Carl Seashore (1938, p. 33) proposed the following definition, "A good vibrato is a pulsation of pitch, usually accompanied with synchronous pulsations of loudness and timbre, of such extent and rate as to give a pleasing flexibility, tenderness, and richness to the tone." Until some intrepid soul finally scales flexibility, tenderness, and richness of tones, this definition leaves much to be desired. The implication is, though, that the presence of vibrato increases these attributes.

Two major studies of vibrato were made in Seashore's laboratory. Harold Seashore (1935) studied vocal vibrato, and Small (1937) violin vibrato. An analysis of the vibrato of musicians acknowledged to be among the best in their field showed a typical rate of six to seven cycles (pulsations) per second, with an average extent of nearly a semit for singers, about half a semit for violinists. However, despite extensive observations on the physical characteristics of vibrato, no study was made of the effect of vibrato on the resultant pitch. Although Carl Seashore (1938, p. 39) stated that, "The mean pitch, that is, the mean between the crest and the trough of the vibrato cycles, coincides fairly with the tone pitch," it is clear from context that he was referring to the objective frequency level instead of pitch, and even then, the method of measuring frequency level was so gross that only large departures (20 to 30 cents) from this rule could be observed.

At the moment, therefore, we have little evidence to indicate just what pitch the listener hears in a tone with vibrato. It may be true that the judged pitch corresponds to that of a steady tone at the mean frequency level. However, we cannot with complete certainty reject even the proposal by Kuttner (1963) that the judged pitch corresponds to the lower excursion of frequency level, although if this statement were true, the singers studied by Harold Seashore would have sounded flat indeed.

Studies matching the pitch of frequency-modulated sinusoids (or of actual musical tones) to that of steady ones are badly needed. However, matching of single tones will need to be augmented by experiments in which the pitch interval of various two-tone combinations, the second of which has vibrato, is judged to be "correct" or not. That is, although the judged pitch of a tone with vibrato heard in isolation may turn out to be the same as that of a steady tone at the mean frequency level, it is possible that an interval will be acceptable if the varying tone merely *includes* the frequency that the listener considers to be the correct one for a particular interval. This notion was expressed by Kock in 1936 (p. 24): "Thus a note originally off pitch may be made acceptable by imparting a frequency vibrato to it, provided the intended pitch is included in the vibrato interval and provided the vibrato interval is not too wide to be objectionable." It is a hypothesis that, if substantiated, will help to reconcile the fact that very few listeners judge the best violinists to be off key despite large individual differences in what pitch these listeners expect (or would prefer) to hear (Ward, 1954). In other words, if a violinist, in striving to play A6 (1760 Hz), oscillates between 1735 and 1785 Hz, then perhaps the tone will satisfy three listeners whose subjective A6s, relative to A5, have been shown to be 1745, 1760, and 1780 Hz, respectively. If so, then since most listeners' scales are tuned sharp (i.e., most people indicate that the octave of 880 is above 1760 Hz), the optimum strategy for the violinist, assuming a fixed average range of vibrato, would be to oscillate about a frequency level slightly higher than the one demanded by the physical scale. In short, he should "think sharp, play sharp, be sharp." A 1965 study by Fletcher *et al.* suggests that, indeed, he does: vibrato excursions were shown to have a 30- to 40-cent amplitude for Gs from 196 to 1570 Hz. The peak frequency was about 40 cents above the target frequency while the minimum was just at it, so that the mean frequency — if that is what determines the pitch — was about 15 to 20 cents sharp. It is also possible that vibrato serves to enhance performance by minimizing the establishment of standing waves in the performance room. This possibility is suggested by a common impression that a vibrato that is acceptable in the concert hall may become intolerable when reproduced over a monaural system in a living room, particularly in the case of singers.

One thing about vibrato is certain — not all peoples regard the vibrato with the esteem given it in our culture. For example, Deva (1959) analyzed the performance of Indian music using an oscillographic trace. He found that in two ragas sung by Indian musicians of acknowledged popularity, there was no vibrato. But then, perhaps Indians do not want their ragas to be flexible, tender, and rich.

V. INTENSITY AND PITCH

Musical performance would be a difficult business indeed if the pitch of a tone of constant frequency were to change very much with intensity. And, according to the best-publicized set of curves showing pitch vs. intensity as a function of the frequency region, it may. Fortunately, however, these curves represent the results of an atypical observer operating in a rather unusual experimental setting.

The functions in question imply a 2-semit or greater change of pitch at 150 and 8000 Hz as the level changes from 40 to 90 dB SPL. In this study by S. S. Stevens (1935), he set two oscillators to different frequencies and had his one and only subject adjust the intensity of one until the two sounded equal in pitch. Now there is nothing intrinsically wrong with this procedure. Theoretically, it should give the same point of equality as when the intensities are set a given distance apart and the frequency of one is adjusted by the listener. However, if the rate of change of pitch with level is small (and it was known even then to be), then one cannot expect precise results with this method. There will be a fairly large range of intensities through which the two stimuli will seem to have the same pitch. Furthermore, there is the possibility that the listener, when given a very large frequency difference, will simply set his intensity control as high as it will go and decide that the pitch match is "close enough" even though he is not able to bracket his final judgment. Certainly no other study dealing with the intensity-pitch function, from the first (Zurmühl, 1930) through the most recent, (Cohen, 1961), has shown as large an average difference.

The typical result shows a nearly complete independence of pitch and intensity of pure tones. At low frequencies, a few listeners show a drop in pitch as the intensity is raised (Morgan *et al.*, 1951). However, even at 50 Hz, the majority of the listeners do not show a statistically significant shift (Cohen, 1961). Similar negative results were obtained by Small and Campbell (1961) using DC and AC pulses in the vicinity of 100 Hz. Consequently, there is no set of curves representing "the pitch-intensity function" because of the wide range of individual differences. Wever (1949) actually went so far as to call it the "pitch-intensity illusion," but he could hardly avoid this position since he had committed himself to a theory of pitch perception based on frequency of neural discharge.

Instead of a set of average curves, therefore, Fig. 2 shows the results of a single typical experiment, using five musicians (Ward, 1953). In this experiment, the subjects adjusted the frequency of a tone in the right ear to match the pitch of a fixed tone of 250 Hz in the left ear, the tones being presented in unending alternate succession. The intensity of the tone in the right ear was systematically varied. The use of the contralateral ear for the standard tone was dictated by the fact that, if the tones to be compared are presented alternately to the same ear with no silent interval between, a very intense variable tone will tend to shift the pitch of the following standard tone. This peripheral interaction of tones probably is linked closely to short-term auditory adaptation, and was probably active in many of the pitch-intensity experiments, although it has not yet been studied systematically. Cohen (1961), at least, minimized it by inserting a quiet period of 0.5 sec between his 0.7 sec variable and comparison stimuli.

Figure 2A shows the average equal-pitch contours from four adjustments by each subject at each level. The ordinate is the frequency of the tone in the right ear, at the level indicated on the abscissa, judged equal to the standard tone of 250 Hz and 62 dB SPL in the left ear. In Fig. 2B these curves have all been shifted slightly in order to coincide at a single point for comparison purposes. This step eliminates individual differences in binaural diplacusis—the differences in tuning between the two ears—and is permissible if one assumes a close similarity between adjacent pitch contours.

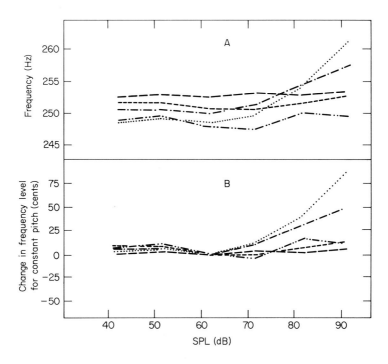

Figure 2 Equal-pitch contours (top set of curves) and changes in frequency level for constant pitch (bottom) for the right ears of five listeners. In all cases the standard comparison tone was a 250-Hz tone at 62 dB SPL in the left ear. (Ward, 1953.)

The differences in frequency level for constant pitch are given in cents on the ordinate of Fig. 2B. Strictly speaking, this ordinate is not "change in pitch level." It is probably *true* that if a 100-cent difference in frequency level were required to produce equal pitch for a 40-dB and 110-dB pair of stimuli, then the listener would judge the two to differ in pitch by about a semit when the frequencies were equal; but this equivalence has not actually been demonstrated for each of the ears concerned.

In this experiment, the typical standard deviation of the four adjustments at each level was about seven cents. Although two of the ears showed a significant drop in pitch at the highest level, the other three indicated no change.

Figure 2B is representative of the results obtained by others using careful monaural techniques. They all show that a change of pitch with intensity is not something that must be explained away in accounting for musical perception, since it is generally negligible even for pure tones at the intensities usually encountered in music. The problem was real, however, during the time that Stevens's (1935) results were thought to be typical. Lewis and Cowan (1936), for example, had four violinists play a set of intervals *pp* and *ff* and demonstrated that the frequencies were not appreciably different in the two cases. However, they only proved that the pitch-intensity function, whatever its form, was invariant over the range of frequencies encompassed by the intervals used, not that it was negligible. That is, even if there had been a 20-cent difference in pitch level between a *pp* and *ff* G3, it would not be discovered by measuring ascending fifths played *pp* and then *ff* starting at G3, if the change at D4 in going from *pp* to *ff* had also been 20 cents.

VI. TIMBRE AND PITCH

Fletcher (1934) also offered a solution to the pitch-intensity problem, namely that the higher partials of ordinary musical tones keep the pitch more constant than that of pure tones. Although the problem has evaporated, Fletcher's suggestion does raise the question of what effect partials have on pitch independent of their effect on timbre (assuming that these effects can be separated). When comparing the pitch of a complex tone with that of a sinusoid, it is often difficult to keep from judging the more complex tone to have a slightly higher pitch even after setting them "equal." (Indeed, the complex tone's average "pitch-extent" in mels *is* somewhat higher.) Jenkins (1961) discussed at some length the problem of separating pitch and timbre in connection with the judgment of the periodicity pitch of recurrent pulses.

For tones similar to those used in music, the meager evidence is ambiguous. In 1941, Lichte had listeners make pitch matches to synthesized tones in which each successive harmonic partial (fundamental frequency 360 Hz) was either one dB higher (rising spectrum) or one dB lower (falling spectrum) than the next lower harmonic. He found that with the rising spectrum, the complex tone was matched tô a 361-Hz pure tone, but with the falling spectrum, a pure tone of 363 Hz had the same pitch, implying that the rising spectrum had a lower pitch. But later, he found just the opposite (Lichte and Gray, 1955). Employing a pulse generator in combination with filters, Lichte and Gray generated tones either with low-order harmonics only or with equal low- and high-order. The tones with only low-order harmonics were judged lower in pitch than those also containing high-order harmonics. Both types appeared higher in pitch than the similar pure tone. However, the *modal* value of each comparison was zero, implying that all stimuli, both complex and pure, had the same pitch when their frequencies were equal. Thus there is a strong suggestion that some of these listeners were not keeping timbre and pitch separate.

Plomp (1967) pitted the frequency of the fundamental against that of higher partials in an ingenious experiment. His listeners were presented first with an ordinary harmonic complex tone (in which all 12 partials were integral multiples of the fundamental), followed by one in which one or more of the lowest of the partials were decreased in frequency but the remainder were increased. The subjects judged whether the "pitch" went up or down. When only the first partial was decreased, then at (fundamental) frequencies of 1000 Hz or below, the pitch appeared to rise (that is, the pitch was determined mainly by the higher partials), while at 2000 Hz it fell (i.e., pitch corresponded to the fundamental); 1400 Hz gave equal numbers of votes "higher" and "lower." With the first two partials dropping and the other ten rising, this "indifference point" was about 700 Hz; with three vs. nine it was 350 Hz; while with four vs. eight the consensus was that all tones dropped in pitch. These results suggest that the frequency of components in the 1000- to 2000-Hz range are exceptionally important in determining pitch, but this interpretation is not unequivocal.

VII. DURATION AND PITCH

How long must a tone be heard in order to be perceived as having an unequivocal pitch? Doughty and Garner (1948) studied this problem using the methods of adjustment and of constant stimuli. They concluded that pitch is unchanging for tones of 25 msec and longer, but that 12-msec and 6-msec tones have a lower pitch. However, Boomsliter *et al.* (1964) emphasize that the transition from "click" to "tone" depends on the intensity. Swigart (1964) has reported a perhaps related phenomenon for repeated short bursts of tone. If one presents successive 8-msec bursts of 1000-Hz tone with 1-msec pauses between (i.e., if one cuts out every ninth cycle), the pitch is significantly lower than that of a continuous 1000-Hz tone. Just why, however, is still unclear. In the context of the place theory of hearing, the observation can be taken as implying that the first few waves travel farther along the basilar membrane than later ones, which seems unlikely. Perhaps a few cycles are necessary to produce stabilization of the neural inhibitory system responsible for transformation of the broad patterns of movement of the basilar membrane into the sharp tuning observed at the cochlear nuclear complex.

VIII. ABSOLUTE PITCH

An aspect of pitch perception that is still regarded as somewhat mysterious despite a goodly amount of experimentation is "absolute" (or "perfect") pitch. Persons possessing this ability are able to give the musical name of a single tone heard in isolation, and can sing, whistle, or otherwise produce at will a given scale note. Their relative pitch grid has, so to speak, an anchor and is not movable. Since there is a recent review of the literature on this topic (Ward, 1963a,b), I shall not attempt a detailed summary here, but instead will confine myself to a recapitulation of the viewpoint of Watt (1917), a viewpoint that has been neglected for nearly 50 years.

Although absolute pitch ordinarily generates some awe, a comparison with analogous phenomena in other sensory modalities removes a good deal of the strangeness. We can identify, on a similar absolute basis—that is, without comparison or reference to a second stimulus of some sort—the color crimson, the smell of camphor, and the taste of salt. In audition itself we can identify musical instruments and voices of acquaintances on the basis of a single tone or word. Indeed, the recognition of C to G as a "fifth" is absolute in a sense, since this pair of tones is not compared to any other tones actually present; instead, a comparison with remembered tone pairs must be made.

The wonder is not that some people have absolute pitch, but that so many do *not* have it. But, as Watt pointed out, the organism is reinforced not for absolute but for relative pitch judgments. "Three Blind Mice" is still "Three Blind Mice" whether it is played in C or in G; transposition is the rule, not the exception. Thus absolute pitch behavior may simply be trained out of us in early life. If so, then the chief theoretical question is if the ability can be "regained" by suitable training. Although previous attempts have met with only slight success (Ward, 1963a,b), perhaps an intensive training program using modern reinforcement techniques would fare better. Lundin and Allen (1962) reported that they were able to improve pitch identification greatly using modern apparatus. But whether or not nearly anyone can be brought (restored?) to a level of proficiency equal to that of the typical "possessor" of absolute pitch—errors of no more than about half a semit—remains to be seen.

IX.   PITCH SATIATION AND AUDITORY FATIGUE

A well-known phenomenon in vision is that of figural after-effects: if a black line on a white field is fixated steadily for several minutes and then removed, a test object whose position on the retina is close to that formerly occupied by the fixation line will appear to be shifted away from the area. Christman and Williams (1963) have reported an analogous phenomenon in audition. They measured the shift in the pitch of a 600-Hz tone produced by 60-sec exposures to higher or lower frequencies at 85 dB SPL, as a function of the time interval between cessation of the adapting stimulus and onset of the test tone. For an interval of 1 sec, the inferred shift in pitch amounted to about 20 cents—upward following a 575-Hz satiating tone and downward following a 625-Hz tone. The effect decreased rapidly with time; after 8 sec of recovery, only a slight amount of shift remained. If the analogy with visual figural after-effects holds, the amount of shift should have been less for satiation tones farther removed from 600 Hz, but their account is unclear on this point.

The Christman and Williams work is probably related to results obtained with ears suffering from auditory fatigue. When a moderate degree of temporary threshold shift, fairly localized in frequency, is induced in an ear, the pitch of tones is shifted away from the locus of maximum fatigue, although the amount of shift is markedly asymmetric (Rüedi and Furrer, 1946). There are slight downward shifts of pitch where fatigue is increasing with frequency and larger upward shifts where it is decreasing. Downward shifts following exposure to simulated gunfire have been observed for test tones as low as 150 Hz, but not at 100 Hz or below (Ward, 1963c).

When auditory fatigue is induced by high intensities, the maximum effect is found about half an octave above the frequency of the fatiguing tone, so the locus of the maximum pitch shift will also occur somewhat above the exposure frequency. At or below the moderate level of exposure tone used by Christman and Williams, however, the maximum fatigue is indeed found at the exposure frequency. All these observations can be accounted for by an hypothesis involving either relatively refractory or completely unresponsive areas of the basilar membrane.

X. PITCH AND MASKING

If a band of noise is introduced into the ear, the pitch of tones near the frequency of this masking noise changes in the same direction as in the presence of auditory fatigue. That is, there is an upward shift in pitch (nearly half a semit) for tones above the area of masking, a slight downward shift for those below (Egan and Meyer, 1950; Webster and Schubert, 1954). The same principle applies to the effects of a broadband noise from which one octave has been rejected ("noise with a hole"); tones just below the upper limit of the "hole" are shifted downward (Webster *et al.*, 1952).

A dissenting voice has been raised on this topic, however — Békésy (1963) claims to have observed exactly the opposite effect. He reports shifts that may amount to three semits or more and are produced by very weak noise bands. For example, he indicates that the pitch of a 600-Hz tone at 40 dB SL shifts downward by 10 percent (1.8 semits) in the presence of a lower-frequency noise (high-frequency cutoff of 300 Hz) at 30 dB SL (Békésy, 1963, p. 603). In verification attempts, all my listeners gave results similar to those of Egan and Meyer (1950) and Webster and Schubert (1954) — a slight upward shift in pitch. Because Békésy gave no details about his psychophysical method, it is not clear how he obtained these strange results.

XI. BINAURAL DIPLACUSIS (MUSICAL PARACUSIS)

The same tone may give rise to different pitches in the two ears of a given observer. When one of the ears has normal hearing, it is generally assumed that this ear is hearing "normal" pitch, and the other is mistuned, so to speak. Unfortunately, this rule is of little help when both ears have normal sensitivity. Diplacusis of half a semit at high frequencies (2000–4000 Hz) can be found in pairs of ears that are both well within normal limits (Kreidl and Gatscher, 1928). In this event, one must study the pitch relations within each ear in order to deduce which (if either) is normal and which has "musical paracusis."

The subjective octave (or any other interval whose reliability is good) can be used for this purpose. In a series of octave measurements, significant departures from the average trend can readily be observed (Ward, 1953, 1954). Suppose a given ear displays about the same disparity (say 10 cents) between the subjective and physical octaves for frequencies up to 1600 Hz. However, when the subject is asked to set the octave of 850 Hz, his final setting is 1800 Hz, implying that 1800 Hz is heard nearly a semit too flat. The only alternative inference, that 850 Hz is heard too sharp, can be rejected because the judgments of "octave of 425 Hz" followed the normal (for that ear) trend. The disturbance of pitch at 1800 Hz will show up again, of course, when the listener is asked to set the octave of 1800 Hz. Because 1800 Hz is heard flat, a subjective octave above is likely to be perhaps only 3500 Hz (unless there happens to be another distortion of pitch at the higher frequency).

Of course, these slight degrees of diplacusis are ordinarily of academic interest only. They certainly do not seem to have much effect on musical perception, or else almost everyone would be complaining of performers being out of tune.

One reason is that most musical performance occurs at lower frequencies than the region in which appreciable musical paracusis is generally found; at least the *fundamentals* of the tones lie within the lower frequency ranges. Perhaps the effect of slight mistuning of higher partials is simply not noticed (jnds for mistuning of partials have not yet been systematically studied).

Secondly, even when there is a solo passage of any length in the upper register, it usually consists of fairly rapid tones. Although they are unlikely to be so short as to have indeterminate pitch, the degree of mistuning that is overlooked or accepted in a musical context is likely to be considerably higher for short tones than for sustained ones.

A third reason why paracusis may not ordinarily influence musical perception is that the disparity is reduced in binaural listening. Liebermann and Révész (1914) noted long ago that when slight diplacusis is present, the pitch heard with the tone presented to both ears is about midway between the pitches heard separately.

Although slight degrees of musical paracusis are usually not noticed, the older German literature (reviewed by Lempp, 1938) is filled with accounts of more severe and/or bilateral cases (e.g., Liebermann and Révész, 1908). One can well imagine that a violinist who hears some intervals a semit or more off in pitch would be in trouble, although a pianist might be able to grit his teeth and endure the cacaphony. It is indeed a startling experience to listen to music with an ear that has been given severe auditory fatigue by exposure to simulated gunfire. Under these conditions, the amount of paracusis increases with frequency so that *everything* sounds flat, harmonics become inharmonic, and consonances become dissonances (Ward, 1963c).

XII.   BINAURAL FUSION AND INTERACTION

Nearly always, when a single frequency is presented to both ears, a single pitch is heard. I know of only one exception to this rule. One listener making binaural octave judgments (with earphones) heard any tone between 2500 and 3800 Hz as being different in each ear; in her own words, "not two different tones, really, but like two different instruments playing the same note." Later investigation showed that she had between 30 and 85 cents of diplacusis in this region. Thus, the claim that the same frequency presented to both ears *always* gives rise to a unitary pitch (van der Tweel, 1956) is incorrect. Another exception to this rule occurs when tonal monaural diplacusis exists (Ward, 1955); with this condition, a single frequency may give rise to several tones in a single ear, so naturally the tone appears multiple when presented binaurally as well.

If a binaurally-presented single frequency usually sounds single despite having a different pitch in each ear, what happens if two different frequencies that sound the same are presented? For example, if 3800 Hz in the right ear is matched to 3700 Hz in the left ear under alternate presentation (as is the case for my own ears), do they fuse when presented simultaneously? The answer seems to be that they do, at least as long as the diplacusis is a semit or less. In the example just given, with 3700 Hz in the left ear, anything from about 3680 to 3820 Hz in the right gives rise to a unitary pitch.

A detailed study of the fusion of dichotic stimuli as a function of degree of diplacusis and of frequency has not yet been reported. However, the agreement among the scattered results using normal listeners is fairly good. The most recent investigation was conducted by Odenthal (1963) on eight "super-subjects" (persons with normal hearing, negligible diplacusis, and low test-test variability). For all frequencies below about 800 Hz, the frequency separation necessary to elicit a report of "two pitches" for tones under 45 dB SL (insuring that no sound from one earphone reached the opposite ear) was constant at about 12 Hz, ranging from 11 to 14 Hz for different listeners. This agrees well with the 11 Hz at 500 Hz reported by Baley (1915) and the 12 Hz at 200 Hz found by Thurlow and Bernstein (1957). The "separation limen" increases as the frequency goes from 900 to about 1500 Hz, and then remains constant at about 4.5 *percent* (not a constant frequency difference) for tones between 1500 and 2400 Hz. With a further increase in frequency, the limen once more rises rapidly to a second plateau of about 9 percent for tones from 3000 to 10,000 Hz. The fact that the absolute limen is constant at 12 Hz for low frequencies is no doubt linked to the phenomenon of binaural beats, which also can be heard only when pairs of dichotic tones are below 800 Hz or so. However, why the relative limen displays two plateaus, one of which is almost exactly twice as high as the other is still unclear.

At very high intensities, the question of monaural vs. binaural pitch is much less clear. In a study using tones at 95 dB LL (loudness level), Thurlow (1943) found that binaural pitch was about half a semit lower than monaural at 200 Hz. At 4000 Hz, binaural pitch was higher than monaural. However, further observations revealed that a 95-dB-LL tone of almost *any* frequency in one ear would raise the pitch of a 4000-Hz tone or lower the pitch of a 200-Hz tone in the other. This phenomenon awaits closer scrutiny.

It may be argued that differences between monaural and binaural pitch are irrelevant to musical perception, since the frequencies arriving at both ears are the same in a real-life situation. But it is only a matter of time before one of the modern composers who deals with electronic music synthesized from tape-recorded sounds comes up with a composition designed for earphone listening only. In such a situation, bizzare effects could be obtained by deliberate matching and mismatching frequencies in the two ears, by having one melody in one ear and another in the other (or switching melodies or instruments from one side to the other), etc. Certainly such composition would provide a challenge to the ingenuity of a composer. Whether it would represent significant progress in music is another question.

XIII. CONSONANCE VS. DISSONANCE

Around the turn of the century, many experiments were designed to elucidate the nature of "consonance" and "dissonance." In the last analysis, as Cazden (1962) points out in an excellent review of the topic, whether two tones sound well together—which is what is usually meant by "consonance"—is a preference judgment from which there is no appeal and which may change from time to time.

This relativistic position is hardly new, since Aristoxenus a couple of millenia ago held the same view about consonance (Cazden, 1959). However, it has been opposed vigorously by certain theorists who either invoke the same small-integer-ratio arguments used in scale construction or else insist that small frequency differences must be avoided because of beats. Now the fact of the matter is that these people simply define consonance in a different way. Instead of asking listeners what is consonant and what is dissonant, they postulate that dissonance is increased by a large-number ratio *per se,* or else that it is determined by the presence of audible beats whose rate lies between perhaps 10 and 100 per second, beats which arise either from interaction between the fundamentals of the tones, between their physically measurable harmonics, or between subjective tones generated in the ear. It can be shown that such audible beats are minimized when the two tones do bear a small-number ratio to each other.

Actually, there should be no argument between the two schools of thought—and there would not be if each camp stuck to its definition. However, the beat theorists, under the leadership of Helmholtz, failed to do so. Forgetting that their definition of consonance was an objective one, they attempted to convince the relativists that it was also subjective—that absence of beats always determines beauty. There is actually a fair correlation between the existence of beats at the rates indicated and judgments of "unpleasantness," "roughness," or other terms implying subjective undesirability of a tonal combination. Thus many musicians were (and are) convinced that the principle is sound and that when there is a disagreement between a judgment of relative pleasantness and the degree of consonance as defined by beats, the value judgment must be "wrong."

The most recent attempt (van de Geer *et al.,* 1962) to untangle the semantics involved here is worth recounting in some detail. Using apparatus that would generate the first 12 harmonics of a fundamental of 85 Hz, a set of 23 pairs of tones was presented to each of

"10 intelligent subjects (all laymen where music is concerned)."
These 23 pairs of tones consisted of all the possible ratios an octave or
less in extent, including all the ordinary "just" intervals of the scale
except the major seventh (8:15) and the minor second (15:16). The
simpler ratios were generated using harmonics that were high enough
to keep the mean frequency of the pairs as nearly constant as possible.
Thus the octave was represented by 5:10 (425 and 850 Hz), the fifth
by 6:9 (510 and 765 Hz), etc. No tone below 340 Hz was used, and this
only once, in the combination 4:7. Each observer listened once to
the sequence of pairs (all at 70 dB SPL, approximately), and then had
to rate each one on 10 successive 7-point scales: high-low, sharp-
round, beautiful-ugly, active-passive, consonant-dissonant, eupho-
nious-diseuphonious, wide-narrow, tense-quiet, rough-smooth, and
unitary-multiple. All listeners judged high-low first, but the order of
the other nine scales (as well as the order of presentation of the individual stimuli) was randomized.

The mean ratings of consonance indicate that there are large differences between consonance as defined by earlier judgments of musicians steeped in beat lore and by laymen in the present experiment.
The octave, that most consonant of intervals to the music theoretician,
got only an average consonance rating of 4.6, being exceeded by 9
others. The intervals judged most consonant, at 5.7, were the ratios
5:7 and 5:8—a 583-cent tritone and an 814-cent minor sixth, respectively. The cellar (2.0) was occupied by the four smallest intervals
(8:9, 9:10, 10:11, and 11:12—204, 182, 165, and 150 cents, respectively). Although in the absence of the raw data one cannot estimate
the statistical significance of the differences, it seems clear that these
results do not agree with the rules of consonance laid down by the
small-integer proponents. It is therefore unnecessary, in explaining
consonance, to appeal to neuromythological structures such as a series
of brain circuits tuned to each frequency, so that "in the case of the
fifth, 3:2, every third wave of the higher note and every second wave
of the lower could use the same circuit, and so on" (Boomsliter and
Creel, 1961, p. 20).

Let us turn to the question of what these particular listeners meant
by consonance. Van de Geer *et al.* (1962) performed a factor analysis
on the intercorrelation matrix, with rotation for oblique factors. They
came up with three factors, which they labeled "pitch" (high, sharp,
tense, narrow, active), "fusion" (rough, multitional, active) and
"evaluation" (euphonious, consonant, beautiful). They concluded,

from the fact that consonance had a high loading only on "evaluation," that the listeners were making an esthetic judgment of the interval when rating consonance, and were not depending on "fusion." However, their argument would be much more convincing if they had actually employed "fused-disparate" as one of their scales. An inspection of the average scores (before factor analysis) shows that the four smallest intervals mentioned above (8:9, 9:10, 10:11, and 11:12) were not only the least consonant, ugliest, and most diseuphonious, but also the sharpest, most tense, and roughest. There is consequently some justification for the hypothesis that roughness was the primary criterion for dissonance. The correlation between roughness and consonance, calculated from their data, is −0.87.

In a later study from the same laboratory, Plomp and Levelt (1962) again had listeners judge the consonance of pairs of pure tones separated by various distances. Five sets of pairs were used; in each set the geometric mean frequency was kept constant at 125, 250, 500, 1000, or 2000 Hz. As in the earlier study, the average consonance ratings for a given center frequency changed rather abruptly from low to high at a particular frequency separation. Plomp and Levelt noted that this change does not occur at a constant frequency difference, but rather when the two tones are approximately one critical bandwidth apart. In other words, sinusoids tend to be judged dissonant if they are separated by less than a critical bandwidth. Combining their own data with some earlier results by Guthrie and Morrill (1928), who asked 380 subjects to give a dichotomous judgment of "consonant" or "dissonant" to pairs of tones composed of 395 and 395+5N Hz (e.g., 395 and 400, 395 and 405, etc.), they arrived at a scale of relative consonance as a function of separation measured in critical bands (Fig. 3).

Since pure tones are seldom found in music, Plomp and Levelt used Fig. 3 to calculate what consonance judgments would be expected for the combination of a 250-Hz-fundamental and a variable-fundamental tone, each composed of the first six harmonics in equal strength. Defining the "consonance of the chord" as one minus the sum of the dissonances (right-hand scale of Fig. 3) of the intervals between two adjacent partials, they calculated the consonance for variable tones with fundamentals from 250 to 500 Hz. It will be interesting to see how well their predictions are confirmed, since they indicate much higher relative consonance when the fundamental frequencies are related by small-integer ratios than when they are

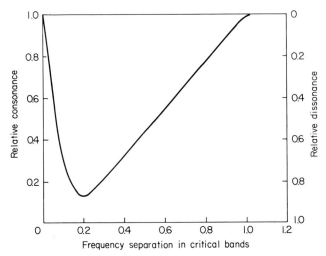

Figure 3 Relative consonance of two tones as a function of the fraction of a critical bandwidth separating their frequencies (Plomp and Levelt, 1962, by permission).

slightly mistuned, supporting the notion that beats tend to determine consonance. But they also show that a rate of beating that is pleasant in one frequency range may be disagreeable in another because of differences in the size of the critical band (a similar idea was expressed by Wever in 1929). It is certain that *some* aspect of desirability is dependent on this critical-band concept; yet whether these particular listeners used as their criterion of consonance what everyone else uses (especially musicians) remains to be seen.

XIV. AURAL HARMONICS AND COMBINATION TONES

For years musicians have been told that the ear is able to separate any complex signal into a series of sinusoidal signals—that it acts as a Fourier analyzer. This quarter-truth, known as Ohm's Other Law, has served to increase the distrust with which perceptive musicians regard scientists, since it is readily apparent to them that the ear acts in this way only under very restricted conditions. True, the partials in a sustained complex tone are separated out on the basilar membrane, and listeners can "hear out" some of them, provided they have been instructed and trained properly, and provided that the partials to be discriminated are more than a critical band apart (Plomp, 1964). But even something as elementary as a simple tone with vibrato, which can be reduced mathematically to three sinusoids of slightly different frequency, is not heard as three sinusoids but as a single tone of fluctuating loudness or pitch. A pulse is not heard as a family of sinusoids. The fact that men study the perception of periodicity pitch is evidence that Ohm's Law is about as far from universal as a law can be. And consider those sustained tones generated by a full orchestra: must we postulate that the aural mechanism analyzes the total complex into a series of several hundred partials and then somehow selectively recombines *some* of them so we can identify — as we do — the parts being played by one particular instrument?

A study of Pollack's (1964) demonstrates an almost unbelievable inability of some listeners to hear elements of a complex tone. His three subjects merely had to determine whether or not a certain frequency had been present in a complex tone presented just before the sinusoid; even when only *two* tones were presented in the complex, no one achieved 100 percent correct! Thus not only does the ear fail to operate as a perfect Fourier analyzer, but it also introduces its own distortion, and this may have had some bearing on the poor performance of Pollack's listeners. That is, at some point (or at several) along the auditory chain, the motion of the structures fails to be exactly proportional to the motion of the air particles striking the eardrum. Of course any system eventually reaches its limit of linearity beyond which successive increases in incoming signal give progressively smaller increments of response, thus producing peak clipping; the aural mechanism introduces distortion at very low levels of stimulation, however.

If the input to a system is a single sinusoid, then the resultant peak-clipped wave can be analyzed into a harmonic series. In the ear, those partials higher than the first are called *aural harmonics*. When two tones are introduced into a nonlinear system, in addition to the harmonics of each, there is generated a series of *combination tones*. If the higher tone has a frequency H and the lower L, then combination tones include the "first difference tone" ($H-L$), the "summation tone" ($H+L$), second-order tones like $2H-2L$, $2H-L$, $2L-H$, $2L+H$, and so on (Wever, 1941, discusses the different systems of nomenclature used for combination tones).

Aural harmonics and combination tones have been studied in two principal ways. In lower organisms, one can first crush the eighth nerve to eliminate nerve potentials and then analyze the remaining cochlear potentials by means of an electronic filter, isolating and measuring the relative intensity of each distortion product (Rawdon-Smith and Hawkins, 1939). The relative strength of each of these components of the cochlear microphonic is assumed to indicate the relative intensity of the percept a cat would have had if his auditory nerve were intact.

In man, however, less drastic measures must be employed. At very high levels, some people can "hear out" aural harmonics; certain combination tones, as well, can be analytically isolated. In general, though, distortion products cannot be heard well by mere listening. Furthermore, we can get only a vague idea of their relative intensity by such a procedure. Therefore, the "probe tone" technique is used. A probe tone about 3 Hz different from the theoretical frequency of the distortion product is introduced at a very low intensity. Then this intensity is raised until 3-Hz beats are heard. As the intensity is increased further, a point can be found where this beating reaches a maximum. After certain corrections (Egan and Klumpp, 1951), the probe-tone intensity that produces the most pronounced beats indicates the effective intensity of the distortion product.

The most recent data on aural harmonics (Egan and Klumpp, 1951) indicate that, for a primary tone of 350 Hz, the second harmonic can first be detected by probe-tone technique when the primary reaches about 55 dB SPL; the effective level of the second harmonic then is some 40 to 45 dB below the fundamental. As the intensity of the fundamental is increased, the harmonic grows more and more rapidly until, at levels of 80 dB SPL or so, it is only a few dB below the fundamental. Third or higher harmonics behave in much the same way, although the higher the order of the harmonic, the higher must be the intensity of the primary tone for detectability. It has always been assumed, though never demonstrated, that the characteristics of aural harmonics are independent of the frequency of the primary tone (Fletcher, 1930), a valid assumption if all distortion were attributable to nonlinearity in the middle ear so that the distortion is a function of amplitude only. However, there is overwhelming evidence that much distortion takes place at the basilar membrane (Wever and Lawrence, 1954, Chapter 9, summarize this evidence), making it likely that a given aural harmonic may grow at different rates for primaries of different frequencies.

The characteristics of combination tones have been studied even more sporadically than aural harmonics. Because of the tediousness of determining best beats for a large number of combination tones, most studies have involved only one pair of frequencies. Thus we have no extensive data bearing on how the magnitude of combination tones is affected by the frequency regions of the two primary tones or by their separation. Wever *et al.* (1940) did show, however, that the level of a 4000 Hz first difference tone depended on whether it was produced by 380 and 4380, by 2300 and 6300, or by 5200 and 9200 Hz. Perhaps, too, quite different laws apply when the primaries are less than a critical bandwidth apart than when they are widely separated (Plomp, 1965).

The combination tone usually described in textbooks as the loudest is the first difference tone, $H-L$. And it may be at extremely high intensities, where middle-ear nonlinearity is producing much of the distortion. However, Moe (1942) using 690 and 950 Hz, found that with 80-dB-SPL primaries, the inferred intensity of $2L-H$ (430 Hz) and $2H-L$ (1210 Hz) was just as great as that of $H-L$ (260 Hz), namely about 17 dB below the level of the primary tones. All three of these were more intense than the second harmonics, $2L$ and $2H$ (1380 and 1900 Hz), which, together with $3L-H$ (1120 Hz) and $3H-L$ (2160 Hz), were down about 25 dB. And about 31 dB below the primaries were $3L$, $3H$, $2L+H$, $2H+L$, $2H-2L$, $2H+2L$, $4L-H$, $4L+H$, and $4H-L$. Notice that only in this third intensity group do "summation tones" first appear; indeed, the "first" summation tone, $H+L$ is even lower, 40 dB down. It is no wonder that difference tones were noticed by musicians long before summation tones.

The fact that $2L-H$ and $2H-L$ are at least as prominent as $H-L$ has been verified by other studies as well (e.g., Newman *et al.*, 1937; Plomp, 1965). More than 50 years ago, Peterson (1915) noticed that the estimated loudness of $2L-H$ was, for certain combinations, even greater than $H-L$. Indeed, because of masking (or at least partly because of it), $2L-H$ may on occasion sound even louder than L itself. If, for example, a 3500-Hz tone is sounding continuously, and periodically a 3000-Hz tone is introduced, most listeners agree that they hear a tone of 2500 Hz being turned on and off.

Thus, owing to the nonlinear characteristics of the system, all manner of tones are produced in the ear. Their intensity, at the levels customarily involved in musical performance, is great enough that they could easily be distinguished using the method of paired comparisons. For instance, Bryan and Parbrook (1960) presented listeners with two successive tones: the first was a 357-Hz pure tone (pure, at least, as it started through the auditory chain), the second was the same tone, but with a variable amount of one particular harmonic added. The listeners judged the two either "same" or "different." Thresholds (criterion not stated) for detection of externally intro- duced harmonic distortion under these conditions were very sensitive: with a 60-dB-SPL fundamental, an 8-dB second harmonic could be detected, representing harmonic distortion of less than 0.3 percent.

In musical performance, happily, one does not have a chance to compare tones in this way. Therefore the detection of distortion is much less likely under ordinary musical conditions. Jacobs and Wittman (1964) had subjects listen alternately to taped music and to disc recordings (made from the tape) with various amounts of dis- tortion added. Although they did not present any details of procedure or data, they concluded that it is practically impossible to determine whether the program is being heard directly from the master tape or from the recorded groove even though harmonic distortion on the order of 5 percent was present in the latter.

XV. CONCLUSION

The outcome of the Jacobs and Wittman experiment underscores the dangers of trying to predict musical perception from simple psychophysical data. Though harmonic distortion of 0.3 percent in a single sustained tone can be detected by suitable techniques, it must be more than ten times greater in order to affect real music. Clearly, we must be most careful in the way we interpret (extrapolate) our results in talking to musicians.

In the same vein, the fact that a change in sound pressure of 0.5 dB can sometimes be perceived does not mean that composers should try to specify performance levels to that degree of precision. Nor does the fact that under optimum laboratory conditions a flutter (frequency vibrato) whose magnitude is about 0.3 percent (5 cents) can be heard (Schecter, 1949) rule out the probability that considerably more may ordinarily go undetected—however, it does seem reasonable to con- clude that reducing flutter and wow below 0.3 percent in a sound reproduction system is a waste of money.

Above all, let us remember that what we can find out in the labora- tory has no bearing on what music should be. The physicist, W. H. George (1961), is most critical of gratuitous and unfounded value judgments by scientists. He takes others to task, for example, for arbitrarily calling strike noises of percussion instruments such as the piano and other noises of real instruments "undesirable." Whether or not they are must be determined by preference tests, not by authoritarian decree. Future studies in musical perception might well keep in mind this observation of George's (1961, p. 423): "The mixing of philosophy with studies in musical acoustics results in nothing but confusion in a subject which is already sufficiently complex by its essential connection with subjective data."

ACKNOWLEDGMENT

Preparation of this chapter was supported by a grant from the National Institute of Health, U.S. Public Health Service, Department of Health, Education and Welfare.

REFERENCES

Baley, S. (1915). Versuche über den dichotischen Zusammenklang wenig verschiedener Töne. *Beitr. Akust. Musikwiss.*, **8**, 57–82.

Barbour, J. M. (1951). *Tuning and temperament.* Michigan State College Press, East Lansing, Michigan.

Beck, J. and Shaw, W. A. (1963). Single estimates of pitch magnitude. *J. Acoust. Soc. Am.*, **35**, 1722–1724.

von Békésy, G. (1963). Three experiments concerned with pitch perception. *J. Acoust. Soc. Am.*, **35**, 602–606.

Boomsliter, P. and Creel, W. (1961). The long pattern hypothesis in harmony and hearing. *J. Music Theory*, **5**, 2–31.

Boomsliter, P. and Creel, W. (1963). Extended reference: an unrecognized dynamic in melody. *J. Music Theory*, **7**, 2–22.

Boomsliter, P. C., Creel, W., and Powers, S. R., Jr. (1964). Time requirements for the tonal function. *J. Acoust. Soc. Am.*, **36**, 1958–1959 (A).

Bryan, M. E. and Parbrook, H. D. (1960). Just audible thresholds for harmonic distortion. *Acustica*, **10**, 87–91.

Cazden, N. (1959). Musical intervals and simple number ratios. *J. Res. Music Educ.*, **7**, 197–220.

Cazden, N. (1962). Sensory theories of musical consonance. *J. Aesth. Art Criticism*, **20**, 301–319.

Christman, R. J. and Williams, W. E. (1963). Influence of the time interval on experimentally induced shifts of pitch. *J. Acoust. Soc. Am.*, **35**, 1030–1033.

Cohen, A. (1961). Further investigation of the effects of intensity upon the pitch of pure tones. *J. Acoust. Soc. Am.*, **33**, 1363–1376.

Corso, J. F. (1954). Unison tuning of musical instruments. *J. Acoust. Soc. Am.*, **26**, 746–750.

Deva, B. C. (1959). The vibrato in Indian music. *Acustica*, **9**, 175–180.

Doughty, J. M. and Garner, W. R. (1948). Pitch characteristics of short tones. II. Pitch as a function of tonal duration. *J. Exp. Psychol.*, **38**, 478–494.

Egan, J. P. and Klumpp, R. G. (1951). The error due to masking in the measurement of aural harmonics by the method of best beats. *J. Acoust. Soc. Am.*, **23**, 275–286.

Egan, J. P. and Meyer, D. R. (1950). Changes in pitch of tones of low frequency as a function of the pattern of excitation produced by a band of noise. *J. Acoust. Soc. Am.*, **22**, 827–833.

Elfner, L. (1964). Systematic shifts in the judgment of octaves of high frequencies. *J. Acoust. Soc. Am.*, **36**, 270–276.

Fletcher, H. (1930). A space-time pattern theory of hearing. *J. Acoust. Soc. Am.*, **1**, 311–343.

Fletcher, H. (1934). Loudness, pitch and the timbre of musical tones and their relation to the intensity, the frequency and the overtone structure. *J. Acoust. Soc. Am.*, **6**, 59–69.

Fletcher, H. (1947). An institute of musical science – a suggestion. *J. Acoust. Soc Am.*, **19**, 527–531.

Fletcher, H., Blackham, E. D., and Geertsen, O. N. (1965). Quality of violin, viola, 'cello, and bass-viol tones, I. *J. Acoust. Soc. Am.*, **37**, 851–863.

van de Geer, J. P., Levelt, W. J. M., and Plomp, R. (1962). The connotation of musical consonance. *Acta Psychol.*, **20**, 308–319.

George, W. H. (1961). Science and music. *Sci. Prog., Lond.*, **49**, 409–426.

Greene, P. C. (1937). Violin intonation. *J. Acoust. Soc. Am.*, **9**, 43–44.

Guthrie, E. R. and Morrill, H. (1928). The fusion of non-musical intervals. *Am. J. Psychol.*, **40**, 624–627.

Harris, J. D. (1952). Pitch discrimination. *J. Acoust. Soc. Am.*, **24**, 750–755.

Harris, J. D. (1963). Loudness discrimination. *J. Speech Hear. Disorders, Monogr. Suppl.*, **11**.

Henning, G. B. (1966). Frequency discrimination of random-amplitude tones. *J. Acoust. Soc. Am.*, **39**, 336–339.

Jacobs, J. E. and Wittman, P. (1964). Psychoacoustics, the determining factor in stereo disc recording. *J. Audio Engng Soc.*, **12**, 115–123.

Jenkins, R. A. (1961). Perception of pitch, timbre, and loudness. *J. Acoust. Soc. Am.*, **33**, 1550–1557.

Kock, W. E. (1936). Certain subjective phenomena accompanying a frequency vibrato. *J. Acoust. Soc. Am.*, **8**, 23–25.

Kolinski, M. (1959). A new equidistant 12-tone temperament. *J. Am. Musicol. Soc.*, **12**, 210–214.

König, E. (1957). Effect of time on pitch discrimination thresholds under several psychophysical procedures; comparison with intensity discrimination thresholds. *J. Acoust. Soc. Am.*, **29**, 606–612.

Kreidl, A. and Gatscher, S. (1928). Über Diplakusis binauralis bei Normalhörigen. *Mschr. Ohrenheilk. Lar.-Rhinol.*, **62**, 694–697.

Kuttner, F. A. (1963). Vibrato, tremolo and beats. *J. Audio Engng Soc.*, **11**, 372–374.

Lempp, O. (1938). Über Diplakusis und musikalisches Falschhören. *Hals- Nas.- u. Ohrenarzt*, **46**, 193–202 and 241–255.

Lewis, D. and Cowan, M. (1936). The influence of intensity on the pitch of violin and 'cello tones. *J. Acoust. Soc. Am.*, **8**, 20–22.

Lichte, W. H. (1941). Attributes of complex tones. *J. Exp. Psychol.*, **28**, 455–480.

Lichte, W. H. and Gray, R. F. (1955). Influence of overtone structure on the pitch of complex tones. *J. Exp. Psychol.*, **49**, 431–436.

Liebermann, P. V. and Révész, G. (1908). Über Orthosymphonie. *Z. Psychol.*, **48**, 259–275.

Liebermann, P. V. and Révész, G. (1914). Die binaurale Tonmischung. *Z. Psychol.*, **69**, 234–255.

Lundin, R. W. and Allen, J. D. (1962). A technique for training perfect pitch. *Psychol. Rec.*, **12**, 139–146.

Mason, J. A. (1960). Comparison of solo and ensemble performances with reference to Pythagorean, just and equi-tempered intonations. *J. Res. Music Educ.*, **8**, 31–38.

Meyer, M. (1898). Zur Theorie der Differenztöne und der Gehörsempfindungen überhaupt. *Beitr. Akust. Musikwiss.*, **2**, 25–65.

Moe, C. R. (1942). An experimental study of subjective tones produced within the human ear. *J. Acoust. Soc. Am.*, **14**, 159–166.

Montgomery, H. C. (1935). Influence of experimental technique on the measurement of differential intensity sensitivity of the ear. *J. Acoust. Soc. Am.*, **7**, 39–43.

Morgan, C. T., Garner, W. R., and Galambos, R. (1951). Pitch and intensity. *J. Acoust. Soc. Am.*, **23**, 658–663.

Newman, E. B., Stevens, S. S., and Davis, H. (1937). Factors in the production of aural harmonics and combination tones. *J. Acoust. Soc. Am.*, **9**, 107–118.

Nickerson, J. F. (1948). A comparison of performances of the same melody played in solo and in ensemble with reference to equi-tempered, just, and Pythagorean intonations. Unpublished doctoral dissertation, University of Minnesota.

Odenthal, D. W. (1963). Perception and neural representation of simultaneous dichotic pure tone stimuli. *Acta Physiol. Pharmacol. Neerl.*, **12**, 453–496.

Peterson, J. (1915). Origin of higher orders of combination tones. *Psychol. Rev.*, **22**, 512–518.

Plomp, R. (1964). The ear as a frequency analyzer. *J. Acoust. Soc. Am.*, **36**, 1628–1636.

Plomp, R. (1965). Detectability threshold for combination tones. *J. Acoust. Soc. Am.*, **37**, 1110–1123.

Plomp, R. (1967). Pitch of complex tones. *J. Acoust. Soc. Am.*, **41**, 1526–1533.

Plomp, R. and Levelt, W. J. M. (1962). Musical consonance and critical bandwidth. *Proc. IV Int. Congr. Acoust.*, paper P 55. Harlang and Toksvig, Copenhagen.

Poland, W. (1963). Theories of music and musical behavior. *J. Music Theory*, **7**, 150–173.

Pollack, I. (1964). Ohm's acoustical law and short-term auditory memory. *J. Acoust. Soc. Am.*, **36**, 2340–2345.

Rawdon-Smith, A. F. and Hawkins, J. E., Jr. (1939). The electrical activity of a denervated ear. *Proc. R. Soc. Med.*, **32**, 496–507.

Révész, G. (1913). *Zur Grundlegung der Tonpsychologie.* Veit, Leipzig.

Rüedi, L. and Furrer, W. (1946). Das akustische Trauma. *Practica Oto-Rhino-Lar.*, **8**, 177–372.

Schecter, H. (1949). Perceptibility of frequency modulation in pure tones. Unpublished doctoral dissertation, Massachusetts Insitute of Technology.

Seashore, C. E. (1938). *Psychology of music.* McGraw-Hill, New York.

Seashore, H. G. (1935). An objective analysis of artistic singing. *Univ. Iowa Stud. Psychol. Music*, **4**, 12–157.

Shackford, C. (1961). Some aspects of perception, Part I. *J. Music Theory*, **5**, 162–202.

Shackford, C. (1962a). Some aspects of perception, Part II. *J. Music Theory*, **6**, 66–90.

Shackford, C. (1962b). Some aspects of perception, Part III. *J. Music Theory*, **6**, 295–303.

Shepard, R. N. (1964). Circularity in judgments of relative pitch. *J. Acoust. Soc. Am.*, **36**, 2346–2353.

Shower, E. G. and Biddulph, R. (1931). Differential pitch sensitivity of the ear. *J. Acoust. Soc. Am.*, **3**, 275–287.

Small, A. M. and Campbell, R. A. (1961). Pitch shifts of periodic stimuli with changes in sound level. *J. Acoust. Soc. Am.*, **33**, 1022–1027.

Small, A. Milroy (1937). An objective analysis of artistic violin performance. *Univ. Iowa Stud. Psychol. Music*, **4**, 172–231.

Stevens, J. C. and Guirao, M. (1964). Individual loudness functions. *J. Acoust. Soc. Am.*, **36**, 2210–2213.

Stevens, S. S. (1934). The attributes of tones. *Proc. Natn. Acad. Sci. U.S.A.*, **20**, 457–459.

Stevens, S. S. (1935). The relation of pitch to intensity. *J. Acoust. Soc. Am.*, **6**, 150–154.

Stevens, S. S. (1959). On the validity of the loudness scale. *J. Acoust. Soc. Am.*, **31**, 995–1003.

Stevens, S. S. (1963). The basis of psychophysical judgments. *J. Acoust. Soc. Am.*, **35**, 611–612.

Stevens, S. S., Volkmann, J. (1940). The relation of pitch to frequency: A revised scale. *Am. J. Psychol.*, **53**, 329–353.

Stevens, S. S., Volkmann, J., and Newman, E. B. (1937). A scale for the measurement of the psychological magnitude pitch. *J. Acoust. Soc. Am.*, **8**, 185–190.

Stevens, S. S., Guirao, M., and Slawson, A. W. (1965). Loudness, a product of volume times density. *J. Exp. Psychol.*, **69**, 503–510.

Stumpf, C. and Meyer, M. (1898). Maassbestimmungen über die Reinheit consonanter Intervalle. *Beitr. Akust. Musikwiss.*, **2**, 84–167.

Swigart, E. (1964). Pitch of periodically interrupted tones. *J. Acoust. Soc. Am.*, **36**, 1027–1028 (A).

Tanner, W. P., Jr. and Rivette, C. L. (1964). Experimental study of "tone deafness." *J. Acoust. Soc. Am.*, **36**, 1465–1467.

Thurlow, W. R. (1943). Studies in auditory theory. I. *J. Exp. Psychol.*, **32**, 17–36.

Thurlow, W. R. and Bernstein, S. (1957). Simultaneous two-tone pitch discrimination. *J. Acoust. Soc. Am.*, **29**, 515–519.

van der Tweel, L. H. (1956). Implication for auditory theory of unitary pitch perception despite diplacusis. *J. Acoust. Soc. Am.*, **28**, 718 (L).

Ward, W. D. (1953). The subjective octave and the pitch of pure tones. Unpublished doctoral dissertation, Harvard University.

Ward, W. D. (1954). Subjective musical pitch. *J. Acoust. Soc. Am.*, **26**, 369–380.

Ward, W. D. (1955). Tonal monaural diplacusis. *J. Acoust. Soc. Am.*, **27**, 365–372.

Ward, W. D. (1963a). Absolute pitch. Part I. *Sound*, **2**(3), 14–21.

Ward, W. D. (1963b). Absolute pitch. Part II. *Sound*, **2**(4), 33–41.

Ward, W. D. (1963c). Diplacusis and auditory theory. *J. Acoust. Soc. Am.*, **35**, 1746–1747.

Warren, R. M. (1963). Are loudness judgments based on distance estimates? *J. Acoust. Soc. Am.*, **35**, 613–614.

Watt, H. J. (1917). *The psychology of sound*. Cambridge Univ. Press, Cambridge, England.

Webster, J. C. and Schubert, E. D. (1954). Pitch shifts accompanying certain auditory threshold shifts. *J. Acoust. Soc. Am.*, **26**, 754–758.

Webster, J. C., Miller, P. H., Thompson, P. O., and Davenport, E. W. (1952). The masking and pitch shifts of pure tones near abrupt changes in a thermal noise spectrum. *J. Acoust. Soc. Am.*, **24**, 147–152.

Wever, E. G. (1929). Beats and related phenomena resulting from the simultaneous sounding of two tones. *Psychol. Rev.*, **36**, 402–418 and 512–523.

Wever, E. G. (1941). The designation of combination tones. *Psychol. Rev.*, **48**, 93–104.

Wever, E. G. (1949). *Theory of hearing.* Wiley, New York.

Wever, E. G. and Lawrence, M. (1954). *Physiological acoustics.* Princeton Univ. Press, Princeton, New Jersey.

Wever, E. G., Bray, C. W., and Lawrence, M. (1940). A quantitative study of combination tones. *J. Exp. Psychol.*, **27**, 469–496.

Young, R. W. (1952). Inharmonicity of plain wire piano strings. *J. Acoust. Soc. Am.*, **24**, 267–273.

Zurmühl, G. (1930). Abhängigkeit der Tonhöhenempfindung von der Lautstärke und ihre Beziehung zur Helmholtzschen Resonanztheorie des Hörens. *Z. Sinnesphysiol.*, **61**, 40–86.

Author Index

Numbers in italics refer to pages on which the complete references are cited.

A

Abraham, O., 4, *53*
Ades, H. W., 230, *251*, 261, 262, 284, 285, *300*, 348, 367, 369, *373*, 377
Adey, W. R., 371, *373*
Adrian, H. O., 364, *375*
Agazzi, C., 397, *403*
Aitkin, L. M., 355, *373*
Allanson, J. T., 347, 351, 354, *373*
Allen, G. W., 235, *250*
Allen, J. D., 430, *444*
Arnold, J. E., 119, 125, *154*

B

Baldwin, R. D., 307, *340*
Baley, S., 434, *443*
Barbour, J. M., 415, 416, *443*
Barlow, H. B., 349, 370, *373*
Batchelor, G. H., 240, *250*
Bauch, H., 161, *198*
Bauman, R. C., 175, *198*
Beament, J. W. L., 337, *340*
Beatty, D. L., 272, *302*
Beck, C., 249, *250*
Beck, J., 411, *443*
Beer, B., 370, *375*
von Békésy, G., 7, 8, 9, 31, 32, 40, 42, 43, 46, 49, *50*, 59, 60, 61, 62, 63, 64, 65, 71, 74, 76, *81*, 109, *112*, 119, 120, 138, 141, 152, *152*, *153*, 176, 177, 184, 187, 188, 195, 196, *198*, 207, 208, 210, 211, 216, 218, 221, 222, 224, 225, 227, 229, 230, 231, 242, 247, *250*, *251*, 272, 274, 275, 276, 277, 278, 280, 282, 283, 284, *300*, 312, 316, 319, 320, 324, *340*, 347, *373*, 392, *402*, 431, *443*

Benson, R. W., 118, *153*, 261, 279, *300*
Bental, E., 351, 371, *373*
van Bergeijk, W. A., 230, *251*
Berger, R., 334, *340*
Bernstein, S., 61, 65, *83*, 434, *446*
Biddulph, R., 32, *53*, 411, *445*
Bihari, B., 351, 371, *373*
Bilger, R. C., 92, *112*, 123, 124, 125, 129, 131, *153*, 175, 184, *198*, *201*
Birdsall, T. G., 103, 105, 106, 107, 108, *112*, *113*, *114*, 184, 185, *199*
Blackham, E. D., 424, *444*
Blodgett, H. C., 108, *112*
Bocca, E., 397, *402*, *403*
de Boer, E., 23, 24, 25, 27, 46, 49, *50*, 75, *81*, 165, 167, 178, 193, *198*, 232, *251*
Bogert, B. P., 211, *253*
Boomsliter, P., 416, 421, 428, 436, *443*
Booten, R. C., Jr., 46, *50*
Boring, E. G., 66, *81*
Bos, C. E., 165, 167, 178, *198*
Boudreau, J. C., 369, *378*
Bouman, M. A., 184, *200*
Bourbon, W. T., 104, *114*
Boyle, A. J. F., 232, 247, *252*
Bramwell, E., 397, *402*
Brandt, J. F., 66, *83*, 185, 187, *201*
Bray, C. W., 271, *303*, 441, *447*
Brecher, G. A., 238, *251*
Bridgman, P. W., 207, *251*, 307, *340*
van den Brink, G., 167, 175, 178, 184, 185, 195, *198*
Broadbent, D. E., 80, *81*
Brodmann, K., 401, *402*
Brogan, F. A., 119, *155*, 264, *303*
Bromiley, R. B., 368, *374*
Brown, G. W., 371, *373*
Brown, R. M., 37, *51*, 362, *375*
Bryan, M. E., 441, *443*

449

Subject Index